The International Handbook of Road Traffic Accidents and Psychological Trauma: Current Understanding, Treatment and Law

The International Handbook of Road Traffic Accidents and Psychological Trauma: Current Understanding, Treatment and Law

Edited by

Edward J. Hickling & Edward B. Blanchard

1999

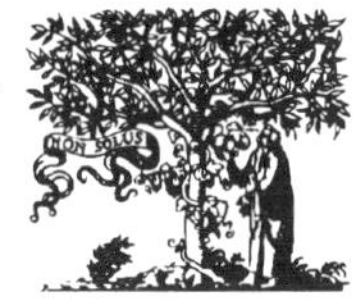

An Imprint of Elsevier Science

Amsterdam – Lausanne – New York – Oxford – Shannon – Singapore – Tokyo

ELSEVIER SCIENCE Ltd
The Boulevard, Langford Lane
Kidlington, Oxford OX5 1GB, UK

First edition 1999

Library of Congress Cataloging-in-Publication Data
The international handbook of road traffic accidents and psychological trauma : current understanding, treatment, and law / edited by Edward J. Hickling & Edward B. Blanchard.
p. cm.
Edited papers originally presented at a conference.
ISBN 0-08-042760-X (hc)
1. Traffic accidents--Psychological aspects. 2. Traffic accident victims--Psychology. 3. Stress (Psychology).4. Post-traumatic stress disorder. I. Hickling, Edward J. II. Blanchard, Edward B.

HE5614.I564 1999
617.1′028′019--dc21

ISBN: 0 08 042760 X

∞ The paper used in this publication meets the requirements of ANSI/NISO Z39.48-1992 (Permanence of Paper).

Printed in The Netherlands.

Dedication

This book is dedicated to the MVA/RTA survivors and the researchers and practitioners who treat the aftermath of this all too common trauma.

Acknowledgements

The editors wish to acknowledge the work, assistance and inspiration of the following people. Without their help, this book would never have been brought to life. First, we would like to thank Mr. Bernie Rowe and his firm of Lyons Davidson, without which there would never have been the opportunity to draw together the collection of world class contributors. Second, we would like to thank the capable Ms. Sandy Agosto, who collated, typed correspondence and made order of the volume of material that made its way across the miles to the Center for Stress and Anxiety Disorders in Albany, NY. Third, we would like to thank the National Institutes of Mental Health, who provide, through grant MH-48476, the funds for the studies and the staff that make possible the research on MVA/RTA done in our Center. We would also like to acknowledge the assistance of Mr. Keith Schockmel for his comments on the legal chapters, and the efforts of Ms. Carol Parsons and Christine Hoosick for their role in completion and coordination of the material.

EJH
EBB
July 7, 1999

Preface

'I know it sounds silly but' is the preface I most frequently encounter in my daily routine of talking to road accident victims. *'I know it sounds silly but I drive 5 miles longer to avoid the junction where I had my accident'; 'It's silly but I grab hold of the seat all the time when I'm a passenger'; 'It's silly but I hardly go out anymore'; 'I'll do almost anything to avoid a long journey'; 'We used to take the children out for trips on the weekend, but now I just can't face it'; 'I haven't been to visit my parents for over a year, I just can't face the journey'; 'I haven't been on a motorway since the accident more than 3 years ago'*.

Why is it *'silly'* to feel this way, and why are road accident victims so often embarrassed to explain their fears and altered behavior after an accident, what could be done to help? This is what I wanted to know and hence the conference in September 1998 on 'Road Accidents and the Mind'.

Although I have received many kind words about the conference that has led to this book, I must confess that the event has its roots in self-interest. I wanted, and needed to understand much more than I did about the problems faced by our road accident clients. My self-interest needed to be enlightened.

I knew I had to organize a conference to gather together all I could find on the subject of road traffic accidents and the mind. My concern and interest was not significant traumatic brain injury, terrible as it is, but with the less obvious 'psychological' injuries if that is what they are.

I wanted to know why it was that so many of my clients felt *'silly'*.

My good fortune is to practice in a law firm that encourages its members to explore issues more widely than just looking at the next case or today's time sheet.

Now for the first time, I asked for, and immediately received, the help and support of my partners in Lyons Davidson to organize an International Conference on the topic.

I would like to express my gratitude to my partners, especially those whose fields of practice have little, if anything, to do with Personal Injury Law, but who have been happy to support this project. Lesser mortals (or even lawyers!) could have so easily cavilled at the budget needed to organize and host a conference that was to last for 3 days.

Partners and financial help are one thing. The detail of planning and organizing the conference is another but, once again, I have been lucky.

Throughout the planning phase I was helped by talking the program through with Richard Mayou, Gordon Turnbull, and Paul Cone. As a result the program was immeasurably better.

Bernie Rowe
Lyons Davidson
June 21, 1999

Introduction

This book began with an innocent idea. The idea came from a conference that took place in the fall of 1998, in Bristol, England, organized by Mr. Bernie Rowe of Lyons Davidson, entitled, *Road Accidents and the Mind: An In-Depth Study of the Psychological Symptoms After Road Accidents*. For the first time ever, the leading experts, researchers, clinicians, lawyers and insurers, were all gathered at the same time and place sharing their work. The mood was electric and the collection of people stimulating. Up until this time the sheer distance of the globe had kept these people from having any face-to-face, in-depth collaboration and sharing of ideas. In fact, the only reason they were brought together now, was the inspiration of one man, Mr. Bernie Rowe. This book is in no small part a credit to him. Special thanks are given to him, from the editors of the book, the contributors, and the individuals who attended that meeting.

The idea of the book was actually finalized at a dinner held in the Lord Mayor's residence in Bristol, England, hosted by Mr. Rowe. The setting seemed very appropriate given the high spirits of the meeting, and the energy it had generated. At that dinner, the participants agreed in principal to the book, and a tentative timetable was outlined.

This edited book was formed, in part, by that conference. It has been updated and added to by even more current work from the contributors that seemed appropriate for inclusion in this text. Several editorial decisions were made regarding the organization of the book which are outlined here. We have also tried to stay with the term road traffic accident (RTA) for most of the chapters, although the words motor vehicle accident (MVA) are more commonly used on the North American side of the Atlantic Ocean. Where we have left the colloquialisms of the author, the reader should feel free to interchangeably apply the terms.

First, in keeping with the international flavor of the contributors, the spelling and language were kept essentially as submitted by the authors. No effort was made to conform to any limitations other than length (with an exception made for a submission by Mr. Rowe and Company). We believe that this allows the reader to join in the distinctly different views and styles of presenting an idea or findings that proved so stimulating for those at the conference.

Second, we organized the material into four loosely connected sections. The first two sections allow for a current understanding of the psychological and medical factors of central importance to the psychological impact of a road traffic accident. The third section involves the legal aspect of the RTA, and attends to concerns both from a legal and psychological framework. The fourth section involves the most current work on psychological treatments. This is an interesting time in the treatment of PTSD following RTAs. At the time this book was being prepared, there are several controlled treatment studies examining the effectiveness of psychological treatments for road traffic accident survivors ongoing throughout the world. This volume allows for a preliminary look at some of that data.

The chapters are quite variable in their length and construction. The longest chapter, in fact, comes from the conference's organizer, Mr. Bernie Rowe, his partners in his firm, and a brave insurer from Lloyd's of London, Mr. Cottington. Their chapter is quite unique in its structure, but we believe it adds considerable insight to the legal side of the RTA, and the issues one needs to deal with as a lawyer and insurer. The role of the expert witness has just been changed in England, and the structure of the change is outlined and explained. Once again, the book seems to be at the cutting edge in terms of timing and information.

The book has been an ambitious undertaking in its scope. We hope it will have a broad impact. The book is written for all professionals that deal with road traffic accidents: it should be of interest to psychologists, psychiatrists, physicians, solicitors, barristers, insurers, and RTA survivors alike. It is the rare book that indeed has something for everyone. The book hopes for more, in that the book is truly international in its scope. Contributors from Australia, Canada, the United States, England, and Europe, all try to add their knowledge to the growing compilation of facts about this all too common event. As editors we have tried to make the book as true a representative of our knowledge at this time as possible. As one of the most common traumas that occur in the modern world, the ability to understand, deal with, and treat this disorder is believed to be of paramount importance.

Edward J. Hickling
Edward B. Blanchard
June 21, 1999

List of Contributors

Professor David A. Alexander, Department of Mental Health, University of Aberdeen, Medical School, Aberdeen, AB25 2ZD, Scotland

Professor David A. Alexander is a graduate of the Universities of Dundee and St Andrews in Scotland, and is a Fellow of the British Psychological Society. He has also undergone postgraduate training at the Universities of Birmingham and Aberdeen and at the FBI Academy, Virginia, USA. He is currently Professor in Mental Health at the Medical School of the University of Aberdeen, and is an honorary consultant clinical psychologist to the Regional Health Board. He is also honorary consultant to the police and fire services, and to the British Transport Police. At Royal Cornhill Hospital, Aberdeen, he runs a Traumatic Stress Clinic, and he is Director of the Centre for Traumatic Research. Regularly he lectures at the Scottish Police College on hostage negotiation and on trauma. He has also been a visiting speaker at the FBI Academy and at the Russian School of Militia in Chelyabinsk.

He has been involved with survivors, victims and rescuers following a number of major incidents, viz., the Piper Alpha oil platform disaster, the sinking of the Estonia ferry, the Lockerbie air disaster, the Chinook helicopter crash, the Urals' train disaster in Russia and the Nairobi terrorist bombing. He is on the editorial Board and panel of assessors for a number of national and international journals, and he sits on several committees which have a responsibility for emergency planning and major incident response.

Dr. Jonathan I. Bisson, BM MRCPsych Dip Clin Psychotherapy, Consultant Liaison Psychiatrist, Gabalfa clinic, 213 North Road, Cardiff, CF4 3AG, UK

Jonathan Bisson qualified as a doctor in 1986 and subsequently spent six years in the British Army training as a psychiatrist and developing his interest in traumatic stress. He has been based in South Wales for the last six years, runs a traumatic stress clinic in Cardiff and continues to pursue traumatic stress related research, particularly into the effectiveness of early interventions in physically traumatised individuals.

Professor Edward B. Blanchard, Center for Stress and Anxiety Disorders, State University of New York, Albany, 1535 Western Avenue, Albany, New York, 12203, USA

Dr. Edward B. Blanchard received his doctoral degree in clinical psychology from Stanford University in 1969. After holding faculty positions at the University of Georgia, the University of Mississippi Medical Center, and the University of Tennessee Center for Health Sciences, Dr. Blanchard went to the University at Albany, State University of New York, in 1977 and has remained there ever since. In 1990 Dr. Blanchard was named Distinguished Professor of Psychology by the University at Albany. He is currently Director of the Center for Stress and Anxiety Disorders at the University at Albany.

Dr. Blanchard began work on PTSD in collaboration with Larry Kolb, MD, at the Albany Veteran's Administration in 1981, focusing primarily on assessment research with Vietnam veterans. In 1990 he began collaborative research on motor vehicle accident survivors with Edward J. Hickling, Psy.D. Current research interests include irritable bowel syndrome, psychological treatments for headache, and psychophysiological assessment.

Dr. Sandra L. Bloom, Executive Director, The Sanctuary, Horsham Clinic, Ambler PA , Hampton Hospital, Rancocas, NJ., Alliance for Creative Development, 200 Apple St., Suite 1, Quakertown, PA, 18951, USA

Dr. Sandra L. Bloom is a board-Certified psychiatrist and founder and Executive Director of The Sanctuary Û , specialized inpatient hospital programs for the treatment of adults traumatized as children, located at two sites, one at Horsham Clinic in Ambler, PA and the other at Hampton Hospital in Rancocas, New Jersey. She is the author of several books on trauma and violence including Creating Sanctuary: Toward the Evolution of Sane Societies published in 1997 by Routledge; Bearing Witness: Violence and Social Responsibility published in the autumn of 1998 by Haworth Press and co-authored with M. Reichert, and she is the editor of Violence: A Public Health Menace and a Public Health Approach published in 1999 by Karnac

Books, London. Dr. Bloom is Immediate Past President of the International Society for Traumatic Stress Studies (ISTSS) and in 1998 was awarded the Sarah Haley Memorial Award for Clinical Excellence from the ISTSS. She is also President of the Philadelphia Chapter of Physicians for Social Responsibility. In May 1998, the Attorney General of Pennsylvania, Mike Fisher, appointed Dr. Bloom top chair a statewide Task force on Family Violence. She holds an academic appointment as Clinical Assistant Professor, Department of Psychiatry, Temple University School of Medicine, Philadelphia, PA. In 1998 she accepted a two-year appointment as the Sol Z. Cohen Chair of the Jewish Board of Family and Children's Services in New York City for the purpose of introducing The Sanctuary Model into their residential facilities for disturbed children and adolescents.

Professor Richard Bryant, School of Psychology, University of New South Wales, Sydney, 2052 Australia

Richard A. Bryant, Ph.D., is Senior Lecturer in Psychology, University of New South Wales, Sydney, Australia and Director of the PTSD Unit, Westmead Hospital, Sydney. He has published over 80 journal articles in the areas of trauma, dissociation, and hypnosis, and has lectured internationally on acute stress disorder.

Dr. Todd C. Buckley, VAMC (116B-2) 150 S. Huntington Avenue, Boston, MA, 02130 USA

Todd C. Buckley, Ph.D. is a research scientist at the Behavioral Science Division of the National Center for PTSD. He is also an Assistant Professor in the Department of Psychiatry at the Boston University School of Medicine. He received his doctorate in clinical psychology from the University at Albany-SUNY. He recently completed his clinical internship at the University of Mississippi Medical Center. His research interests include the psychophysiology of anxiety disorders and treatment outcome research.

Mr. Norman Cottington, Highway Motor Policies, Kelting House, Southernhay, Basildon, SS14 1NT, UK

Mr. Norman Cottington has worked in the insurance industry for the past 35 years, having spent 23 years as a Claims Manager in both the company and Lloyd's markets. He is presently Claims Manager at Highway Motor Policies at Lloyd's. He is past Chairman of Claims Managers, Lloyd's Underwriters Association, Lloyd's Legal Expense sub-Committee and Lumacare Management Committee. He was a founding member and past Chairman of the Advisory Committee to the Disability Assessment Unit.

Norman Cottington joined The Injury Care Clinics as Managing Director on 26 April 1999. His career spans a period in excess of 35 years attending to motor claims including 7 years with Plaintiff solicitors and 25 years as a Motor Insurance Claims Manager. His last appointment was as Claims Manager of Highway Motor Policies, the largest of the Lloyd's motor syndicates and the seventh largest motor insurer in the United Kingdom.

He remains as Chairman of the UK Bodily Injury Claims Management Group which counts amongst its number members of APIL, MASS and FOIL. He remains a member of the IUA Rehabilitation Working Party, part of the UK Bodily Injury Awards Study. Mr. Cottington now joins the Injury Care Clinics Ltd. He intends to provide a complete approach to rehabilitation to assist in bridging the adversarial barriers and providing services that will work toward best possible recovery at the earliest opportunity.

Mr. Trishul Devineni, Center for Stress and Anxiety Disorders, University at Albany-SUNY, 1535 Western Avenue, Albany, New York, 12203 USA

Trishul Devineni received his BS in Psychology and BA in Philosophy from the University of Pittsburgh in 1996. There he conducted research on the socioeconomic correlates of cardiovascular reactivity to stressful life events. Presently he is a doctoral student in the Clinical Psychology program at the University at Albany, State University of New York. He is currently serving as research assistant under the direction of Dr. Edward Blanchard at the Center for Stress & Anxiety Disorders. His current research interests include the emotional Stroop effect in PTSD and Panic Disorder, and Internet-based applications of self-help treatments for headache and PTSD.

Mr. Kevin S. Douglas, Department of Psychology, Simon Fraser University, Burnaby, B.C. V5A 1S6, Canada

Kevin S. Douglas is currently in the Graduate Program in Law and Psychology at Simon Fraser University in Burnaby, British Columbia. He is in the joint Ph.D./LL.B. program, completing the final year of law school at the University of British Columbia, and working on a Ph.D. in clinical-forensic psychology at Simon Fraser University. Interests include the overlap between psychology and law, and the application of psychological principles to legal phenomena. He is involved in research on posttraumatic stress disorder and motor vehicle accidents. He also has carried out research and published in the areas of violence risk assessment, forensic assessment, the relationship between mental illness and violence, jury decision-making, and public knowledge of and attitudes toward sentencing.

Professor Anke Ehlers, Department of Psychiatry, University of Oxford, Warneford Hospital, Oxford OX3 7JX, UK

Anke Ehlers is a clinical psychologist and Wellcome Trust Principal Research Fellow at the Oxford University Department of Psychiatry. She obtained the degree of Diplom-Psychologin and her Ph.D. from the University of Tubingen, Germany, and a post-doctoral degree in clinical psychology and psychophysiology (Habilitation) from the University of Marburg, Germany. Her previous posts include Research Scholar at Stanford University, CA, USA, Assistant Professor (Hochschulassistent) at the University of Marburg, and Professor of Clinical Psychology at the University of Gottingen, Germany. Her research and clinical work focus on anxiety disorders (panic disorder, posttraumatic stress disorder, social phobia) and psychological aspects of cardiovascular and dermatological problems.

Dr. George Everly, International Critical Incident Stress Foundation, Inc., 10176 Baltimore National Pike, Unit 201, Ellicott City, MD 21042, USA

George S. Everly, Jr., Ph.D.,C.T.S., is CEO and cofounder of the International Critical Incident Stress Foundation, Inc. and is Professor of Psychology at Loyola College in Maryland. Dr. Everly is a Fellow of the American Institute of Stress and a Fellow of the Academy of Psychosomatic Medicine and has held faculty appointments at Harvard University, Harvard Medical School and Johns Hopkins University. He is the author or co-author of ten textbooks including: CISD: An Operations Manual, Second Edition (Revised); Personality and Its Disorders; Controlling Stress and Tension; Psychotraumatology; and the critically acclaimed A Clinical Guide to the Treatment of the Human Stress Response. Dr. Everly has lectured in eleven countries on four continents on the topics of stress and post-trauma syndromes. Dr. Everly is past President of the Maryland Psychological Association and developed the disaster mental health network for the Central Maryland branch of the American Red Cross.

Dr. Ingrid Fedoroff, St. Paul's Hospital, Pain Clinic, Burrard St., Vancouver, BC, Canada

Dr. Ingrid C. Fedoroff completed the research described in this book during a post-doctoral fellowship in the Department of psychiatry at the University of British Columbia. She is currently a clinical psychologist at St. Paul's Hospital, Vancouver. She received her Ph.D. in clinical psychology at the University of Toronto.

Dr. Christopher Fox BSc (Hons) MB BS MRCPsych MMedSci , Department of Old Age Psychiatry, Warneford Hospital, Oxford OX3 7JX, UK

Dr Christopher Fox served in the RAF for 7 years. He is presently a Specialist Registrar in old age psychiatry in Oxford. He is continuing research into the psychophysiology of PTSD.

Dr. Allison Harvey, Department of Experimental Psychology, University of Oxford, South Parks Rd., Oxford OX1 3UD, UK

Allison G. Harvey, BSc. Psychol.(Hons), MClinPsych., Ph.D., is Lecturer in Abnormal Psychology at the Department of Experimental Psychology, University of Oxford, United Kingdom and Fellow of St. Anne's College, Oxford. She has published over 40 journal articles in the areas of trauma, dissociation and insomnia and has received the Chaim Danielle Early Career Award from the International Society for Traumatic Stress Studies.

Dr. Edward J. Hickling, Center for Stress and Anxiety Disorders, State University of New York- Albany, 1535 Western Avenue, Albany, New York, 12203, USA and The Sage Colleges, Department of Health & Rehabilitation Sciences, Troy, NY 12180 USA

Edward J. Hickling received his PsyD in clinical psychology from the University of Denver, School of Professional Psychology in 1982. He is an Assistant Professor in the Department of Health and Rehabilitation Sciences at Russell Sage College in Troy, New York. In addition he has a practice specializing in the treatment of trauma survivors, anxiety and affective disorders, behavioral medicine and psychological assessment. Since 1990 he has been the Co-Principal Investigator on several NIMH grants with Dr. Edward Blanchard. He has published numerous scientific articles and chapters in books. He is the co-author with Dr. Blanchard of the book, After the Crash: Assessment and Treatment of Motor Vehicle Accident Survivors, published by APA in 1997. His current research interests include the assessment and treatment of PTSD, the detection of malingering in a clinical setting, the psychological impact of physical illnesses, and sports psychology.

Mr. Nicholas Hill, Sqn Ldr Nicholas Hill MB BS MRCPsych RAF. Duchess of Kent Psychiatric Hospital. Horne Road. Catterick Garrison. North Yorkshire DL9 4DF, UK

Sqn Ldr Nicholas Hill is a Consultant General Adult Psychiatrist who has served in the RAF for 9 years. He maintains a keen interest in PTSD research and is currently investigating noradrenaline cortisol ratios as a diagnostic measure.

Mr. Matthew T. Huss, Department of Psychology, University of Nebraska - Lincoln, Lincoln, Nebraska, 68588 USA
Matthew T. Huss, M.S., is currently a Doctoral Candidate in the Law/Psychology (Clinical) Program at the University of Nebraska-Lincoln. He will be a Predoctoral intern at the Palo Alto VA Health Systems in Palo Alto, CA during the1999-2000 academic year. His research interests generally focus on domestic violence and the assessment of risk in various populations and he has received external funding from the National Institute of Mental Health and the Guggenheim Foundation for his work examining the expression of psychopathy among domestic violence perpetrators.

Dr. Grant Iverson, Department of Psychiatry, University of British Columbia, 2255 Wesbrook Mall, Vancouver, BC, V6T 2A1, Canada
Grant Iverson received his Ph.D. in Clinical Psychology from the University of West Virginia. He is currently an Assistant Professor of Psychiatry at the University of British Columbia, and a clinical psychologist at Riverview Hospital. He is well published in neuropsychology, the assessment of malingering, and behavioural medicine.

Dr. Robin Jacobson, St George's Hospital Medical School, Department of Psychiatry, Jenner Wing, Cranmer Terrace, London, SW17 ORE, UK
Dr. Robin Jacobson trained in medicine and neurology before switching to psychiatry at the Maudsley Hospital in London. He was awarded a Wellcome Fellowship at the Institute of Psychiatry in Neuropsychiatric research. He moved to St. George's Hospital Medical School, (London, UK) in 1986, where he runs Mood and Neuropsychiatric clinics. His research interests are head injury, bipolar mood disorders and psychopharmacology. He lectures in Evidence-Based Medicine and Mental Health.

Dr. Sue Jeavons, Psychological Science, La Trobe University, PO Box 199, Bendigo, VIC 3552, Australia
Dr. Sue Jeavons is an Australian clinical psychologist working part time as a lecturer at La Trobe University's Bendigo campus and part time in private practice. She did her clinical training (M Phil) at the University of Edinburgh and her Ph.D. at the University of Melbourne. She has worked with road accident victims for 10 years in a hospital rehabilitation unit, in private practice and through research. She has also been involved with the Road Trauma Support Team, a voluntary support organisation for people affected by road trauma.

Dr. William J. Koch, Health Psychology Clinic, UBC Hospital, 2211 Wesbrook Mall, Vancouver, BC V6T 2B5, Canada

William J. Koch received his Ph.D. in Psychology from the University of Alberta in 1981. He is currently Director of Internship Training and Director of the Health Psychology Clinic at UBC Hospital. He is also Clinical Professor of Psychiatry at the University of British Columbia and Adjunct Professor of Psychology at Simon Fraser University, where he teaches the graduate course in civil forensic psychology. He has a practice in forensic consultation with respect to emotional injuries attributed to motor vehicle accidents, sexual assault, or sexual harassment, among other areas. He has published articles and chapters, and given presentations primarily with respect to posttraumatic stress, professional practice, and the intersection of psychology and the law. His research interests include the psychological effects of motor vehicle accidents, sexual assault, and sexual harassment, and the clinical judgement of psychologists. Dr. Koch currently holds two grants from the Insurance Corporation of British Columbia to develop clinical practice guidelines for the assessment and treatment of emotional disorders stemming from motor vehicle accidents, and to conduct a controlled trial for prevention of PTSD from such accidents.

Professor Richard Mayou, University Department of Psychiatry, Warneford Hospital Oxford, OX3 7JX, UK

Professor of Psychiatry, Oxford University. Trained in medicine and psychiatry Oxford and Bethlem Royal and Maudsley hospitals and the Institute of Psychiatry, London. Research interests CL psychiatry, psychological aspects of heart disease, diabetes, RTA and unexplained physical symptoms. Founder chairman of Royal College Group for CL Psychiatry.

Mr. Douglas Mitchell International Critical Incident Stress Foundation, Inc., 10176 Baltimore National Pike, Unit 201, Ellicott City, MD, 21042 USA

Douglas J. Mitchell, MPA, is a recent retiree from the New York City Fire Department. He retired as a Lieutenant with 28 years in the service. Doug Mitchell has earned an Associate Degree in Applied Science, in Fire Sciences; a Bachelor of Science Degree in Fire Science and Administration and a Master's Degree in Public Administration. He has taught Fire Science, Fire Protection, Fire Prevention and Fire Investigation Courses at the college level and within FDNY. He has also taught extension courses for John Jay College at the United States Military Academy at West Point. Mr. Mitchell has conducted Critical Incident Stress Debriefings (CISDs) for Emergency Response personnel within FDNY and participated in many other highly stressful events for disaster workers involved in the following events: The World Trade Center Bombing; The Oklahoma City Bombing; the TWA Flight 800 Crash; and the Flooding Disaster in Kentucky.

Dr. Jeffrey Mitchell, International Critical Incident Stress Foundation, Inc., 10176 Baltimore National Pike, Unit 201, Ellicott City, MD, 21042 USA

Jeffrey T. Mitchell, Ph.D., is a Clinical Associate Professor of the Emergency Health Services Dept. at the University of Maryland. He developed the Critical Incident Stress Debriefing (CISD) process which is utilized by over 300 communities throughout the United States and in five other nations. He founded the International CISD network. He is a well-known speaker who has lectured to emergency personnel in all fifty states and seven countries. He is the senior author of the following books: Human Elements Training; CISD: An Operations Manual, Second Edition (Revised); Emergency Response to Crisis and Emergency Services Stress. He has over sixty other publications on critical incident stress, crisis intervention and the treatment of stress in emergency personnel.

Dr. Margaret Mitchell, Police Research Unit, Department of Psychology, Glasgow Caledonian University, Glasgow G4 0BA, Scotland

Dr. Margaret Mitchell, Ph.D. is the Director of Research for the Police Research Unit, Glasgow Caledonian University and has researched police practice and post traumatic stress disorder for the past ten years. Her previous publication, The Aftermath of Road Accidents: Psychological, Social and Legal Consequences, was published by Routledge UK, in 1997.

Ms. Elizabeth Mundy, Center for Stress and Anxiety Disorders, State University of New York- Albany, 1535 Western Avenue, Albany, New York, 12203 USA

Elizabeth Mundy received her BS in Psychology from the University of Massachusetts at Amherst in 1991. Since that time she has worked at Massachusetts General Hospital in the Pediatric Psychopharmacology Unit as a research fellow with Joseph Biederman, M.D.. There she conducted research on bipolar disorder and ADHD in pre-pubertal children. She is currently enrolled at the University at Albany, State University of New York as a doctoral candidate in clinical psychology. At the present time she is working as a research coordinator under the direction of Dr. Edward Blanchard, at the Center for Stress and Anxiety disorders. Her current research interests include PTSD secondary to MVAs and medical illnesses such as breast cancer and prostate cancer.

Ms. Lynda L. Murdoch, Department of Psychology, Simon Fraser University, Burnaby, B.C. V5A 1S6, Canada
Lynda L. Murdoch is currently a graduate student in the Law and Psychology program in the Psychology Department of Simon Fraser University in Burnaby, B.C. Canada. Before entering graduate school, Ms. Murdoch was a civil litigation lawyer in private practice. She is also a former judicial law clerk of the British Columbia Court of Appeal.

Wg Cdr Leigh Neal, MB. BCh. MRCPsych. MRCGP. DRCOG. RAF. Consultant Psychiatrist and Commanding Officer of the Duchess of Kent's Hospital, Horne Road, Catterick Garrison, North Yorkshire, UK. DL9 4DF
Wg Cdr Neal is the Commanding Officer of the Duchess of Kent's Military Hospital and the Head of the UK Defence Medical Services Psychological Injuries Unit. He has published mainly in the area of military PTSD assessment and has acted as an expert witness in many civilian road traffic accident claims. The Psychological Injuries Unit is tasked with refining protocols for the multi-modal assessment of psychological injuries from clinical, behavioral, psychometric and psychophysiological perspectives in order to minimise the effect of exaggeration and deception on disability claims.

Mr. David O'Neil Washington, Department of Psychology, University of Nebraska - Lincoln, Lincoln, Nebraska, 68588 USA
David O'Neill Washington has an MA in clinical psychology (forensic emphasis) and a Masters in Legal Studies (workplace violence emphasis), both from the University of Nebraska - Lincoln (UNL). He is currently completing his Ph.D. in clinical-forensic psychology program at UNL. He has received a grant from the National Institute of Justice for workplace violence. Mr. Washington completed his bachelor degree at Yale University, and spent a year at Oxford University in the Junior Year Abroad program. His current research is on workplace violence, particularly with respect to risk factors and legal implications. He has been involved in the threat assessment of threatening letters to members of the U.S. Congress, and is a Legislative Aid to Nebraska State Senator Ernie Chambers.

Ms. Carol Parsons, Lyons Davidson, Solicitors, Bridge House, 48-52 Baldwin Street, Bristol, BS1 1QD, UK
Carol Parsons LL.B. (Hons). Carol completed her academic training in 1998 and is in the final stages of her vocational training. She will qualify as a Solicitor in December 1999. Before completing her Law Degree, Carol worked for six years as a Paralegal, specializing in personal injury cases. Her interest in Whip-

lash Associated Disorders developed when she joined Lyons Davidson in 1994 and she has co-authored an article on the subject which has recently been published in a number of UK law journals.

Carol has also been involved in organizing two International Conferences; Road Accidents and the Mind Conference in 1998 and Whiplash Associated Disorders in 1997.

Mr. Mark Rivers. Lyons Davidson, Solicitors, Bridge House, 48-52 Baldwin Street, Bristol, BS1 1QD, UK

Degree: BA (Hons) from Bristol Polytechnic in 1985.Qualified as a solicitor 1987.Worked in Bath as a partner in Macfarlane Guy solicitors conducting Personal Injury cases for both Plaintiffs and Defendants.He has experience of road traffic, employers and public liability cases and has conducted many inquests and fatal accident cases as well as some clinical negligence actions. He joined Lyons Davidson in 1997 and was appointed as a partner in 1998.He speaks at a number of conferences and approximately 50% of his caseload has a psychological element to it.

Mr. Bernie Rowe, Lyons Davidson, Solicitors, Bridge House, 48-52 Baldwin Street, Bristol, BS1 1QD, UK

Bernie Rowe is a Partner with Lyons Davidson Solicitors, Bristol and is Head of their Insurance and Personal Injury Department.

Bernie spent nine years in partnership in Hull before moving to Bristol in 1986 to build the personal injury and insurance practice of Lyons Davidson. The firm has a total of 240 staff, 105 of whom are involved in personal injury work, making Lyons Davidson the largest Personal Injury and Insurance Practice in the South West. Bernie and his colleagues believe that lawyers should practice on both sides of the fence and the Department acts for a number of well-known Liability and Legal Expense Insurers handling both plaintiff and defendant work. The Firm organised a highly successful three-day conference on whiplash injuries in 1997, attracting speakers and delegates from the USA, Canada, Europe and the UK. The conference took an in-depth study of the biomechanics and medical issues surrounding the whiplash epidemic.

Bernie Rowe was a founder member of MASS, the Motor Accident Solicitor's Society, and served as its first Chairman. Bernie in fact was Chairman of MASS from 1991 - 1993. Bernie continues his involvement as a member of its National Management Committee and as Treasurer. Elsewhere Bernie continues to campaign for the introduction of Windscreen Insurance Discs to combat the problem of uninsured driving. Bernie has also recently served on a working party leading to the formation of the Disability Assessment Unit by Rehab UK. The Disability Assessment Unit provides a fresh approach to rehabilitation assessment by plaintiffs and defendants co-operating in the early stages of a claim. He is an active speaker and writer with a particular interest in reforming claims processing procedures to become quicker and cheaper.

Mr. Regan Shercliffe, Department of Psychology, Simon Fraser University, Burnaby, B.C. V5A 1S6, Canada
Regan Shercliffe, M.A. is a doctoral student in Clinical Psychology at Simon Fraser University. His research interests include premorbid factors and correlates related to the development of PTSD, as well as cognitive deficits associated with schizophrenia. He has conducted research and presented papers with respect to PTSD, Schizophrenia, and using statistical methods in predicting World Series winners.

Dr. Daniel J. Silverman, Capital Neurological Associates, 650 Warren Street, Albany, New York, 12208 USA
Dr. Daniel Silverman received his Doctorate in Medicine from the University of Vermont College of Medicine 1981. He completed his residency in Neurology from Albany Medical Center 1985 and became Board Certified in Neurology in 1987. He is presently the Chief of Neurology at St Peter's Hospital, Albany NY. Clinical interests include acute stroke management, headache and minor head trauma with published research in headache. He presently heads the Stroke Team at St.Peter's Hospital. Dr. Silverman has served as a consultant for several pharmaceutical companies. He is an advisor for a local not-for-profit managed health company. Dr. Silverman continues to actively practice Clinical Neurology in Albany New York.

Mr. Paul Stallard, Department of Child and Family Psychiatry, Royal United Hospital, Combe Park, Bath, BA1 3NG, UK
Mr. Paul Stallard is a Chartered Clinical Psychologist with the Avon and Western Wiltshire Mental Health Care NHS Trust. He has been working with children and young people for the past 19 years and has recently completed a study examining the psychological effects of everyday road traffic accidents upon children.

Professor Ann E. Taylor, The Sage Colleges, Department of Health & Rehabilitation Sciences, Troy, New York, 12180 USA
Ann E. Taylor received her training in clinical psychology from the University at Albany. She has worked at the Center for Stress and Anxiety Disorders on several clinical research projects. Her involvement with PTSD and Motor Vehicle Accidents began in 1990 with the initial assessment study. Her main

contributions have been with psychophysiological assessment and data analysis. She is currently an Assistant Professor at the Sage Colleges, in the Department of Health and Rehabilitation Sciences.

Dr. Steven Taylor, Department of Psychiatry, University of British Columbia, 2255 Wesbrook Mall, Vancouver, BC, V6T 2A1, Canada
Dr. Steven Taylor is an Associate Professor in the Department of Psychiatry at the University of British Columbia. He received his Ph.D. in clinical psychology at the University of British Columbia.

Dr. Gordon Turnbull, Consultant Psychiatrist, Ticehurst House Hospital, Ticehurst, Wadhurst, East Sussex, TN5 7HU, UK
Dr. Gordon Turnbull, BSc MB FRCP FRCPsych, is a Consultant Psychiatrist with a background in Internal Medicine, Neurology, Neuropsychiatry and Psychosomatics in the Royal Air Force Medical Branch. He first became involved in the management of traumatic stress reactions following the Lockerbie Air Disaster in 1988, when he led the RAF team which conducted the psychological debriefings of the RAF Mountain Rescue Teams involved. Wing Commander Turnbull was deployed to the Gulf War in 1991 as RAF Psychiatric Advisor in the Field and led the team which debriefed the released British prisoners-of-war. Later in 1991 he led the teams which debriefed the released hostages from Beirut, John McCarthy, Jack Mann and Terry Waite. He left the RAF in 1993 after setting up a PTSD treatment centre and was appointed Clinical Director of a new Traumatic Stress Unit at Ticehurst House Hospital in East Sussex- notably an innovative treatment approach to the oldest independent psychiatric hospital in England (208 years). He was also appointed Consulting Psychiatrist to the Civil Aviation authority. Awards include Fellowship of the Royal Geographical Society and the Royal Society of Arts, and People of the Year (1993). He has written extensively on the subject of Traumatic Stress and published research and lectures nationally and internally. Ambitions, apart from reduction of his golf handicap, include reduction of stigma surrounding PTSD generally, but especially among emergency service personnel, by improving awareness that PTSD represents a normal survival reaction, not psychopathology.

Ms. Connie H. Veazey, Center for Stress and Anxiety Disorders, State University of New York- Albany, 1535 Western Avenue, Albany, New York, 12203 USA
Connie Veazey received her BS in psychology from the University of Southwestern Louisiana in 1996. Presently she is a doctoral student in the Clinical Psychology program at the University at Albany, State University

of New York. She is currently serving as a research assistant under the direction of Dr. Edward Blanchard at the Center for Stress and Anxiety Disorders. Her current research interests include the psychophysiology of PTSD.

Dr Nigel H Walton MA Ph.D. Head, Department of Clinical Neuropsychology, The Burden Neurological Hospital, North Bristol NHS Trust, Stapleton, UK

BA (Hons) in Psychology, MA (Clinical Neuropsychology) The University of Melbourne, Australia, Ph.D. The University of Bristol, UK.

Dr Walton studied clinical neuropsychology at Melbourne University and has worked in head injury rehabilitation, epilepsy surgery and general neurology settings in Australia and the UK. He has an extensive experience of the neuropsychological assessment of head injury and a special interest in the neuropsychological sequelae of mild traumatic brain injury. He holds a lecturing post in the Department of Experimental Psychology at the University of Bristol.

Mr. David Watson BSc (Hons) Medeci Developments. St Andrews Lodge, 7 Southdown Rd, Harpenden, Hertfordshire AL5 1PB, UK

David Watson is a post graduate clinical scientist at the Department of Medical Electronics at St Bartholemews Medical College London. He is completing a Ph.D. thesis into the assessment of workloads and fatigue in aerospace medicine. He has 20 years experience in clinical measurements technology. He will shortly be moving to a new post in the Department of Biological and Medical systems at Imperial College London.

Professor William Yule, University of London, Institute of Psychiatry, de Crespigny Park, London, SE5 8AF, UK

William Yule Ph.D., F.B.PsS, trained as a clinical psychologist at the Institute of Psychiatry/Maudsley Hospital in London where for many years he was Head of Clinical Psychology Services. He is Professor of Applied Child Psychology in the University of London and has wide research interests, having published on epidemiology, reading disorders, the effects of lead on children's development, parent training, childhood autism. For the past decade he has concentrated on studying PTSD in children both in civilian and war situations. He is Director of the Child Traumatic Stress Clinic at the Maudsley Hospital.

Table of Contents

Section 3: Legal Issues

Section 4: Psychological Treatment

Section 1: Overview and Background

1

The Presentation of Adult Symptoms

DAVID A ALEXANDER, MA, CPsychol, PhD, FBPS

Professor in Mental Health, Medical School, University of Aberdeen, Scotland; Director, Centre for Trauma Research, Royal Cornhill Hospital, Aberdeen, Scotland

Preface

This chapter addresses the kind of normal and pathological reactions shown by survivors of trauma. In addition, it describes some of the historical background, our knowledge of post-traumatic reactions and those factors leading to poor adjustment after trauma. Finally, it provides some guidelines for identifying those individuals who are not coping following a traumatic experience.

A Historical Perspective

The psychological impact of traumatic events has been well documented, particularly in the annals of military combat, dating back to the Trojan and Graeco-Roman Wars (Babington, 1997). Unfortunately, until very recently, each new military campaign had tended to ignore the lessons painfully learned from previous ones. Moreover, again until relatively recently, there was an unwillingness to acknowledge that these widely reported medical conditions and the oddities of behaviour, associated with combat, were due to psychological factors. The pre-eminence of the physical sciences ensured that psychological causes were rarely postulated, as will be seen below.

Historically, civilian trauma has not added much to our understanding of the impact of traumatic events on the emotional well-being of victims. This is surprising in view of the fact that for centuries mankind has been the victim of many natural phenomena, including floods, earthquakes and the visitations of the plagues. However, one of the best known autobiographical accounts of the personal impact of a major catastrophe is that provided by Samuel Pepys in his diary. It is worth reading his own report of how he was affected by the Great Fire of London in the 17th Century.

The Industrial Revolution generated new potential hazards particularly in the fashion of industrial and transportation disasters. A Swiss investigator, Stierlin, studied the victims of mining disasters, and an English surgeon, Erichsen, introduced the concept of "Railway Spine"; a condition reported after railway collisions characterised by memory impairment, irritability and nightmares. (Probably the most famous victim of this condition was the author Charles Dickens.) Although Stierlin proposed that fright was the main factor underlying the symptoms reported by survivors of mining tragedies, Erichsen and most of his contemporaries still favoured explanations in physical terms, including, a disturbance of the spinal bone marrow (Beveridge, 1997).

Throughout much of the 19th Century there was considerable scepticism about the authenticity of the symptoms reported by survivors of accidents. This was probably due to the availability of compensation through the Compensation Laws. Such concerns about simulation and artifice still prevail in the wake of contemporary accidents even when there is little evidence to suggest that symptoms remit once compensation has been paid out (Tarsh & Royston, 1985).

More Recent Developments

Although there persisted ignorance and scepticism about the cause of so-called "shell-shock" described among the victims of the Great War (in which over 200,000 men were exempted on psychiatric grounds from further combat), there was a growing awareness, perhaps even unease, that the psychological trauma of combat might be the main cause of the varied and at times extraordinary symptoms associated with that condition. Unfortunately, the War Office and even some medical authorities argued that only those individuals with "weak" personalities would succumb to such pressures. Regrettably, this pejorative view still persists.

In the Second World War the earlier diagnosis of "shell shock" yielded to that of "battle fatigue" or "combat exhaustion". Therein there is some acknowledgement that combat itself was the source of soldiers' symptoms rather that some physical factor, ie, such as carbon monoxide poisoning, diarrhoea, excessively tight equipment and altered atmospheric pressure due to exploding artillery shells. This view was reinforced by the severe and prolonged reactions reported among the survivors of the Nazi concentration camps. This kind of evidence moved our thinking towards the conclusion that there may be some stressors which are so intense and pervasive that almost anybody is likely to develop post-traumatic reactions.

Order Out of Chaos

Because of the uncertainty about the causes of reactions to trauma, and because of some prejudice against such victims, by the 1970s the literature was awash with diagnostic terms, including:

Soldier's Heart
Railway Spine
Spinal Concussion
Shell Fever
Hysterical Hemianaesthesia
Hysterical Sympathy with the Enemy
Burial-alive Neurosis
Neurocirculatory Asthenia
War Psychoneurosis
Gross Stress Reactions
Concentration Camp Syndrome

Clearly, this situation could not persist, and the classification of reactions to combat and other trauma had to be revised.

A landmark in this revision followed the Vietnam War, when the American Psychiatric Association coined the term "Post-traumatic Stress Disorder", a term which clearly identifies the pre-eminent role of the trauma in the aetiology of the symptoms. This term was introduced in 1980 into the 3rd edition of the Diagnostic and Statistical Manual of Mental Disorders This important condition will be dealt with more fully in Chapter 12, but below it will be defined, along with other conditions associated with trauma.

Currently there are two principal classification schemes relating to psychiatric symptoms, namely, the aforementioned Diagnostic and Statistical Manual of Mental Disorders (DSM-IV) and the International Classification of

Mental and Behavioural Disorders (ICD-10). The latter is the one most commonly used in the United Kingdom, thus consideration will now be given to the trauma-related disorders recognised by the ICD-10.

(i) *Post-traumatic Stress Disorder (PTSD)*

This may follow a "stressful event or situation of an exceptionally threatening or catastrophic nature, which is likely to cause pervasive distress in almost anyone ... ". The characteristic symptoms are intrusive experiences involving flashbacks[1] and nightmares, against a background of a sense of numbness and emotional blunting, detachment from others, unresponsiveness and avoidance.

'Commonly' there is fear and avoidance of reminders of the trauma, and "often" there is hyperarousal and hypervigilance (these phenomena are associated with an exaggerated reaction to sudden noises, irritability, insomnia and exaggerated awareness of personal threat and risk to safety).

These symptoms normally appear within a few weeks of the trauma, and the diagnosis is not normally made unless it can be shown that the symptoms arose within six months of the trauma.

In its "pure" form PTSD is relatively uncommon; it is most frequently associated with comorbid conditions of anxiety, depression and alcohol abuse.

(ii) *Acute stress reaction*

This is often a precursor to Post-traumatic Stress Disorder. It is a transient condition which normally remits within hours or days after the trauma. It includes a miscellany of symptoms (often fluctuating), including anger, anxiety, despair, depression, withdrawal, numbness and overactivity.

(iii) *Adjustment disorders*

These are characterised by distress and emotional disturbance of a severity which interferes with normal adjustment. The onset is within one month of the trauma, and the conditions do not last for more than six months (with the exception of prolonged depressive reaction which can last for up to about two years).

There are six sub-categories each of which reflects the primary nature of the disturbance:

[1] 'Flashbacks' are the vivid and involuntary re-living of the event accompanied by the emotional and sensory experiences originally associated with that event. Flashbacks are mostly visual but may involve any sensory modality.

- Brief depressive reaction
- Prolonged depressive reaction
- Mixed anxiety and depressive reaction
- With predominant disturbance of other emotions
- With predominant disturbance of emotion and conduct
- With other specified predominant symptoms

(iv) *Dissociative disorders*

These disorders include: dissociative amnesia, dissociative fugue and dissociative disorders of mobility, sensation and function. (These used to be described as "hysterical conversion disorders"; a misleading and pejorative diagnosis.)

The characteristic feature of these conditions is a partial or complete loss of the normal integration between memories of past events, an awareness of one's identity and sensations and bodily control. These conditions can result in, for instance, paralysis, blindness, a loss of sensation in part of the body or major lapses of recall. Although there is nothing physically wrong, the patient genuinely believes there is. Thus, these conditions are not due to conscious deception. In a "fugue" patients may wander off for hours or even days without knowing why and who they are.

The onset of such phenomena is usually acute, in response to some overwhelming or threatening event. They tend to remit spontaneously within a few weeks or months after the trauma, although, in certain instances following exceptionally traumatic events, they may become chronic.

(v) *Enduring personality change after a catastrophic experience*

Certain trauma, either because of their intensity or duration, may be so devastating in their impact that they cause a permanent change in the survivor's personality. Most commonly these changes result in:

- a hostile and suspicious attitude
- social withdrawal
- a feeling of personal "emptiness" and/or hopelessness
- a chronic feeling of always being on edge

The kind of circumstance which may induce such profound changes are major disasters, being taken hostage, being tortured and being held captive under conditions of extreme deprivation and brutality (such as occurred in Concentration Camps).

Prognosis Following Trauma

There is no single event or situation which inevitably gives rise to psychiatric disorder in the survivors. Even after the worst imaginable trauma certain individuals will come through without any obvious symptoms. Why this should be so is not fully understood, but we do know that there are certain factors which are more likely to lead to psychopathology and problems of adjustment.

These can be classified under three headings: (a) the trauma, (b) the survivor, and (c) the environment.

(a) *The trauma*

- prolonged exposure (eg, being trapped in a motor vehicle)
- (perceived) threat to life (it does not matter if the survivor's life was not objectively at risk)
- multiple death and/or mutilations
- sudden and unexpected (because there is no time to prepare emotionally)
- special meaning (the involvement of children in trauma always gives it a "special meaning". Tragedies at, for example, Christmas time also carry a special poignancy.)

(b) *The survivor*

- Severity and significance of personal injury. (Generally, the more serious the injury the worse the psychological reactions. We need to remember it may also be the personal significance of the injury in terms of its effect on the individual's self-esteem, relationships and work capabilities which may make the injury a devastating experience even although in objective or surgical terms the scale of tissue damage may not be extensive.)
- Extreme initial stress reactions. (Those who subsequently develop PTSD are more likely to have shown extreme reactions in the immediate aftermath of the trauma.)
- Previous trauma. (This relationship is complex. For some victims previous experience of trauma may help them to cope with a subsequent one. For others the outcome may be the opposite in that the effect is cumulative or sensitising, thus, it makes it harder for them to cope with subsequent trauma. Key factors may be the time interval between the events and how well the individuals believed they had coped with the previous ones.)
- Miscellaneous factors. (Early parental loss, personal history of psychiatric ill health, low educational level and female gender commonly

but certainly not universally correlate with poor outcome after trauma.)

(c) *The environment*

- Concurrent life stressors. (Sometimes the survivors' ability to cope with the most recent trauma is poor only because their emotional resilience has already been compromised by other pressures on them, eg, family, health, accommodation or employment problems. Instead of asking victims of road traffic accidents (RTAs), before they are discharged from hospital, "have you someone to go home to?" perhaps we should ask, "what are you going home to?")
- Lack of support from others (including family, friends and colleagues).

"Ripple Effect" (Raphael, 1986)

Following a serious RTA it is fairly obvious that those who survive the incident are entitled to be called "victims". However, in the same way that a pebble dropping in a pool of water produces not just one ripple but a series, accidents may affect many individuals apart from drivers and passengers.

The author recently had to deal with the victims of an RTA in which four young people were killed. The driver of the vehicle was badly injured and obviously guilty about his role in the accident. He was the "primary victim". However, a pedestrian witnessed this horrific accident in which two of the deceased were decapitated and subsequently incinerated in front of her. Clearly, although not personally involved in the RTA, the impact on her of this horrific scene justifies her being described as a "secondary" victim. Also, we need to remember the possible impact of dealing with carnage on this scale on the rescuers and other helpers. There are occasions when emergency personnel and trauma staff may themselves become "tertiary" victims, even when they are very experienced (Alexander & Atcheson, 1998).

Normal Reactions to Trauma

With very few exceptions, "normal" and "pathological' reactions to trauma differ only in degree rather than in kind. Consequently, there is a degree of arbitrariness about the distinction; there is no absolute cut-off point or threshold. In general terms, we regard reactions as pathological if they are so severe as to render the survivors "dysfunctional" in that they are unable to fulfil the usual demands of their lives, eg, maintaining relationships, working and looking after themselves.

These points should be borne in mind when considering the following list of reactions which are commonly seen in the short term following traumatic incidents.

- *Numbness, shock, denial and dissociation*
  Nature has devised ways to shield us from the immediate impact of horrific events. Survivors of RTAs commonly report feeling perfectly calm during the incident and feeling rather detached or as though it had been a bad dream. Some even behave as though it had not happened.

- *Fear*
  This often sets in after an RTA when survivors realise what has happened or what might have happened. Fear is a normal biological response of great survival value as it initiates the "fight/flight" response.

- *Depression*
  Probably all trauma involve a loss of something (eg, loss of life, loss of a vehicle, loss of a limb, loss of one's looks and loss of a future). Depression is the most common reaction to loss. It may be coupled with a sense of grieving over that which has been lost.

- *Elation*
  This is less common. It is probably due to psychological relief at having survived, for example, a serious RTA and/or to neuroendocrinal changes. (These may lead to a surprising ability to tolerate pain following injury in an accident.)

- *Anger*
  Survivors commonly feel angry. Their anger may be directed at others involved in the accident or believed to be the cause of the accident. Sometimes the anger has no obvious legitimate target, and it is therefore "displaced" on to others, including rescuers, helpers, relatives and hospital staff.

- *Helplessness*
  Trauma nearly always give rise to at least a temporary sense of helplessness when the victims suddenly feel they have no control over whether they will live or die or be injured or escape unscathed. This sense of being out of control may persist in hospital, particularly if they are badly injured and require specialist care as is available in an Intensive Treatment Unit.

- *Guilt*
  "Survivor" guilt was seen, for example, in the case of a father whose child was killed in the vehicle he was driving, even although he was not in any way responsible for the accident. Such individuals commonly are heard to say "I wish I had died instead'.
  Another example occurred when two young daughters died in a bus crash after their mother had sent them down to visit relatives. She now commonly berates herself for arranging this trip. "If only I hadn't... ".

- *Irritability*
  This is not a dramatic reaction but it can have a pernicious effect on the families, friends and colleagues of survivors of RTAs. It is probably associated with autonomic hypersensitivity and anger at the fact that the accident happened.

- *Cognitive changes*
  Survivors of RTAs commonly have difficulty in describing consistently and accurately what happened. When there are several survivors of the same incident they quite often give differing accounts of the event. This is very rarely because of lying or attempting to cover up what happened.
  Particularly sudden and dramatic incidents cause misperceptions in terms of the apparent speed at which events occur (usually everything seems to be slowed down) and of the order in which they occurred. Also, survivors often report "tunnel vision", ie, they have focused on one particular aspect of the accident and, therefore, have little or perhaps even no recollection of other aspects. Other cognitive changes commonly seen after trauma are impaired concentration and problems of short term memory.

- *Impaired sleep*
  This is associated with autonomic hyperarousal and hypervigilance such that the individual often claims, "I can't switch off my brain" or "I just feel too alert and hear everything".
  Sleep may also be interrupted by nightmares or prevented by "flashbacks'. This can be particularly distressing as is evident in the case of the badly burned patient who, despite being in great pain, refused to take his self-administered morphine. This puzzled the nursing staff. On enquiry the explanation was perfectly rational. If the patient took his analgesic he would become sleepy. If he fell asleep he had horrific nightmares of the accident in which he had been burned. So distressing were these that he decided he would rather lie awake in pain.

- *Flashbacks*
  As described earlier these are vivid re-enactments of the incidents or features of it, and may involve any of the sensory modalities or emotions implicated in the initial trauma. It is like reliving the event.

- *Autonomic hyperarousal and hypervigilance*
  A serious trauma overstimulates the autonomic nervous system, and this effect may endure for weeks or even months. During this period patients report feeling particularly "jumpy" and "on edge". They also seem to be much more aware of risk, eg, in motor vehicles, such that they may over-react to horns blowing or to the sound of brakes screeching.

- *Avoidant behaviour*
  Survivors of RTAs may initially avoid talking about the incidents, reading about them, getting into vehicles (or even something reminiscent of a vehicle such as a lift) or going past the scene of the accident.
  NB: These last three reactions are of course the hallmarks of PTSD.

- *Alcohol (or other substance misuse)*
  Alcohol is a powerful drug which *temporarily* reduces anxiety and helps people to blot out unpleasant memories. Thus, it is not uncommon to find an increased use of alcohol after RTAs as survivors attempt to self-medicate. This is not effective in the long term, and it most commonly gives rise to a series of secondary health and social problems.

A World of Assumptions (Janoff-Bulman, 1989)

Most of us share a number of assumptions about life which allow us to proceed without being preoccupied or even paralysed about the possibility of things going wrong. These assumptions are:

- the world is largely benevolent
  thus: dreadful events should not happen
- the world is meaningful
  thus: it is predictable and not random or capricious
- we are fairly decent individuals
  thus: we deserve justice and fairness, and we do not deserve dreadful things to happen to us

When we drive our cars we do not seriously expect to have an accident at any moment. Accidents, we believe, happen to others. Modern cars may reinforce our assumptions about invincibility. Cars have become increasingly comfortable; they have seats similar to those we might sit in at home; there are various comforts available, ie, we can eat, drink and listen to a stereo or radio. Technically, cars are now easier to drive because of high technology, automatic gears and computers. All these factors conspire to make us feel safe, secure and comfortable.

The need to maintain these assumptions may also account for the lack of sympathy and concern sometimes shown towards victims of trauma, including RTAs. The accounts of survivors of bad accidents threaten our assumptions because, unless we can reassure ourselves that the circumstances relating to their accidents are different from our own, there is an uneasy realisation the same fate could await us. Perhaps that is why one hears dismissive allegations and assertions such as these.

(i) Said to a young male who suffered a traumatic amputation of his lower limb following a collision on his motor bike.
"Well, if you will go around on bikes like that that's what you can expect to happen."

(ii) Said of a young female driver who lost control of her car on a bend and suffered serious internal and orthopaedic injuries.
"I'll bet you she would have been chattering to her pal about something – probably didn't even see the bend."

(iii) Said of a driver of a military vehicle who was blinded in one eye after a crash.
"Well, I'm not surprised he complains all the time – tasty bit of compensation is coming his way."

These assumptions may also help to explain why so many people fail to prepare a will until they are in their later years, and why safety guidelines and road traffic laws are so commonly breached.

However, once we have been involved in a serious RTA, these assumptions are rudely challenged, perhaps even shattered. The world is no longer seen as such a safe and benevolent place; cars and their drivers are not to be trusted, and we now feel vulnerable and at risk. It may take considerable time and, in some cases, expert psychological treatment may be required, before once more these working assumptions can be re-established on a more realistic basis.

If we are really to understand the reactions of victims of RTAs then we need to come to terms with our own sense of vulnerability which their experiences highlight, and we cannot dismiss their experiences as merely due to their incompetence, foolhardiness or quest for sympathy and financial gain.

How do we Know when Somebody is Not Coping?

Most survivors do not develop PTSD, and most survivors do eventually adjust even after the most horrific accidents. However, we can identify those who need help even when they themselves appear not to be aware of the need or when they deny it.

Guidelines to Identify Who is Not Coping

- *Excessive denial and numbness*
  In the face of contrary evidence some survivors (perhaps through pride, guilt or anxiety) consistently claim, "I'm fine'. On the other hand, even weeks after the accident, some look like automata, mechanically acting out their lives with no obvious emotion or self-reflection; they seem as though they are in a daze.

- *Repeated carelessness*
  A common time to have an accident is in the wake of one which has just occurred. Survivors may display a regular tendency to have mishaps. Even if these are minor ones, it may suggest impaired concentration and adjustment.

  Occasionally, unresolved guilt about an accident may lead survivors to have accidents, perhaps as a form of self-punishment. This may be of an unconscious motivation although it can be due to a conscious effort to self-harm.

- *Reduced work performance*
  Even in the most diligent and conscientious individuals one can see a chronic decline in their performance at work (including housework in the case of those who work at home).

- *Overindulgences*
  The sustained and excessive misuse of alcohol, tobacco, food or even work may suggest an individual is not coping after an RTA.

- *'Russian roulette'*
  It has been noted that some survivors of trauma begin to take unnecessary and uncharacteristic risks with their lives. This may reflect their view that they are now invincible, having survived a major, life-threatening trauma. Alternatively, this tendency may also relate to an enduring sense of guilt about an accident. Perhaps there is an unconscious need to be punished by having another accident (as described above).

This phenomenon can be seen in survivors of RTAs who drive too fast, may even buy bigger and more powerful cars or "drink and drive'.

A Positive Outcome

It is remarkable how well individuals do cope with even the most dreadful RTAs; events which appear initially to have destroyed lives. It is important therefore to bear in mind how adaptable we are. Moreover, it is also comforting to note how often some good can derive from tragedy and adversity (Raphael, 1986).

Survivors of RTAs (particularly following those in which there was a genuine threat to life) may become much more appreciative of what they have in life; family and marital bonds may become strengthened; new relationships may develop, and the survivors may gain in self-esteem and self-respect through their recognition of previously unrecognised strengths and ability to cope.

Conclusions

A trauma such as a road traffic accident is a violation of our sense of security and invincibility. Suddenly, we may become very aware of our vulnerability.

In addition, such an event may give rise to a constellation of emotional, behavioural, physiological, social and cognitive changes.

In most cases these are no more than normal reactions but, in the case of some survivors, these may be so acute, widespread or chronic, that the individuals may not be able to cope with the demands of living. Consequently, they may be described as suffering from one of a number of post-traumatic conditions.

Accidents will affect a "primary" victim, but the effects of accidents extend to others, eg, bystanders, the families of the primary victims and those who rescue or render help to the victims.

Fortunately, despite the major unpleasant and otherwise adverse effects of trauma, one often observes positive reactions, such as a fuller appreciation of life, during the recovery and rehabilitation phase. These reactions never compensate for all the emotional scars which a bad accident is likely to leave but it is important to facilitate and to identify any positive changes in order that survivors can transcend their suffering and retrieve their sense of hope and purpose in life.

References

Alexander, D. A. & Atcheson, S.F. (1998). Psychiatric aspects of trauma care: survey of nurses and doctors. *Psychiatric Bulletin*, *22*, 132–136.

Babington, A. (1997). *Shell–Shock. A history of the changing attitudes to war neurosis*. London: Lee Cooper.

Beveridge, A. (1997). On the origins of post–traumatic stress disorder. In: *Psychological Trauma. A developmental approach*. (eds. D. Black, M. Newman, J. Harris-Hendriks, and G. Mezey), pp 3–9. London: Gaskell.

Janoff-Bulman, R. (1989). The benefits of illusions, the threat of disillusionment, and the limitations of inaccuracy. *Journal of Social and Clinical Psychology*, *8*, 158–175.

Raphael, B. (1986). *When disaster strikes*. New York: Basic Books.

Tarsh, M. & Royston, C. (1985). A follow up study of accident neurosis. *British Journal of Psychiatry*, *146*, 18–25.

Further Reading

Alexander, D. A. (1996). Trauma research: a new era. (editorial) *Journal of Psychosomatic Research*, *41*, 1–5.

Diagnostic and Statistical Manual of Mental Disorders, 4th Edition (1994). Washington, DC: American Psychiatric Association.

Gibbon, M. (1998). *Order from Chaos* (2nd edition). Birmingham: Venture Press.

Giller, E. L. & Weisaeth, L. (1996). *Post-traumatic Stress*. Disorder. Baillière Tindall London.

International Classification of Mental and Behavioural Disorders (ICD-10), (1992). World Health Organisation. London, Churchill Livingstone.

Kinchin, D. (1994). *Post Traumatic Stress Disorder. A practical guide to recovery*. London: Thorsons.

O'Brien, L. S. (1998). *Traumatic Events and Mental Health*. Cambridge: Cambridge University Press.

2

Survival, Fear, Post-Traumatic Stress Disorder and All That

Dr GORDON TURNBULL, BSc, FRCP, FRCPsych, FRGS

Clinical Director, Tramatic Stress Unit, Ticehurst House Hospital, East Sussex, UK.
& Consultant Psychiatrist to the Civil Aviation Authority

Introduction

In ancient times, evil spirits bent on mischief were believed to be responsible for many illnesses. Perhaps the best example of this philosophy is *epilepsy* where demons invaded the brain and charged around with all the resultant, convulsive chaos. The only answer was to release them by opening the skull. This was, however, in keeping with the times.

Nowadays "*stress*" is believed to be the cause of many medical conditions. The solution is generally thought to be to release it. Despite the remarkable advances in physiology and its sister science, psychology, the subject of "stress" is still bedevilled by myth and controversy. The general aim of this chapter is to look at the reactions which are the result of being exposed to overwhelmingly stressful events in the light of present knowledge and to exorcise the mythology. In particular, the aim is to look at the potential of one of the most common of such reactions, Post-Traumatic Stress Disorder (PTSD), to enhance positive and adaptive mental processes in survivors.

This piece of doggerel by Jonathan Swift helps to remind us that living is an eternal struggle of survival:-

"Big Fleas have little fleas
Upon their backs to bite 'em.
And little fleas have smaller fleas
And so on, 'ad infinitum'.
Thus every poet, in his kind
Is bit by him that comes behind".

Our physiological and psychological defence mechanisms are always "on duty", vigilantly protecting us from competitive influences. We may be at war occasionally with other members of our own species but we are constantly in conflict with representatives of all of the other major divisions of the animal kingdom with which we share the planet. And, if we are not vigilant, even the lowest orders of micro-organisms are bent on seizing supremacy. Sometimes they win. Human beings have to be resilient. We have to be good at surviving. After all this time it would be surprising if we did not come ready-equipped with instincts which help us to survive amongst all the competition.

An *instinct* is defined as *"an innate propensity to certain seemingly rational acts performed without conscious intention"* or, more simply put, *"an innate, usually fixed pattern of behaviour especially in response to certain simple stimuli"* or, best *"an unconscious skill" (Collins Dictionary & Thesaurus, 1987)*. There is a strong case to be made in favour of "stress reactions" being adaptive and instinctual; for example, depressive reactions as "learned helplessness" (Seligman, 1992). There is an even stronger case to be made for Post-Traumatic Stress Disorder actually representing a survival instinct, in response to the supreme challenge ... threat to life itself.

Stress

"Stress" is a word borrowed from the world of Newtonian physics. It is defined as a *force that moves or distorts objects*. Biological stresses put pressure on biological objects (organisms) and tend to induce change. Organisms are complex systems which are dedicated to homeostasis. When an imbalance develops between *demands* exerted by external and internal environments and the *resources* required to meet them then a *"stress reaction"* will occur.

Adrenaline and other hormones (the body's chemical messengers) broker the adjustments in function to keep metabolism in "tune" with demand. This has upper and lower limits and the adrenaline works just like a spanner on a carburettor to keep things working smoothly. Adrenaline plays such a pivotal role that it has earned a reputation as the "fight or flight" hormone.

Reasonable amounts of stress are necessary just to keep going but an over-accumulation of too much over too long is exhausting. Before exhaustion actually occurs stress-related *symptoms* develop which are really advance warning signals to announce that energy is running low and that, if a major decompensation of the whole system is to be averted, a rest needs to be taken. Ignore the "smoke-signals" and the *symptoms* become more intense and persistent and serious interference of normal physical and emotional functioning will develop. Most stress-reactions are undifferentiated, wispy clouds of free-floating *symptoms* but, if they are allowed to gather, they will form a dense fog which will subsequently take on the shape of a familiar syndrome, such as depression, phobic anxiety etc. Once that threshold has been crossed, active intervention and not simply rest and the passage of time is usually required.

Disorders which develop a gradual accumulation of stress are quite different from Post-Traumatic Stress Disorder (PTSD). The stresses which cause PTSD are extreme and are generated extremely rapidly. No meaningful resistance can possibly be mounted. The normal trickle of stimulating adrenaline suddenly turns into a ranging torrent as if a dam has broken or a barrier breeched and even the defences of the most robust personality or of the best-trained and talented individuals are swamped. The only circumstances which produce the catharsis are survival situations.

Post-Traumatic Stress Disorder (PTSD)

PTSD is a serious psychological reaction in overwhelmingly frightening events that strike suddenly and with such brutal force that it is impossible to fight back at the time. A *trauma* is the word used to describe such an event. *Trauma* is an Ancient Greek word that means to *"pierce"* or to *"puncture"*. It is a very telling way to describe the real meaning of a traumatic experience, because such an event not only has to be powerfully forceful in itself but it also has a powerful effect.

Traumatic Events

The word *trauma* is not the only significant contribution that has been made in the understanding of PTSD by the Ancient Greeks. Homer's *Iliad* (Homer, circa 850 BC: Shay, 1994) described changes in the behaviour of Achilles in the aftermath of the Trojan Wars indistinguishable from the modern definition of Post-Traumatic Stress Disorder. There have been many historical descriptions of the condition which are, in reality, documented antecedents of PTSD (Trimble 1981; Parry-Jones & Parry-Jones 1994). The most striking is from William Shakespeare's *The First Part of King Henry IV*, Shakespeare 1598). He appears to have a complete grasp of the condition now known as PTSD and encapsulated this in his speech from Lady Percy to the extent that she appears to be reading the definition from DSM-IV (Diagnostic & Statistical Manual of the American Psychiatric Association, 1994) as she describes the changes in her husband, the Knight Hotspur, during the Wars of the Roses in England, four hundred years ago.

" '*O, my good lord! why are you thus alone?*
For what offence have I this fortnight been
A banish'd woman from my Harry's bed?
Tell me, sweet lord, what is't that takes from thee..
Thy stomach, pleasure, and thy golden sleep?
Why dost thou bend thine eyes upon the earth,
And start so often when thou sitt'st alone?
Why has thou lost the fresh bood in thy cheeks.
And given my treasures and my rights of thee
To thick-eyed musing and curst melancholy?
In they faint slumbers! by thee have watch'd
Any heard thee murmur tales of iron wars
Speak terms of manage to thy bounding steed
Cry, 'Courage! to the field!' And thou has talk's.
Of sallies and retires, of trenches, tents
Of palisadoes, frontiers, parapets,
Of basilisks, of cannon, culverin.
Of prisoners' ransom, and of soldiers slain,
And all the currents of a heady fight.
They spirit within thee hath been so at war,
And thus hath so bestirr'd thee in they sleep,
That beads of sweat have stood upon thy brow.
Like bubbles in a late-disturbed stream,
And in thy face strange motions have appear'd,
Such as we see when met restrain their breath
On some great sudden hest. O! what portens are these?
Some heavy business hath my lord in hand,
And I must know it, else he loves me not."

A trauma is a powerful event that involves *direct personal experience* of threatened death, of serious injury or *witnessing* threatened death in others. It is also the experience of learning about unexpected or violent death or serious harm in family members or close friends. A trauma induces a powerful reaction as evidence of it having *pierced* psychological defences. These characrteristics are embraced by Criterion A of the DSM-IV Classification of PTSD which has earned its reputation as "*The Gatekeeper*" because it must be satisfied before the other features of PTSD can develop.

Some examples of traumatic events:–

- military combat
- violent personal asssault (sexual assault, physical attack, abuse, robbery, mugging)
- being taken hostage
- being a prisoner-of-war
- natural or man-made disasters
- being diagnosed with a life-threatening illness

By far the moment common traumatic event in developed countries is the serious road traffic accident (Mayou et al 1993, Blanchard et al, 1995). Published research has shown that the *traumagenicity* of the accident depends upon what it has meant to the victim and cannot always be predicted accurately from the extent of damage at the scene, the degree of physical injury or the opinion of the examining physician or the judgement of the lawyer if personal injury litigation is entered into subsequently. This is one medical field in which the patient definitely knows more about the subject than the doctor, whose role is first to listen, next to listen again and learn and last to advise.

The most traumatic events are sudden and unexpected, involve close and long-exposure (such is being trapped), are man-made (there is nobody to blame if the trauma is natural), and involves multiple deaths and/or mutilation. Events are especially traumatic when children are involved. Survivors who *dissociate* at the time of the trauma tend to develop chronic and disabling post-traumatic stress reactions. These are the most significant *primary* features of a trauma.

Secondary factors such as not being supported or even receiving a hostile reaction from others reinforce the primary impact of the trauma. Some individuals and organisations still believe that post-traumatic reactions is a sign of weakness of character or even that the victim is to blame for having become involved in the trauma or, most unreasonable of all, that the victim is inventing the reaction for compensation reasons. These are examples of defensive reactions to the anticipated discomfort of discussing events which might be gruesome, horrifying or unimaginable and from which listeners seek protection for themselves.

Characteristic Features of PTSD

PTSD has been recognised formally since 1980, since it was first identified in the Third Edition of the Diagnostic and Statistical Manual of the American Psychiatric Association (DSM-III 1980) and has undergone two slight revisions in DSM-III-Revised (DSM-III-R, 1987) and DSM-IV (DSM-IV, 1994). Extensive research has upheld the initial concept. When it is established that a person has been traumatised three major symptom clusters develop.

The first symptom cluster is called the *re-experiencing* symptoms in which the trauma essentially continues to have a life of its own in the form of recurrent and intrusive thoughts, in nightmares, or in dissociative states called flashbacks, or any combination of all three. These phenomena are based upon actual memories of the trauma and may be spontaneous or triggered by stimuli that resemble or are reminiscent of the trauma. They may be so realistic that the trauma may seem to be happening all over again. Reminders can be very obvious or might be very subtle. Anniversaries are example of obvious reminders but weather such as fog or rain or snow might trigger memories of traumatic events such as a road traffic accident or a flood or an avalanche respectively.

The second cluster is called the *avoidance-numbing* cluster. This is because individuals suffering from PTSD find the re-experiencing symptoms so intolerable and so difficult to deal with that a variety of cognitive strategies and behavioural adjustments are brought into play to reduce the frequency and the intensity of the flashbacks. Included are *avoidance* symptoms such as avoiding situations that are reminiscent of the trauma and *numbing* symptoms which include shutting down emotional expression, dissociation, psychogenic amnesia, reduction of general responsiveness, social withdrawal and blunted affect. Effective communication ceases, personal and work relationships are jeopardised or lost and the sufferer from PTSD becomes cocooned into a private world, creating a barrier against the emotional pain.

The third cluster of symptoms closely resembles most anxiety disorder symptoms such as irritability, insomnia etc, but unique to PTSD is the degree of *hypervigilance* (being on guard). Those who have been traumatised never want to be traumatised again in some situations, the degree of hypervigilance can be so extreme that it resembles (and may be mistaken for) a paranoid state.

PTSD is the reaction to the near-loss of "*the self*" and is a normal reaction just as *grieving* is the normal reaction at the actual loss of a strong attachment figure. In effect, PTSD seems to be a unique anxiety disorder involving many of the cognitive, psychological and psychobiological mechanisms that are important in coping and adaptation.

PTSD as a Survival Instinct

In the early stages of a post-traumatic reaction the three characteristic symptom clusters appear to be making an attempt to repair the damage done by the impact of the trauma to three core beliefs that the great majority of people need to have to feel secure in the world. These are that life is reasonably *fair,* reasonably *safe* and that there is a place for us in the world (Janoff-Bulman, 1992).

Flashbacks facilitate repetitive re-examination of the traumatic experience so that survival tactics can be learnt. Distortions of perception are less likely to persist and fairness and security are more likely to be restored.

Avoidance keeps the number of replays down to a manageable level. This facilitates the assimilation of newly learned impressions.

Hyperarousal maintains alertness to the possibility of further trauma (for example, a second earthquake) and supplies the adrenaline to field the repair work that needs to be done.

Grief, depression, anxiety, guilt and anger are commonly found companions to the three main symptom clusters. In most cases, the repair work is completed quickly but if this is not possible the memory-processing pathways in the brain becomes "jammed" and "stuck". Although most survivors successfully resolve acute post-traumatic stress reactions, a significant minority (20–40%) go on to develop chronic, disabling stress reactions which persist beyond three months after the traumatic exposure.

The Trauma "Rocket"

The trauma reaction is like a rocket carrying a satellite on its nose-cone. The "right stuff" has to gather together for the launching pad to be "ignited". The trauma and its impact must both be very powerful to achieve "lift off". ("The Gatekeeper" Criterion A must be satisfied). Once the rocket is under way, it has enough fuel on board to keep climbing for about one month, before it reaches orbital altitude. If the trauma reaction *"fizzles out"* within that critical month then the rocket will fall back to Earth and the satellite will not be released. In such a case a short-lived "Acute Stress Reaction" has occurred. This is characterised by powerful emotions mixed with flashbacks, avoidance tactics and shock.

Even more powerful fuel *"mixes"* will carry the rocket to its full altitude, release the satellite into orbit. Only about 20–40% of acute stress reactions go on to the stage of releasing a "satellite". The unresolved, raw traumatic stress reaction becomes "encapsulated" and will just keep on going, round and round in its orbit, until an opportunity comes along to repair the damage.

At least, the awareness of the orbiting satellite can be minimised when it is in orbit. This is chronic *Post-Traumatic Stress Disorder* which can last for several months or even many years. Instead of seeing this as a permanent state it is more accurately viewed as a *postponement of opportunity* to organise resolution of the impact of the trauma until a suitable time arrives. Effective management of the "satellite" involves opening the capsule and then processing the contents. Once achieved, the satellite will fall gently back to Earth by parachute nd *"re-entry"* will be accomplished.

The Key Role of Memory in PTSD

All frightening events are laid down in memory. This is probably designed to be adaptive, to facilitate learning about survival. Survivors who have been traumatised recover when they understand what it is that has happened to them, assimilate the information and integrate it into memory. Those survivors who cannot interpret meaningfully what happened to them, or at least, put it into words, continue to remain bewildered and perplexed. It is very difficult to come to terms with something if it does not make sense. Often trauma engenders a trance-like state (dissociation) which can produce partial psychogenic amnesia which reinforces the bewilderment. Perplexity may be enormously increased if dissociation defences extend to *depersonalisation* or *out-of-body experiences (OOBE)* /Blacmore, 1988.

"Ordinary fear" has a rational basis. *Conditioned fear* is a special type of memory. Unlike most memories, it does not need to be consciously recalled to be effective. Fear information entering the brain travels to the sensory information gathering centre the *thalamus*. From the thalamus the information is sent to appropriate information processing areas of the brain. Emotional stimuli provides two streams of information which travel down two separate pathways. Both pathways end up in the *amagdyla* which is the alarm system in the brain and the initiator of emotional responses. The longer of the two pathways takes the information to the visual cortex at the back of the brain initially and next to the recognition areas which releases stored knowledtge about the object from long-term memory. These elements of information are then congregated together and the synthesised congruent message is sent to the amagdyla to stir the body into action. This is a relatively slow pathway and would be of limited usefulness in emergencies when a much quicker system is required. This is provided by a second pathway which emerges from the thalamus. Fast connections between the thalamus, amagdyla, limbic system and hypothalamus allow information to pass from eyes to body – eliciting the "fight or flight" response – almost instantaneously. Conditioned fear seems to be mainly composed of information that takes the short-cut, the emergency pathway.

It is known that most recently-acquired memories are encoded and collected in the hippocampus (a nucleus in the limbic system). This especially applies to recent *conscious* memory. It is from the hippocampus that conscious memory information is despatched to the long-term memory stores. Serious damage to the hippocampus leads to severe impairment of recent memory and an inability to lay down memories in the long-term store.

The hippocampus does not seem to be responsible for all memory acquisition because recent research has demonstrated that *unconscious* memories are stored in the amagdyla. The amagdyla are thought to lay down *unconscious* memories in much the same way that the hippocampus lays down *conscious* ones. Therefore, when an event is recalled the hippocampal system will provide the conscious recollections of what was seen, what was heard, where it took place, who was present – the orientating factors, while the amagdyla will provide a reminiscence of the body's state at the time of the event (body memory), reconstituting the emotional and physical reactions that arose with the original experience (palpitations, sweating, nausea, feelings of fear etc).

The amagdyla permits full and faithfull recollections of emotional reactions as they occurred during a traumatic experience. When a conditioned memory is *burnt into* the amagdyla with enough force then it may become almost uncontainable, and trigger reactions that a trauma victim may re-experience the precipitating trauma, complete with full sensory replay. Therefore, a flashback memory not only has the power to re-kindle intensly clear replay of the factual elements of a truma but also brings back the full cargo of sensations and emotions as well (Le Doux, 1992: Van der Kolk & Van der Hart, 1989: Van der Kolk & McFarlane, 1996).

Unconscious memories are particularly likely to be formed during stressful events because the neuro-transmitter chemicals released at such times make the amagdyla more excitable (Yehuda & Harvey, 1998). Super-sensitivity of the amagdyla is the result of its exposure to particularly powerful events, such as traumatic experiences. It is as if the amagdyla are on a "hair-trigger" and the direct reminders are not essential to fire-off a full flashback response; even oblique or unconscious cues will do.

The painful sensations from a chronic whiplash injury to the neck sustained in a road traffic accident, for example, will provide sufficient stimulus to excite the amagdyla to produce a flashback memory to the original trauma. Once the physical tissue damage has settled down and resolved, however, movements of the neck might continue to excite the amagdyla-sponsored flashbacks (Turnbull, 1997). These will necessarily include the pain sensations which accompanied the original injury. This helps to explain the well-recognised phenomena of the chronically-painful injury which does not seem to have adequate explanation in terms of ongoing tissue-damage without resorting to traditional psychiatric interpretations that such phenomena are *hysterical,* the result of *abnormal illness behaviour, plumbum oscillans* or *compensationitis.* This area of research will have a very significant contribution to make in both clinical and medico-legal work.

The Issue of Pre-Vulnerability to PTSD

In the light of the new understanding of the key role of memory systems and the sensitised amagdyla to the development of PTSD, it is clear that PTSD is linked to particularly powerful experience. Previous traumatic exposures may leave a legacy of sensitivity in the amagdyla to future exposure to trauma. Successful resolution of PTSD seems to depend on *de-conditioning* of the conditioned, unconscious memory of the trauma. Unresolved traumatic reactions will leave the amagdyla in a hypersensitive state. Future exposure to frightening events will lead to the laying down of more conditioned fears and more material for flashback re-experiences.

The issues of pre-vulnerability was addressed in the definition of PTSD in the International Classificiation of Diseases, Tenth Edition (ICD-10, 1992) before research unveiled much of the new information about memory-processing. Remarkably, the ICD-10 comment on pre-vulnerability is very compatable with the more recent biological dimension of understanding. ICD-10 states:–

> *"Predisposing factors such as personality traits (eg compulsive, asthenic) or previous history of neurotic illness may lower the threshold for the development of the syndrome or aggravate its course, but they are neither necessary nor sufficient to explain its occurrence".*

Barriers to Diagnosing PTSD

While hallmark symptoms of PTSD are pathognomonic, the detection of PTSD is often difficult and is frequently missed, even by mental health professionals (Davidson, 1992) Reasons include:–

- reluctance to talk about unpleasant events and sensations
- embarrassment at admitting symptoms because of anxiety about being thought to be "weak" or, worse, "mentally unstable".
- physician discomfort in discussing events which might be gruesome, horrifying or beyond imagination.

- the fact that PTSD often presents with misleading symptoms such as headache,
- insomnia, irritability, depression, tension, substance abuse or even family or work-related problems.

Children and PTSD

PTSD can develop at any age, including childhood. In younger children distressing dreams of the actual trauma they have been involved in may change into nightmares of monsters. Young children do not seem to sense that they are re-living the past in dreams but they often re-live the trauma through repetitive play. Children who have been involved in a serious road traffic accident might repeatedly re-enact the crash with toy cars. Parents and teachers might report loss of interest in previously relished activities. The sense of a foreshortened future might take the form of the child not believing that it is possible to become an adult. Stomach aches and headaches are frequent physical symptoms. Children are often the forgotten victims of trauma (Yule, 1994). In terms of their exposure to trauma, children seem to be as absorptive as sponges.

PTSD Criteria

DSM-IV

A. The person has been exposed to a traumatic event in which **BOTH** of the following were present:

(1) the person experienced, witnessed, or was confronted with an event or events that involved actual or threatened death or serious injury, or a threat to physical integrity of self or others.
(2) the person's response involved intense fear, helplessness, or horror. (The Gatekeeper)

B. The traumatic event is persistently re-experienced in one (or more) of the following ways:

(1) recurrent and intrusive distressing recollections of the event, including images, thoughts, or perceptions.
(2) recurrent distressing dreams of the event.

(3) acting or feeling as if the traumatic event were recurring (includes a sense of reliving the experience, illusions, hallucinations, and dissociative flashback episodes, including those that occur on wakening or when intoxicated).
(4) intense psychological distress at exposure to internal or external cues that symbolise or resemble an aspect of the traumatic event.
(5) physiological reactivity on exposure to internal or external cues that symbolise or resemble an aspect of the traumatic event.

C. Persistent avoidance of stimuli associated with the trauma and numbing of general responsiveness (not present before the trauma), as indicated by three (or more) of the following:

(1) efforts to avoid thoughts, feelings, or conversations associated with the trauma.
(2) efforts to avoid activities, places, or people that arouse recollections of the trauma.
(3) inability to recall an important aspects of the trauma.
(4) markedly diminished interest or participation in significant activities.
(5) feelings of detachment or estrangement from others.
(6) restricted range of affect (eg. being unable to have loving feelings).
(7) sense of foreshortened future (eg does not expect to have a career, marriage, children or a normal life span).

D. Persistent symptoms of increased arousal (not present before the trauma), as indicated by two (or more) of the following.

(1) difficulty falling or staying asleep.
(2) irritability or outbursts of anger.
(3) difficulty concentrating.
(4) hypervigilance.
(5) exaggerated startle response.

E. Duration of the disturbance (symptoms in criteria B, C and D) is more than one month.

F. The disturbance causes clinically significant distress in impairment in social, occupational, or other important areas of functioning.

Conclusions

Post-traumatic stress disorder (PTSD) is a serious psychological reaction to very frightening experiences which are known as "traumatic". Although only formally classified in 1980 in DSM-III, the features of what is now known as PTSD have been observed on many occasions down through the ages in the literature of many nations.

There is a strong case to be made for PTSD to be regarded as a survival instinct, at least in its early stageds, with adaptive advantages for the survivor of trauma. Recent advances in the understanding of the neurobiology of memory has strongly reinforced the impression that memory-processing has a fundamentally important role in the generation of the features of PTSD, thus adding a further validation of the criteria which are at the core of the syndrome.

All those who have professional responsibility for the management of the victims of trauma, in all its aspects, need to maintain a high level of awareness that their patients or clients may have been traumatised, that PTSD can often account for a variety of common symptoms, and that it may also be at the root of a persisting, treatment-resistant depression or anxiety state.

Road traffic accidents are the most common precipitating cause of PTSD in developmed countries. Children are often the forgotten victims. Thorough assessment of accident victims will lead to improved identification of PTSD (Mayou et al, 1993) and reduction of suffering and persistent morbility from a condition which is eminently treatable (Busuttil & Turnbull, 1995)

References

American Psychiatric Association (1980). *Diagnostic & Statistical Manual of Mental Disorders* (3rd edn) (DSM-111). Washington, DC : APA

American Psychiatric Association (1987). *Diagnostic & statistical Manual of Mental Disorders* (3rd edn, revised) DSM-III-R). Washing, DC: APA

American Psychiatric Association (1994). *Diagnostic & Statistical Manual of Mental Disorders* (4th. edn) DSM-IV). Washington,DC: APA.

Blackmore, S. J. (1988) Visions from the dying brain. *New Scientists*, *118*, 1611, 43–46.

Blanchard, E. B., Hickling, E. J., Taylor, A. E. et al. (1995). Psychiatric morbidity associated with motor vehicle accidents. *Journal of Nervous and Mental Diseases*, *183*, 495–504.

Busuttil, E, Turnbull, G. J., Neal, L. A., Rollins, J., West, A. G., Blanch, N. & Herepath, R. (1995). Incorporating psychological debriefing techniques within a brief group psychotherapy programme for the treatment of post-traumatic stress disorder. *British Journal of Psychiatry, 167*, 495–502.

Davidson, J. (1992). Drug therapy of post-traumatic stress disorder. *British Journal of Psychiatry, 160*, 309–314.

Homer, (circa 850 BC). *The Illiad.*

Janoff-Bulman, R. (1992). *Shattered Assumptions: Towards a New Psychology of Trauma*. New York: Free Press.

Le-Doux, J. E. (1992). Brain mechanisms of emotion and emotional learning. *Current Opinions in Neurobiology*, *2*, 191–1997.

Mayou, R., Bryant, B. & Duthrie, R. (1993), Psychiatric consequences of road traffic accidents, *British Medical Journal, 307*, 647–651.

Parry-Jones, B. & Parry-Jones, W. L. (1994). Post-traumatic stress disorder: supportive evidence from an eighteenth century natural disaster. *Psychological Medicine, 24*, 15–28.

Seligman, M. E. P. (1992). *Helplessness: On Development, Depression and Death.* New York: Freeman.

Shakespeare, William (1598). *The First Part of King Henry IV.*

Shay, J (1994). *Achilles in Vietnam: Combat Trauma and the Undoing of Character.* New York: Atheneum.

Swift, Jonathan (1733). *On Poetry.*

Trimble, M. R. (1981). *Post-Traumatic Neurosis: From Railway Spine to the Whiplash.* Chichester: John Wiley.

Turnbull, G. J. (1997). Lyons Davidson medico-Legal Conference 1987, "*Medico-Legal Aspects of Whiplash Injury*". Bristol, England.

Van der Kolk, B. A. & McFarlane, A. C., (1996). The black hole of trauma. In B.A. Van der Kolk, A.C.McFarlane, & L Weisaeth. *Traumatic Stress: The Effects of Overwhelming Experience on Mind, Body and Society.* New York: Guildford Press.

World Health Organisation (1992). *The ICD-10 Classification of Mental and Behavioural Disorders: Clinical Descriptions and Diagnostic Guidelines.* Geneva: WHO

Yehuda, R. & Harvey, H. (1998). Relevance of neuroendocrine alteration in PTSD to cognitive impairments of trauma survivors. In *Recollections of Trauma: Scientific Research and Clinical Practice*: Proceedings of the 1996 NATO Conference on Trauma and Memory in Port Bourgenay, France, New York: Plenum.

Yule, W. (1994). Post traumatic stress disorders. In *Child and Adolescent Psychiatry: Modern Approaches.* (eds. M. Rutter, E. Taylor, & L. Hersov) (3rd edn) 392–406. Oxford: Blackwell

3

Acute Stress Disorder Following Motor Vehicle Accidents

RICHARD A. BRYANT, PhD

School of Psychology, University of New South Wales, Sydney, Australia

ALLISON G. HARVEY, PhD

Department of Experimental Psychology, University of Oxford, Oxford, United Kingdom

In 1994 the fourth edition of the *Diagnostic and Statistical Manual for Mental Disorders* (DSM-IV; American Psychiatric Association, 1994) introduced acute stress disorder (ASD) as a new diagnostic category to describe posttraumatic stress reactions that occur in the initial month after a trauma. A major reason for the inclusion of this diagnosis was that the 1-month minimum duration criterion of posttraumatic stress disorder (PTSD) precluded description of the significant distress observed in the initial weeks after a trauma. Since its initial description, this new diagnosis has variably elicited enthusiastic support or strong criticism. Despite the varying opinions about the ASD diagnosis, its introduction has resulted in a surge of empirical investigation into acute trauma reactions. In this chapter we will review the major rationales for ASD, the extent to which recent research supports the current conceptualization of the diagnosis, and the relevance of ASD to motor vehicle accident (MVA) survivors.

Definition of ASD

DSM-IV stipulates that ASD can occur after a fearful response to experiencing or witnessing a threatening event (Cluster A). The requisite symptoms to meet ASD include three dissociative symptoms (Cluster B), one reexperiencing symptom (Cluster C), marked avoidance (Cluster D), marked anxiety or increased arousal (Cluster E), and evidence of significant distress or impairment (Cluster F). The disturbance must last for a minimum of two days and a maximum of four weeks (Cluster G), after which time a diagnosis of PTSD should be considered. The primary difference between the criteria for ASD and PTSD is the former's emphasis on dissociative reactions to the trauma. The diagnosis of ASD requires that the individual has at least three of the following: (a) a subjective sense of numbing or detachment, (b) reduced awareness of one's surroundings, (c) derealization, (d) depersonalization, or (e) dissociative amnesia (for a review, see Bryant & Harvey, 1997).

Rationale of ASD

The ASD diagnosis was driven by the notion that acute dissociative reactions are a crucial mechanism in posttraumatic adjustment. This view stems from the early theorizing of Janet (1907), who argued that trauma led to attempts to minimize discomfort by dissociating awareness. Janet proposed that this dissociation resulted in diminished psychological well-being because it drained mental resources that were required for other processes. On the basis of this theory, Janet argued that adaptation to a traumatic event involved integrating the fragmented memories into awareness. Recent adaptations of Janet's (1907) views hold that acutely traumatized individuals will have impaired recovery if their dissociative responses impede access to and resolution of their traumatic experience (van der Kolk & van der Hart, 1989). Specifically, this perspective has stimulated the rationale that the ASD criteria (and most particularly, the dissociative symptoms) will predict chronic PTSD (Koopman, Classen, Cardeña & Spiegel, 1995). The ASD diagnosis was criticized, however, on several grounds. First, it was argued that this diagnosis potentially pathologizes normal and transient responses to trauma (Solomon, Laor & McFarlane, 1996). Second, at the time of its introduction it possessed virtually no empirical justification to warrant its description (Bryant & Harvey, 1997). Third, the strong emphasis on dissociation was contrary to one view that conceptualized acute dissociation as a protective mechanism that could potentially facilitate adaptation (Horowitz, 1986).

Incidence of ASD

Six studies have now been conducted which have specifically investigated the incidence of ASD; two of which were conducted with individuals who survived a MVA. Harvey & Bryant (1998a) assessed 92 MVA survivors who did not sustain a traumatic brain injury between 2-days and 1-month posttrauma for ASD. Full criteria for ASD were met by 13%, and 21% presented with subclinical ASD. These latter participants were predominantly characterized by meeting all criteria except for dissociation. Bryant & Harvey (1998a) also assessed a sample of 79 MVA survivors who had sustained a mild traumatic brain injury (MTBI). Although the brain injury resulted in these people being unable to recall some aspects of their trauma, ASD was diagnosed in 14% of patients and 5% had a subclinical diagnosis. These rates for ASD following MVAs are comparable to rates reported following other traumatic events. For example, Harvey & Bryant (1999a) assessed 120 individuals who survived MVAs, assaults, burns, or industrial accidents for the presence of ASD. The observed incidence of ASD was 11%, and this rate was comparable across the trauma groups. Another study that assessed survivors of assault reported that 19% met criteria for ASD (Brewin, Andrews, Rose & Kirk, 1999). In a sample of 36 bystanders to a mass shooting, 33% were diagnosed with ASD (Classen, Koopman, Hales & Spiegel, 1998). In a study of 47 survivors of an industrial accident, Creamer & Manning (1998) reported that 6% of their sample met criteria for ASD. Overall, these initial studies indicate that the incidence of ASD is lower than previously reported incidence rates of posttraumatic stress in the acute posttrauma phase (see Bryant & Harvey, in press for a review). This pattern probably reflects the more stringent criteria of ASD.

Relationship Between ASD and PTSD

A major reason proposed for the inclusion of ASD in DSM-IV was its purported ability to predict PTSD (Koopman et al., 1995). At the time ASD was introduced into DSM-IV, however, there was no evidence that ASD actually predicted PTSD. At that time prospective studies indicated that most people who were symptomatic in the acute posttrauma phase remitted in the following months. For example, Riggs, Rothbaum & Foa (1995) reported that 70% of women and 50% of men were diagnosed with PTSD an average of 19 days posttrauma. However, at 4-months posttrauma the rate of PTSD had dropped to 21% for women and zero for men. Rothbaum, Foa, Riggs, Murdock & Walsh (1992) reported that 94% of rape victims interviewed an average of two weeks posttrauma met criteria for PTSD and that three weeks later this proportion dropped to 64%, and then to 47% at eleven weeks post-assessment. Similarly, half of a sample meeting criteria for PTSD following a MVA had remitted by 6-months and two-thirds had remitted by one year posttrauma (Blanchard, Hickling, Barton et al., 1996). These patterns highlighted the need for different criteria to distinguish between those acutely traumatized individuals who will remit and those who will subsequently develop PTSD.

Five prospective studies employing the ASD criteria have now been completed. Harvey & Bryant (1998a) found that 78% of MVA survivors who were initially assessed for ASD were diagnosed with PTSD 6-months posttrauma. Interestingly, 60% of those who satisfied all ASD criteria except dissociation were diagnosed with PTSD 6-months posttrauma. These participants were subsequently re-assessed for PTSD 2-years after their MVAs (Harvey & Bryant, in press[a]). At this assessment, 75% of those who were initially diagnosed with ASD still had PTSD. In a sample of MVA survivors who had sustained a mild traumatic brain injury, Bryant & Harvey (1998) reported that 82% of those who initially had ASD met criteria for PTSD 6-months posttrauma. In a subsequent study that re-assessed this sample 2-years after the trauma, Harvey & Bryant (in press[b]) found that 80% of those who initially met ASD criteria still suffered PTSD. Brewin et al. (1999) found that 83% of assault victims who initially satisfied ASD criteria were subsequently diagnosed with PTSD at 6-months follow-up. Other studies have investigated the relationship between ASD symptoms and subsequent posttraumatic stress (rather than PTSD status). In a prospective study of firestorm survivors, it was observed that three acute dissociative symptoms combined with reexperiencing, avoidance, and arousal symptoms best predicted subsequent distress (Spiegel, Koopman, Cardeña & Classen, 1996). A further study of survivors of a mass shooting reported that a diagnosis of ASD within 8-days of the trauma was found to be a significant predictor of the level of posttraumatic stress symptoms at 7 to 10 months posttrauma (Classen et al., 1998).

Overall, these initial studies provide partial support for the ASD diagnosis because they indicate that a significant proportion of people who initially meet criteria for ASD subsequently display persistent PTSD. However, initial evidence indicates that the current emphasis on dissociative symptoms in the ASD definition needs to be questioned because a significant proportion of individuals who initially present with acute stress reactions that lack dissociative symptoms can also subsequently develop PTSD.

Predictive Power of ASD Symptoms

The studies by Harvey & Bryant (1998a) and Bryant & Harvey (1998) found that numbing and depersonalization had reasonably strong positive predictive power compared to the other dissociative symptoms for MVA samples. These results are consistent with earlier studies with a range of samples suggesting that acute dissociation predicts subsequent PTSD (Koopman, Classen & Spiegel, 1994; Marmar, Weiss, Schlenger, et al., 1994; McFarlane, 1986; Shalev, Orr & Pitman, 1993) and with evidence that emotional numbing best distinguishes individuals with and without PTSD following assault (Foa, Riggs & Gershuny, 1995). There is evidence to question whether the emphasis placed on acute dissociation is warranted, however. First, the findings that many people who meet all ASD criteria except dissociation subsequently develop PTSD (Harvey & Bryant, 1998a) suggests that the requirement that three dissociative symptoms be present may result in people who are at risk of developing PTSD not being identified. Second, there is considerable overlap between the acute dissociative symptoms stipulated by the ASD criteria. In the study by Harvey & Bryant (in press[c]), of those participants who reported derealization, 85% also reported reduced awareness, 79% also reported numbing, and 80% also reported depersonalization. This degree of overlap has been reported in other studies (Bremner, Krystal, Putnam, Southwick, Marmar, Charney & Mazure, 1998). These findings question the extent to which the dissociative symptoms specified by the ASD criteria are distinct reactions. Third, in the 2-year follow-up study by Harvey & Bryant (in press[a]) it was found that requiring emotional numbing rather than the other dissociative symptoms markedly improved the predictive power of the ASD diagnosis.

Harvey & Bryant (1998a) found that in terms of nondissociative ASD symptoms, a sense of reliving the trauma, avoidance of thinking and talking about the trauma, and motor restlessness also strongly predicted subsequent PTSD. These findings point to the utility of including symptoms from the range of symptom clusters stipulated in the ASD criteria. However, the positive predictive power of the ASD diagnosis was markedly improved by modifying the criteria so that three arousal symptoms are required rather than only one (Bryant & Harvey, 1998; Harvey & Bryant, 1998a). Consistent with this proposition, Spiegel et al. (1996) reported that three anxiety symptoms resulted in the best sensitivity (89%) and specificity (69%).

In summary, the preliminary work on ASD indicates that this diagnosis has utility in predicting those acutely traumatized people who will later develop PTSD. It should be noted, however, that the current criteria are not optimal because many people who do not meet the criteria can also develop PTSD. Initial evidence suggests that there are multiple pathways to developing PTSD, and these may or may not involve acute dissociation.

Cognitive Processes in ASD

Management of Traumatic Memories

There is increasing recognition of the important role of cognitive strategies in the acute posttrauma. This interest has been stimulated by the theoretical proposal that impaired access to traumatic memories in the acute phase may impede resolution of the traumatic experience (Foa & Hearst-Ikeda, 1996). In an initial study of the acute management of traumatic memories, Harvey & Bryant (in press[d]) audiotaped the narratives of MVA survivors who either did or did not develop ASD. These narratives were subsequently coded in terms of dissociative content, disorganized structure, and perception of threat. The narratives of ASD individuals included more dissociative content and more disorganized structure than those without ASD. The notion that posttraumatic psychopathology is associated with poorly organized trauma memories is consistent with findings that resolution of PTSD symptoms is associated with increased organization of trauma memories following treatment (Foa, Molnar & Cashman, 1995).

In a study that directly assessed the accessibility of trauma memories in the acute phase, Harvey, Bryant & Dang (1998) requested ASD and non-ASD MVA survivors to provide memories in response to either positive or negative cue words. ASD participants reported fewer specific memories than non-ASD participants. Further, poor retrieval of specific memories in the acute phase of the trauma accounted for 25% of the variance of PTSD severity 6-months posttrauma. This finding is consistent with the proposal that impaired access to trauma memories in the acute phase can impede activation of the fear network, and contribute to chronic PTSD.

Coping Strategies

There is considerable evidence that coping strategies play a significant role in posttraumatic adjustment. Specifically, strategies that result in avoidance of the traumatic experience tend to contribute to long-term dysfunction (Bryant & Harvey, 1995; Solomon, Mikulincer & Flum, 1988). In an initial investigation of cognitive avoidance in ASD, Harvey & Bryant (1998b) instructed ASD and non-ASD participants to monitor the frequency of their trauma memories during three successive 5-minute periods: (a) when they were told to think about anything, (b) when they were administered suppression or non-suppression instructions, and (c) when they were again asked to only monitor their memories. Participants who were instructed to suppress their memories displayed a delayed increase in the frequency of their memories when the suppression instructions were terminated. This finding indicates that cognitive avoidance can lead to increased traumatic intrusions. In a replication of this design that studied the effects of attempted suppression over three 24-hour periods, Guthrie & Bryant (in press) did not find a delayed increase in intrusions. Interestingly, they observed that efforts to suppress, anxiety levels, and frequency of intrusions were related to participants' tendencies to use worry and punishment as coping strategies. This finding accords with reports that people with ASD utilize punishment and worry more often than non-ASD participants to manage their traumatic memories (Warda & Bryant, 1998a). Further, resolution of ASD following treatment is associated with a reduction in worry and punishment strategies (Bryant, Guthrie & Moulds, 1999).

Cognitive Bias

Recent attention has also focused on the content of the cognitive responses of ASD survivors of MVAs. There is evidence that people with ASD exaggerate both the probability of future negative events occurring and the adverse effects of these events than non-ASD participants (Warda & Bryant, 1998b). These findings accord with previous reports of cognitive bias in other anxiety disorders (Butler & Mathews, 1983; Foa, Franklin & Perry, 1996). Interestingly, panic disorder patients display cognitive biases that are specific to physiological arousal and not to events that are unrelated to arousal (McNally & Foa, 1987), and social phobia patients tend to exhibit higher probability estimates of negative social events but not of negative nonsocial events (Foa et al., 1996). In contrast, ASD trauma survivors with ASD display exaggerated estimates about threats pertaining to external harm, somatic sensations, and social situations (Smith & Bryant, in press). This finding accords with theoretical propositions that posttraumatic anxiety is characterized by fear networks that are more pervasive than other anxiety disorders (Foa, Steketee & Rothbaum, 1989). The importance of cognitive responses in the acute phase after a MVA has also been underscored by the finding that MVA survivors who attribute responsibility for their MVA to others in the acute phase suffer more severe PTSD 12 months later (Delahanty, Herberman, Craig, Hayward, Fullerton, Ursano & Baum, 1997).

Biological Processes

In recent years there has been increasing attention to biological processes that can mediate acute stress reactions. One major line of research has implicated elevated arousal in the acute phase as a primary mediator of subsequent PTSD. One recent study reported that heart rates of civilian trauma survivors were higher in those that later developed PTSD than those who did not when they arrived at a hospital emergency department and also 1-week later; they did not differ at 1- or 4-months follow-up (Shalev, Sahar, Freedman, Peri, Glick, Brandes, Orr & Pitman, 1998). Similarly, Bryant and colleagues found that heart rates obtained before people were discharged from hospital following a MVA were significantly higher in those who later developed PTSD than those who did not (Bryant, Harvey, Guthrie & Moulds, in press). Interestingly, this study also found that participants who had acute stress reactions but no acute dissociation had higher heart rates than those whom either had ASD or no ASD. This finding suggests that the dissociative mechanisms displayed by ASD participants may have lead to suppression of arousal. These findings are consistent with reports that rape victims in the acute posttrauma phase who are highly dissociative are less physiologically reactive to trauma reminders than those who are not dissociative (Griffin, Resick & Mechanic, 1997).

Another intriguing development in our understanding of ASD has been findings of lowered cortisol levels in acutely traumatized people who subsequently develop PTSD. In a sample of MVA survivors who were assessed in the acute posttrauma phase, those who subsequently developed PTSD had lower serum cortisol levels than those who did not develop PTSD and those who later developed depression (McFarlane, Atchison & Yehuda, 1997). This finding is consistent with an earlier report that found that acute cortisol levels following rape were lower in those who had been previously traumatized (Resnick, Yehuda, Pitman & Foy, 1995). These findings have been understood in terms of dysfunction in the feedback mechanism of the hypothalmic-pituitary-adrenal axis in PTSD populations (Yehuda, 1997). Specifically, it is proposed that cortisol functions as an antistress hormone that counters a series of biological reactions initiated by a stressful event. Consequently, reduced cortisol in the acute phase may contribute to dysfunctional elevated arousal.

Predictors of ASD

Only a few studies have assessed the predictors of ASD. In a study of MVA survivors, Barton, Blanchard & Hickling (1996) found that individuals diagnosed with ASD showed more psychiatric dysfunction (both Axis-I and Axis-II) prior to the MVA than a group who did not meet criteria for ASD but later were diagnosed with PTSD. There was also a trend suggesting that ASD survivors had higher rates of prior PTSD and previous exposure to traumatic events. Similarly, Harvey & Bryant (1998c, 1999b) reported that history of psychiatric treatment, history of PTSD, and previous trauma were significant predictors of ASD severity, and accounted for 61% of the variance.

In terms of predictors of acute symptom clusters, acute dissociative symptoms have been associated with level of trauma exposure, being female, inappropriate coping behaviors, and previous stressful events (Koopman Classen & Spiegel, 1996). Acute intrusive symptoms have been predicted by fear, trait anxiety, and absence of traumatic brain injury, and avoidance symptoms have been predicted by fear, trait anxiety, death of a loved one, and financial difficulty (Bryant & Harvey, 1996). In contrast, a study by Solomon and colleagues reported no significant predictors of avoidance, but reported that intrusions were predicted by the degree of threat, exposure to injury, and property loss (Solomon, Laor, Weiler, et al., 1993). In general, predictors of ASD are consistent with the predictors of PTSD (see Blanchard, Hickling, Taylor, Loos, Forneris & Jaccard, 1996; Blanchard, Hickling, Taylor, Loos & Gerardi, 1994).

Treatment of ASD

The finding that the majority of people who meet criteria for ASD subsequently develop chronic PTSD represents an exciting opportunity for early intervention in order to reduce the risk of PTSD. There is convergent evidence that chronic PTSD can be difficult to treat because of the complex disorders that develop over time (Frueh, Turner & Beidel, 1995). Moreover, the ASD criteria provide for a stringent test of early intervention because whereas most people with initial PTSD symptoms remit without formal intervention, remission is less common after ASD. In the first study of treatment of ASD, MVA survivors were allocated to either cognitive behavior therapy (CBT) or supportive counseling (SC) within 2-weeks of their MVA (Bryant, Harvey, Sackville, Dang & Basten, 1998). CBT comprised education, prolonged imaginal exposure, cognitive therapy, and anxiety management. SC involved education, problem-solving, and nondirective support. All participants met criteria for ASD, as indexed by the Acute Stress Disorder Interview (Bryant, Harvey, Dang & Sackville, 1998). Fewer participants in CBT (8%) than SC (83%) met criteria for PTSD at posttreatment. There were also fewer cases of PTSD in the

CBT (17%) than SC (67%) conditions 6-months posttrauma. At follow-up there were greater statistically and clinically significant reductions in intrusive, avoidance, and depressive symptomatology in the CBT than SC participants. The results of this study suggest that PTSD can be effectively prevented in many cases by provision of CBT. Further, this study highlights that the provision of supportive counseling is largely ineffective in assisting those people who are at risk of long-term disorder. In a subsequent study, Bryant and colleagues investigated the components of CBT that are effective in preventing PTSD (Bryant, Sackville, Dang, Guthrie & Moulds, in press). Forty-five civilian trauma survivors (either MVA or nonsexual assault) with ASD were given 5 sessions of either (a) prolonged exposure (PE), (b) a combination of PE and anxiety management (PE+AM), or (c) supportive counseling (SC) within two weeks of their trauma. Fewer patients allocated to the PE (14%) and PE+AM (20%) conditions, compared to the SC (56%) condition, met criteria for PTSD at posttreatment. At 6-months follow-up, there were fewer cases of PTSD in the PE (15%) and PE+AM (23%) than SC (67%) conditions. These findings suggest that the combination of imaginal exposure and cognitive therapy may be the critical ingredients in treating ASD. It should be noted, however, that early intervention is not a panacea for all acutely traumatized people. Bryant, Sackville, Dang, et al. (in press) reported that 20% of their sample dropped out of treatment, and the drop-outs were characterized by more severe ASD than the completers. This pattern suggests that not all trauma survivors are amenable to early intervention, and that further controlled studies are required to delineate the optimal interventions for people presenting with ASD.

Concluding Comments

Although the introduction of the ASD diagnosis was premature because of the lack of empirical data to justify its criteria, its establishment as a descriptor of acute stress reactions has stimulated considerable research. However, it appears that the current criteria of ASD are not optimal, and that the present emphasis on acute dissociative symptoms needs to be modified. Further, it appears that there may be multiple pathways to PTSD; whereas a subset of trauma survivors who will develop PTSD will display acute dissociative symptoms, many others will not. Future revisions of ASD need to give greater attention to the role of nondissociative symptoms. It is possible that acute arousal reactions may be particularly useful in identifying those who subsequently develop PTSD. Most of the research on ASD has focused on MVA survivors, and these findings need to be replicated in other trauma populations. Perhaps the most beneficial feature of this new diagnosis has been the opportunity to provide early intervention for those trauma survivors who are at risk of developing PTSD. Although this research is in its infancy, the initial evidence points to the potential efficacy of CBT in ameliorating the symptoms of ASD. Considering the lack of empirical basis for the ASD diagnosis when it was introduced, there is still a significant need for well-controlled research. Specifically, this fledgling diagnosis requires further prospective studies, validation of measurement tools of ASD, and controlled outcome studies of treatments of ASD. Ensuring that our understanding and management of ASD is based on empirical standards will facilitate more effective and responsible assistance for acutely traumatized survivors.

References

American Psychiatric Association. (1994). *Diagnostic and statistical manual of mental disorders* (4th ed.). Washington, DC: Author.

Barton A., Blanchard E. B. & Hickling E. J. (1996). Antecedents and consequences of acute stress disorder among motor vehicle accident victims. *Behaviour Research and Therapy, 34*, 805–813.

Blanchard E. B., Hickling E. J., Barton K. A., Taylor A. E., Loos W. R. & Jones-Alexander J. (1996). One-year prospective follow-up of motor vehicle accident victims. *Behaviour Research and Therapy*, 34, 775–786.

Blanchard, E. B., Hickling, E. J., Taylor, A. E., Loos, W. R., Forneris, C. A. & Jaccard, J. (1996). Who develops PTSD from motor vehicle accidents? *Behaviour Research and Therapy, 34*, 1–10.

Blanchard E. B., Hickling E. J., Taylor A. E., Loos W. & Gerardi R. J. (1994). Psychological morbidity associated with motor vehicle accidents. *Behaviour Research and Therapy, 32*, 283–290.

Bremner, J. D., Krystal, J. H., Putnam, F. W., Southwick, S. M., Marmar, C., Charney, D. S. & Mazure, C. M. (1998). Measurement of dissociative states with the Clinician-Administered Dissociative States Scale (CADSS). *Journal of Traumatic Stress, 11*, 125–136

Brewin, C. R., Andrews, B., Rose, S. & Kirk, M. (1999). Acute stress disorder and posttraumatic stress disorder in victims of violent crime. *American Journal of Psychiatry. 156*, 360–366.

Bryant, R. A., Guthrie, R. & Moulds, M. (1999). *Cognitive strategies and the resolution of acute stress disorder*. Manuscript submitted for publication.

Bryant, R. A. & Harvey, A. G. (1995). Avoidant coping style and post-traumatic stress following motor vehicle accidents. *Behaviour Research and Therapy, 33*, 631–635.

Bryant, R. A. & Harvey, A. G. (1996). Initial post-traumatic stress responses following motor vehicle accidents. *Journal of Traumatic Stress, 9*, 223–234.

Bryant, R. A. & Harvey, A. G. (1997) Acute stress disorder: a critical review of diagnostic issues. *Clinical Psychology Review, 17*, 757–773.

Bryant, R. A. & Harvey, A. G. (1998). Relationship of acute stress disorder and posttraumatic stress disorder following mild traumatic brain injury. *American Journal of Psychiatry, 155*, 625–629.

Bryant, R. A. & Harvey, A. G. (in press). *Acute stress disorder: A handbook of theory, assessment, and treatment.* Washington, DC: American Psychological Association.

Bryant, R. A, Harvey, A. G., Dang, S. & Sackville, T. (1998). Assessing acute stress disorder: Psychometric properties of a structured clinical interview. *Psychological Assessment, 10*, 215–220.

Bryant, R. A., Harvey, A. G., Guthrie, R. & Moulds, M. (in press). A prospective study of acute psychophysiological arousal, acute stress disorder, and posttraumatic stress disorder. *Journal of Abnormal Psychology.*

Bryant, R. A, Harvey, A. G., Sackville, T., Dang, S. & Basten, C. (1998). Treatment of acute stress disorder: A comparison of cognitive-behavioral therapy and supportive counseling. *Journal of Consulting and Clinical Psychology, 66*, 862–866.

Bryant, R. A, Sackville, T., Dang, S., Guthrie, R. M. & Moulds, M. (in press). Treatment of acute stress disorder: A evaluation of cognitive-behavioral and supportive counseling techniques. *American Journal of Psychiatry.*

Butler, G. & Mathews, A. (1983). Cognitive processes in anxiety. *Advances in Behavior Research and Therapy, 5*, 51–62.

Classen, C., Koopman, C., Hales, R. & Spiegel, D. (1998). Acute stress disorder as a predictor of posttraumatic stress symptoms. *American Journal of Psychiatry, 155*, 620–624.

Creamer, M. & Manning, C. (1998). Acute stress disorder following an industrial accident. *Australian Psychologist, 33*, 125–129.

Delahanty, D. L., Herberman, H. B., Craig, K. J., Hayward, M. C., Fullerton, C. S., Ursano, R. J. & Baum, A. (1997). Acute and chronic distress and posttraumatic stress disorder as a function of responsibility for serious motor vehicle accidents. *Journal of Consulting and Clinical Psychology, 65*, 560–567.

Foa, E. B. & Hearst-Ikeda, D. (1996). Emotional dissociation in response to trauma: An information-processing approach. In L. K. Michelson & W. J. Ray (Eds.), *Handbook of dissociation: Theoretical and clinical perspectives* (pp. 207–222). New York: Plenum Press.

Foa, E. B., Franklin, M. E. & Perry, K. J. (1996). Cognitive bias in generalized social phobia. *Journal of Abnormal Psychology, 15*, 433–439.

Foa, E. B., Molnar, C. & Cashman, L. (1995). Change in rape narratives during exposure therapy for posttraumatic stress disorder. *Journal of Traumatic Stress, 8*, 675–690.

Foa, E.B., Riggs, D.S. & Gershuny, B. (1995). Arousal, numbing, and intrusion: Symptom structure of posttraumatic stress disorder following assault. *American Journal of Psychiatry, 152*, 116–120.

Foa, E. B., Steketee, G. & Rothbaum, B. O. (1989). Behavioral/cognitive conceptualizations of post-traumatic stress disorder. *Behavior Therapy, 20*, 155–176.

Frueh, B. C., Turner, S. M. & Beidel, D. C. (1995). Exposure therapy for combat-related PTSD: A critical review. *Clinical Psychology Review, 15*, 799–815.

Griffin, M. G., Resick, P. A. & Mechanic, M. (1997). Objective assessment of peritraumatic dissociation: Psychophysiological indicators. *American Journal of Psychiatry, 154*, 1081–1088.

Guthrie, R. M. & Bryant, R. A. (in press). *Thought suppression over prolonged periods in acute stress disorder.* Behaviour Research and Therapy.

Harvey, A. G. & Bryant, R. A. (1998a). Relationship of acute stress disorder and posttraumatic stress disorder following motor vehicle accidents. *Journal of Consulting and Clinical Psychology, 66*, 507–512.

Harvey, A. G. & Bryant, R. A. (1998b). Attempted thought suppression in acute stress disorder. *Behaviour Research and Therapy, 36*, 583–590.

Harvey, A. G. & Bryant, R. A. (1998c). Predictors of acute stress disorder following mild traumatic brain injury. *Brain Injury, 12*, 147–154.

Harvey, A. G. & Bryant, R. A. (1999a). Acute stress disorder across trauma populations. *Journal of Nervous and Mental Disease.*

Harvey, A. G. & Bryant, R. A. (1999b). Predictors of acute stress following motor vehicle accidents. *Journal of Traumatic Stress, 12*, 519–525.

Harvey, A. G. & Bryant, R. A. (in press[a]). The relationship between acute stress disorder and posttraumatic stress disorder: A two-year prospective evaluation. *Journal of Consulting and Clinical Psychology.*

Harvey, A. G. & Bryant, R. A. (in press [b]). *A two-year prospective evaluation of the relationship between acute stress disorder and posttraumatic stress disorder following mild traumatic brain injury.* American Journal of Psychiatry.

Harvey, A. G. & Bryant, R. A. (in press[c]). Dissociative symptoms in acute stress disorder. *Journal of Traumatic Stress.*

Harvey, A. G. & Bryant, R. A. (in press[d]). A qualitative investion of traumatic memories. *British Journal of Clinical Psychology.*

Harvey, A. G., Bryant, R. A. & Dang, S. T. (1998). Autobiographical memory in acute stress disorder and posttraumatic stress disorder. *Journal of Consulting and Clinical Psychology, 66*, 500–506.

Janet, P. (1907). *The major symptoms of hysteria.* New York: Macmillan.

Koopman, C., Classen, C. & Spiegel, D. (1994). Predictors of posttraumatic stress symptoms among survivors of the Oakland/Berkeley, Calif., firestorm. *American Journal of Psychiatry, 151*, 888–894.

Koopman, C., Classen, C., Cardeña, E. & Spiegel, D. (1995). When disaster strikes, acute stress disorder may follow. *Journal of Traumatic Stress, 8*, 29–46.

Koopman, C., Classen, C. & Spiegel, D. (1996). Dissociative responses in the immediate aftermath of the Oakland/Berkeley firestorm. *Journal of Traumatic Stress, 9*, 521–540.

Marmar, C. R., Weiss, D. S., Schlenger, W. E., Fairbank, J. A., Jordan, K., Kulka, R. A. & Hough, R. L. (1994). Peritraumatic dissociation and posttraumatic stress in male Vietnam theater veterans. *American Journal of Psychiatry, 151*, 902–907.

McFarlane, A. C. (1986). Posttraumatic morbidity of a disaster. *Journal of Nervous and Mental Disease, 174*, 4–14.

McFarlane, A. C., Atchison, M. & Yehuda, R. (1997). The acute stress response following motor vehicle accidents and its relation to PTSD. In R. Yehuda & A.C. McFarlane (Eds.), *Psychobiology of posttraumatic stress disorder* (pp. 437–441). New York: New York Academy of Sciences.

McNally, R. J. & Foa, E. B. (1987). Cognition and agoraphobia: Bias in the interpretation of threat. *Cognitive Therapy and Research, 11*, 567–581.

Resnick, H. S., Yehuda, R. K., Pitman, R. K. & Foy, D. W. (1995). Effect of previous trauma on acute plasma cortisol level following rape. *American Journal of Psychiatry, 152*, 1675–1677.

Riggs, D. S., Rothbaum, B. O. & Foa, E. B. (1995). A prospective examination of symptoms of posttraumatic stress disorder in victims of non-sexual assault. *Journal of Interpersonal Violence, 10*, 201–213.

Rothbaum, B. O., Foa, E. B., Riggs, D. S., Murdock, T. & Walsh, W. (1992). A prospective examination of post-traumatic stress disorder in rape victims. *Journal of Traumatic Stress, 5*, 455–475.

Shalev, A. Y., Orr, S. P. & Pitman, R. K. (1993). Psychophysiologic assessment of traumatic imagery in Israeli civilian patients with posttraumatic stress disorder. *American Journal of Psychiatry, 150*, 620–624.

Shalev, A.Y., Sahar, T., Freedman, S., Peri, T., Glick, N., Brandes, D., Orr, S.P. & Pitman, R.K. (1998). A prospective study of heart rate responses following trauma and the subsequent development of PTSD. *Archives of General Psychiatry, 55*, 553–559.

Smith, K. & Bryant, R.A. (in press). The generality of cognitive bias in acute stress disorder. *Behaviour Research and Therapy.*

Solomon, Z., Laor, N. & McFarlane, A. C. (1996). Acute posttraumatic reactions in soldiers and civilians. In B. A. van der Kolk, A. C. McFarlane, & L. Weisaeth (Eds.), *Traumatic stress: The effects of overwhelming experience on mind, body, and society* (pp. 102–114). New York: Guilford Press.

Solomon, Z., Laor, N., Weiler, D., Muller, U. F., Hadar, O., Waysman, M., Koslowsky, M., Yakar, M. B. & Bleich, A. (1993). The psychological impact of the Gulf war: A study of acute stress in Israeli evacuees. [Letter to the editor]. *Archives of General Psychiatry, 50*, 320–321.

Solomon Z., Mikulincer M. & Flum H. (1988). Negative life events, coping responses, and combat-related psychopathology: A prospective study. *Journal of Abnormal Psychology, 97*, 302–307.

Spiegel, D., Koopman, C., Cardeña, E. & Classen, C. (1996). Dissociative symptoms in the diagnosis of acute stress disorder. In L.K. Michelson & W.J. Ray (Eds.), *Handbook of dissociation: Empirical, theoretical, and clinical perspectives* (pp. 367–380). New York: Plenum.

van der Kolk, B. A. & van der Hart, O. (1989). Pierre Janet and the breakdown of adaptation in psychological trauma. *American Journal of Psychiatry, 146*, 1530–1540.

Warda, G. & Bryant, R. A. (1998a). Thought control strategies in acute stress disorder. *Behaviour Research and Therapy, 36*, 1171–1175.

Warda, G. & Bryant, R. A. (1998b). Cognitive bias in acute stress disorder. *Behaviour Research and Therapy, 36*, 1177–1183.

Yehuda, R. (1997). Sensitization of the hypothalamic-pituitary-adrenal axis in posttraumatic stress disorder. In R. Yehuda & A. C. McFarlane (Eds.), *Psychobiology of posttraumatic stress disorder* (pp. 57–75). New York: New York Academy of Sciences.

4

Medical, Social and Legal Consequences

RICHARD MAYOU

Oxford University Department of Psychiatry, U.K.

Introduction

Until recently psychiatrically and psychologically determined problems following motor vehicle accidents were regarded as uncommon complications largely associated with seeking compensation. It is now apparent that they are frequent. Since they result from frightening events which can have major financial, medical and legal consequences and whose prevalence and characteristics depend upon individual psychological vulnerability and circumstances, as well as the nature of any injuries. This book is convincing evidence that the subject is now increasingly regarded as being of clinical, legal and economic importance and a substantial public health problem.

This chapter gives an overview illustrated with findings from our own recent published and yet to be published recent work (Ehlers et al., 1998) (Table 1). It aims to be comprehensive by emphasising epidemiology in representative populations and by considering both the whole range of physical injury severity and in the range of physical, psychological, social and legal outcomes that are important to accident victims. Many of the issues are discussed more fully in other chapters.

It is important at the outset to acknowledge that there are major limitations to our present understanding (Blaszczynski et al., 1998). Although psychiatry and psychology have become much interested in the consequences of all

Table 1. Oxford research on the consequences of road traffic accident injury

1.	Long-term follow-up of travel problems amongst consecutive emergency department attenders (Mayou et al., 1991).
2.	Prospective study of consecutive multiple injury and whiplash attenders at an emergency department (Bryant et al., 1997; Mayou et al., 1996; Mayou et al., 1994; Mayou et al., 1993).
3.	Prospective study of all consecutive attenders at an emergency department with follow-up at three months, one year and three years (Ellis et al., 1998; Ehlers et al., 1998).
4.	Randomised controlled trial of critical incident debriefing (Hobbs et al., 1996).
5.	Studies of dissociation in emergency department attenders (admitted and not admitted) (Murray, 1997).
6.	Prospective study of children attending a hospital emergency department (to be published).
7.	A randomised trial of Cognitive Behavioural Therapy (in progress).

trauma, they have focused largely on Post-Traumatic Stress Disorder (PTSD) in following combat and disasters. There has been much less interest in what could be the commonest cause of major frightening trauma (Blaszczynski et al., 1998; Mayou et al., 1993; Taylor et al., 1995; Blanchard et al., 1997; Bryant & Harvey, 1995). The main sources of evidence on the psychological and social consequences of road accidents are the large and unsatisfactory literatures on whiplash and compensation and, more recently, a number of reports on PTSD. The total amount of research is still small and much of it relates to highly unrepresentative populations; even samples which are representative of hospital attenders, tell us little about those who do not attend hospitals because they are uninjured or only slightly injured, about bystanders and about consequences for close relatives. Not only has outcome been considered too narrowly, many of the measures that have been used have been unsatisfactory and others unstandardised. This is true even of PTSD, where very minor differences in the interpretation of criteria can have substantial effects on prevalence.

Despite the serious shortcomings of the evidence and the literature, we now know the nature and scale of the consequences of road accidents, have a good understanding of possible aetiological factors and can demonstrate that they have large implications for medical treatment, social policy and legal proceedings.

The Scale of the Problem

Road traffic accidents are extremely frequent and only a minority involve medically significant injury. Most injuries seen in emergency departments or primary care are medically minor and only small proportions result in admission or in major medical or surgical treatment. A large minority are diagnosed as suffering whiplash neck injury. Not all those injured seek medical attention, which may be at an accident and emergency department or in primary care. An unknown proportion of those who are uninjured suffer frightening experiences which may result in the problems described in this chapter and the rest of this book. Whilst most accounts concentrate on vehicle occupants, road accidents also involve motorcyclists, pedal cyclists and pedestrians. There may also be consequences for bystanders and those involved in providing help at the site of the accident. The implications for families may be as great as for the victims themselves. Although there is no evidence about the psychological consequences of accidents in less developed countries, it is likely they are considerable in that road traffic accidents and injury are frequent in all countries.

Physical Consequences

Most road accident injuries are minor and physical recovery is rapid. In a minority, physical problems persist for months or years and a small proportion suffer permanent physical disability, for example brain damage, spinal injuries, severe disability in walking and other basic activities, disfiguring facial scars and late whiplash syndrome. In addition, some are at increased risk of late complications such as progress of arthritis.

Acute medical care. Is usually both efficient and effective, even with the more severe injuries, but treatment has important limitations. This is especially evident in long-term care, for example in the lack of multidisciplinary rehabilitation for patients with severe brain damage and for those who have both disabling physical problems and disabling pain and distress. Care is especially unsatisfactory for those with minor injuries in that there is explanation, encouragement and reassurance and this results in considerable "medically unnecessary" disability. Any consideration of patients' behaviour that does not take into account these limitations of medical care and the possibility of iatrogenic complications is likely to be misleading. For example, many of post-traumatic musculoskeletal problems, such as whiplash neck injury, are poorly understood (and even controversial) and doctors in emergency departments and primary care often find them difficult to assess and treat. Their uncertainty and bewilderment may be reflected in ambiguous, contradictory advice, excessive caution and over investigation. Thus it is now widely accepted that the standard treatments of whiplash neck injury and back pain have been harmful and that more active mobilisation is much more effective.

Psychological Consequences

The consequences of road traffic injury (Table 2) are in many ways identical to those described for other acute medical problems (Mayou, 1995a); anxiety, depression and psychologically-determined behavioural and social complications. *There is no standard, normal or appropriate response to being physically unwell; there is a range of response with individual variation in the consequences over a wide range of outcomes.* Individual outcome depends on the nature of the physical problem, psychological vulnerability and past and continuing circumstances. It also depends of course on medical treatment - the physical treatment itself, explanation, advice about prognosis and convalescence and on practical social support both for the patient and the family. The principal determinants are shown in Table 3.

In those with previous psychological problems or who have suffered a series of stresses or social difficulties, it may be difficult to disentangle aetiology. The very considerable research on the aetiological significance of stressful life events and chronic personal difficulties shows that they can have a cumulative effect. Emotional disorders may be exacerbated or prolonged by other adverse events, but they may improve following positive events. Inevitably, some people are inclined to see chronic problems or dif-

Table 2. Psychologically-determined consequences of road traffic accidents

Cognitive impairment – acute and chronic
Acute Stress Disorder
Anxiety
Depression
Post-Traumatic Stress Disorder
Phobic Travel Anxiety
Chronic medically unexplained symptoms and pain
Adverse effects on quality of life
Consultation, compliance and use of resources
Effects on families

Table 3. Determinants of outcome of physical disorder

Nature and severity of physical disorder
Nature, efficacy and side-effects of treatment
Psychological vulnerability
Social circumstances
Family reactions

ficulties associated with quite independent causes as being due to the road accident. Formulation of treatment and medicolegal assessment both depend on taking a careful history from the subject, and if possible a relative, to identify the extent to which psychosocial problems appear to have been precipitated by the accident.

There are three general conclusions for those writing medicolegal reports and for those planning the treatment of road accident victims:

- There is wide individual variation in reaction to having a road accident as to any physical disorder, whether or not compensation is an issue.
- It is wrong to assume that all those who describe problems which are apparently medically unjustified are consciously simulating, exaggerating or suffering from "functional overlay". Even so, there is a small minority in which the pursuit of maximum compensation is a major and conscious motivation; such people may be disproportionately prominent in the highly selective, practice of some doctors and lawyers.
- Although most psychological problems become apparent soon after the accident but their subsequent course may be exacerbated by adverse aspects of medical care, legal problems and social difficulties associated with the road traffic accident, as well as by entirely independent events. This emphasises the need for the earliest possible recognition and for relatively simple interventions which may prevent longer-term chronic difficulties.

The various psychological consequences or road accidents described in the following section are best considered as independent outcomes, even though they overlap. Each outcome has a rather different prevalence and course during the year after the accident and there are also differences in baseline and early predictive factors (Mayou,, Bryant, Ehlers, to be published). The pattern in any individual reflects the meaning of the accident and any injuries to that particular individual.

Cognitive impairment: Delirium and Dementia. Head injury occurs in a minority of accidents; most are medically minor with only brief unconsciousness and initial amnesia. More severe injuries are followed by acute delirium and significant risk of permanent impairment: dementia. It must always be kept in mind that even minor brain injury may have prolonged effects on cognitive function; effects which are particularly important for those whose jobs and interests are dependent on acute intellectual function. The greatest difficulty occurs in assessing alleged post-concussional symptoms whose causes may be both psychological and physical. There is good evidence that even those who have been unconscious may later suffer from the post-traumatic complications described below.

Acute reaction. Acute Stress Disorder was only recently introduced in classifications and unfortunately is defined rather differently in DSM and ICD (Bryant and Harvey, 1997). It is best considered (as in DSM) as the immediate equivalent of PTSD which can only be diagnosed with a minimum time period. The post-traumatic symptoms of intrusion, avoidance, emotional arousal or dissociation are very commonly reported immediately after an accident and recent work suggests that Acute Stress Disorder occurs in a substantial proportion. At later follow-up many patients are improved but those who do have Acute Stress Disorder are at high risk of continuing Post-Traumatic Stress Disorder (Murray, 1997; Bryant & Harvey, 1995). The immediate psychological reaction to a road traffic accident may indicate the need for emotional and practical support but is also a sign of significantly increased risk of later psychiatric complications.

Anxiety. General anxiety is similar to those seen following other acute medical problems, and indeed other forms of life event, and are associated with evidence of previous psychological vulnerability and adverse social circumstances.

In addition to general anxiety, two other more specific forms of anxiety Post-traumatic Stress Disorder and Travel Anxiety – are common.

Post-Traumatic Stress Disorder. PTSD has been described in between 1 – 40% of victims and review suggests a probable incidence of 10 – 20%. The variation in the literature undoubtedly reflects the nature of samples and the changes in methodology. Small differences in the ways in which the criteria are applied may lead to large variations in case identification.

Our large study of a representative sample suggests a prevalence in the middle range (Ehlers et al., 1998). We found that post-traumatic symptoms are very common soon after an accident but then become less frequent in the early weeks with some degree of improvement between three months and one year. In a minority of cases there is delayed onset of between three months and one year. At three years PTSD remains a significant problem.

Who gets PTSD? It is not substantially related to the severity of the accident or to the type of accident. The large numbers of people seen once with no more than minor injuries have almost the same risk as people admitted with life-threatening problems. In recent analysis of our large prospective series (Ehlers et al., 1998) we have been able to identify predisposing and maintaining factors as summarised in Table 4. In general, these are very similar to

Table 4. Determinants of the occurrence of PTSD

Pre-accident characteristics:
Female gender
Previous emotional problems
Accdent:
Perceived threat
Immediate emotional reaction:
Dissociation
Later cognitive variables:
Negative interpretation of intrusions
Rumination
Thought suppression
Anger cognition
Other later variables:
Continuing health problems
Litigation

Table 5. Travel anxiety

Increased caution
Increased awareness of behaviour of other drivers
Use of safer vehicles
Loss of pleasure in travel
Anxiety about travel by means used in road traffic accident
Avoidance of travel by means used in road traffic accident
Generalisation of anxiety of other travel
Concern about family member's travel

those described by Blanchard and colleagues in their smaller and more selective study using more detailed measures (Blanchard et al., 1997) which are reported elsewhere in this book.

Travel anxiety. Travel anxiety (Table 5) has generally attracted less attention but it is common (Mayou et al., 1994; Mayou et al., 1991). Not only does it affect vehicle drivers and passengers; it is just as common amongst cyclist and pedestrian accident victims. Although greater caution and awareness of road safety may be benefits, travel anxiety is often the most disabling and important psychological consequence of a road accident. It can also be more persistent. It overlaps with PTSD but it is not the same condition.

Who gets Phobic Travel Anxiety? The factors predicting travel anxiety are similar to those of PTSD but they are not the same. Previous emotional problems, nervousness about driving or being a passenger, and gender are prominent determinants.

Depression. Major depression, satisfying standard diagnostic criteria, is not common but in clinical and medicolegal practice it is a frequent cause of long-term difficulties. It is often associated with complaints of pain and other physical symptoms and of disability and often remains unrecognised. The successful treatment of depression has benefits not only for mood but for other psychological outcomes and for physical status.

Other Psychologically-Determined Complications

Anger. Anger is prominent amongst those who are innocent victims, especially if they feel that they have suffered significant medical or other problems, and their distress has not been recognised by others or the legal system. It is an emotion which may impair convalescence and is associated with an increased risk of psychological complications. It is difficult to live with and to treat in that sufferers very often have considerable reason to feel aggrieved about their predicaments.

A general feeling of vulnerability may affect day-to-day confidence and views about the future. This is a feeling which is also encountered in those who suffered unexpected acute illness and other events.

Chronic unexplained physical symptoms. A more difficult group to understand are those who have chronic physical symptoms and pain which appear disproportionate to any objective medical findings. I have already indicated that these complications occur following any major illness and the explanation may be due to an interaction of physical and psychological variables (Mayou et al., 1995c).

The commonest example following road accident injury is the problem of late whiplash syndrome. Our two studies suggest that whiplash is very little different to other types of injuries in its consequences (Mayou et al., 1996b) (Mayou & Bryant, to be published). It is medically less serious than those injuries which result in admission but appears to be associated with a consistent physical syndrome. Its psychological and social outcome is comparable to soft tissue injuries.

It is not uncommon, especially in preparing medico-legal reports, to meet patients who have long histories of physical symptoms, largely negative medical investigation and considerable consultation, who describe physical symptoms and restrictions which appear to have bewildered those responsible for treatment and aroused the suspicions of at least some of those who have already written reports. Whilst it is undeniable that there are victims who exaggerate and simulate for deliberate gain, this is almost certainly less common than symptoms which result from original pathology, psychological

Table 6. Social consequences

Financial
Limitation of work
Limitation of leisure and social activities
Limitation of family activities
Effects on family members
Economic cost – direct and indirect

factors and psychological variables and are frequently complicated by conflicting, ambiguous or over-cautious advice. In many instances, the psychiatrists and psychologists may believe that a behaviourally-planned, comprehensive rehabilitation approach would be useful. Unfortunately it is often extremely difficult to arrange such care and, in any case, the prognosis several years after an accident is probably poor whatever the treatment.

Social Consequences

Road accidents will inevitably have many consequences for everyday life (Table 6). They are associated with injury and disability, post-traumatic psychological complications, financial consequences and legal and compensation proceedings. Changes in the health and behaviour of the victim and the extra demands and consequences for the family mean that changes are often for the worse. In a minority of cases there are clear improvements in marital and family relationships.

A comprehensive view of outcome must place considerable emphasis on changes in quality of life for the victim and those around him. Narrow concern with a diagnosis of objective physical disorder or with the criteria of psychiatric disorder is inappropriate and may miss changes of profound significance.

Legal Consequences

A proportion of victims are subsequently prosecuted for driving offences, such as careless or dangerous driving and driving whilst above the legal limit for alcohol. Overall, the psychological and social outcome for those convicted seems to be similar, or slightly better, than for those not involved in proceedings.

We have followed-up compensation victims in our two studies (Mayou, 1996a; Mayou, 1995a; Bryant et al., 1997a). In the first, we followed-up those seeking compensation for six years and in the second study we have rather less information over a period of three years. It is striking that outcome for those seeking compensation is very similar to those who do not seek it. Detailed examination suggests that many of those who do not seem to have been responsible for accidents are not notably keen to pursue compensation and that only a very small number appear to be in any way behaving so as to maximise their chances of financial gain. At the same time, we need to be aware that there is general evidence following any sort of trauma that disability seems to be somewhat greater in those who see a specific external cause than in those who do not. I would see causation and financial factors as being amongst the many social factors that always influence reaction to physical disorder.

Type of Accident

Most evidence has related to vehicle occupants but our study of all consecutive attenders suggests that there are substantial similarities in those who are drivers and passengers in vehicles, motorcyclists, cyclists and pedestrians. Despite the differences in the injuries experienced in these situations, psychological consequences are broadly similar. Inevitably the content of travel anxiety reflects the nature of the accident itself. It is also apparent that vehicle passengers, especially if they are women, are at particular risk of travel anxiety.

Severity and Type of Injury

There have been few indications that the psychological consequences are substantially related to the severity or type of injury. We have been able to look at the whole range of injury severity in our consecutive series. Severity of injury did not emerge as a significant predictor of any aspect of psychological outcome at three or twelve months.

Although there is no overall association between the type of injury and psychological consequences, it is important to recognise that there are small sub-groups who may be particularly at risk. Examples include those with major leg fractures who suffer continuing pain, limitation and the risk of arthritis, and those with disfiguring facial injuries who may become markedly fearful of social situations to a disabling extent.

Whiplash neck injuries are extremely common and remain controversial (Mayou et al., 1996b; Mayou et al., 1996b). Late whiplash physical symptoms have often been seen as psychologically determined and as being substantially attributable to compensation-seeking. Such conclusions have mainly been derived from highly selected samples and there is little evidence from prospective studies that whiplash is not basically a syndrome with a physical basis. Even so, as with any other painful and limiting musculoskeletal problem, psychological and behavioural factors are substantial determinants of subjective distress and handicap.

Children

Recognition of problems for adult victims has led to consideration of whether problems are as great for children involved in accidents. As with adults, there has been a particular emphasis on PTSD and recent studies have reported prevalences of up to 45% in the months following an accident (Stallard et al., 1998; Mirza et al., 1998; Di Gallo et al., 1997; Ellis et al., 1998).

Our own current experience with a detailed study of consecutive child victims is that previous studies have probably somewhat over-estimated PTSD because of the use of somewhat unsatisfactory criteria. They have also probably under-estimated the variety of psychological and behavioural consequences that occur for children and also the effects on families, which may be considerable.

Implications

There is convincing evidence that road accidents have a wide range of psychologically determined consequences, that these in the past have been under-recognised and often wrongly attributed to conscious exaggeration or to chronic neurosis. We are faced with an extremely expensive problem. This is not just a medical problem, it is also a social and a legal problem. The answers lie only partly within the scope of clinical medicine, psychiatry and psychology.

Theoretical implications. Prospective evidence about the common trauma of being in a road traffic accident provides an important model for trauma in general. Whilst there are specific features, such as the particular prominence of travel anxiety and avoidance, psychological research can be expected to have wide relevance to our understanding of epidemiology, aetiology and treatment.

Clinical implications. We need to consider more efficient medical care with better advice and information so as to minimise iatrogenic problems which appear to be common in whiplash and some other late complications. What can we do to improve psychological treatment? There are several issues:

- What can we do immediately?
- Is there a role for immediate "debriefing"?
- How can we recognise problems early?
- What interventions are useful in early convalescence?
- How should we treat chronic problems?

The answers to these problems are very similar to those for the management of psychological complications of any physical illness. We require a "stepped" approach. There should be a combination of early routine information and advice, together with support for those who are distressed, followed by early recognition of problems and the use of standard proven treatments. A particular difficulty with road accident victims is that many of those who consult initially, at emergency departments or elsewhere, are seen on the one occasion and not offered follow-up. We need a much greater awareness which will lead to early recognition of those with persistent problems. This means a greater awareness amongst accident victims as well as among doctors. It also perhaps means a greater awareness and willingness to encourage treatment amongst lawyers, insurers and all others who may be involved.

Our evidence suggests that Critical Incidence Debriefing is unhelpful, and indeed harmful (Hobbs et al., 1996) (Mayou, Ehlers, Hobbs; submitted for publication). A three year follow-up of subjects in a randomised controlled trial found that intervention subjects who initially had high Impact of Events scores had very considerably poorer outcomes in terms of Post-traumatic Stress Disorder, travel anxiety and other measures than did untreated controls. It would be more appropriate to offer immediate supportive care to those in need and then to concentrate on the recognition of the problems described above early in convalescence. This must depend upon greater awareness amongst hospital and primary care doctors, lawyers and others who may be involved of the importance of recognition and early treatment. Simple handouts in emergency departments and elsewhere encouraging those who have problems to consult and reassuring them that there is effective treatment, would be useful. As described in other chapters, there are encouraging findings about a number of specialist psychological and other treatments. Further research is needed as to efficacy and also to delivery but, overall, the findings are encouraging.

The greatest difficulties are those of chronic patients with pain, physical symptoms, disability, emotional distress. Doctors find them difficult to treat and they are often involved in frustrating compensation proceedings. There can be no simple answers; rather we require recognition of the problem and of the likelihood that multidisciplinary programmes could be helpful and cost-effective.

Legal implications. There can also be no doubt that many difficulties arise from the inadequacies and extremely prolonged course of compensation proceedings in many jurisdictions (Law Commission, 1995). Even where there is no dispute about liability it may be difficult to obtain financial compensation and almost impossible to do so soon after the accident when it is likely to be most needed. An extremely expensive system results in few participants being satisfied. There remain problems for many accident victims in whom evidence about liability is not available. It is only in no fault systems that it may be possible to fund the medical and social interventions which may be necessary to prevent chronic difficulties which require very expensive medical and other resources.

Social implications. Social implications overlap with the legal consequences. They relate to financial difficulties and the effects on employment and activities of road accident victims, many of whom are in early adult life.

Conclusion

Road traffic accidents pose major problems for public policy, public health and the legal system. In the past, inadequate evidence and highly selective experience have led to erroneous conclusions. Better understanding will depend upon the contributions of all the disciplines represented by contributors to this book and by the willingness of their disciplines to learn from each other.

Bibliography

Blanchard E. B. & Hickling, E. J. (1997). *After the crash: assessment and treatment of motor vehicle accident survivors.* American Psychological Association. Washington DC.

Blaszczynski, A., Gordon, K., Silove, D., Sloane, D., Hillman, K. & Panasetis, P. (1998). Psychiatric morbidity following motor vehicle accidents: a review of methodological issues. *Comprehensive Psychiatry, 39*(3), 111–121.

Bryant B, Mayou, R. & Lloyd-Bostock, S. (1997). Compensation claims following road accidents: a six-year follow-up study. *Medicine, Science and The Law, 37*: 4, 326–336.

Bryant, R. A. & Harvey, A. G. (1995). Psychological impairment following motor vehicle accidents. *Australian Journal of Public Health, 19*, 185–188.

Bryant, R. A. & Harvey, A. G. (1997). Acute Stress Disorder: a critical review of diagnostic issues. *Clinical Psychology Review, 17*(7), 757–773.

Di Gallo A, Barton, J. & Parry-Jones, W. (1997). Road traffic accidents: early psychological consequences in children and adolescents. *British Journal of Psychiatry, 170*, 358–362.

Ehlers, A., Mayou, R. A. & Bryant, B. (1998). Psychological predictors of chronic posttraumatic stress disorder after motor vehicle accidents. *J. Abnormal Psychol, 107*(3), 508–519.

Ellis A, Stores, G. & Mayou, R. (1998). Psychological consequences of road traffic accidents in children. *European Child & Adolescent Psychiatry, 7*, 61–68.

Hobbs, M., Mayou, R., Harrison, B. & Worlock, P. (1996). A randomised controlled trial of psychological debriefing for victims of road traffic accidents. *British Medical Journal, 313*, 1438–1439.

Law Commission. (1995). *Damages for personal injury: non-pecuniary loss.* Consultation Paper No 140. HMSO. London

Mayou R. (1996a). Accident Neurosis revisited. *British Journal of Psychiatry, 168*, 399–403.

Mayou, R. & B. Bryant. (1996b). Outcome of whiplash neck injury. *Injury, 27*: 9, 617–623.

Mayou, R. & Radanov, B. P. (1996c). Whiplash neck injury. *Journal of Psychsomatic Research, I40D: 5, 461–474.*

Mayou, R. A., Simkin, S. & Thelfall, J. (1991). Effects of road traffic accidents on driving behaviour. *Injury, 22*, 365–368.

Mayou R. A., Bryant, B. & Duthie, R. (1993). Psychiatric consequences of road traffic accidents. *British Medical Journal, 307*, 647–651.

Mayou, R. A. & Bryant, B. M. (1994). Effects of road accidents on travel. *Injury, 25*, 457–460.

Mayou, R. A. (1995a). Introduction: the relationship between physical and psychiatric pathology. In *Psychiatric aspects of physical disease* (A. House, R. A. Mayou, & C. Mallinson). pp. 3–8. The Royal College of Physicians and Royal College of Psychiatrists. London

Mayou, R. A. (1995b). Medico-legal aspects of road traffic accidents. *Journal of Psychosomatic Research, 39*, 789–798.

Mayou, R. A., Bass, C. & Sharpe, M. (1995c). *Treatment of functional somatic symptoms.* Oxford University Press, Oxford.

Mirza, K. A. H., Bhadrinath, B. R., Goodyer, I. M. & Gilmour, C. (1998). Post-traumatic stress disorder in children and adolescents following road traffic accidents. *British Journal of Psychiatry, 172*, 443–447.

Murray, J. *Trauma and dissociation.* DPhil thesis. Oxford. (unpublished)

Stallard P, Velleman, R. & Baldwin, S. (1998). Prospective study of post-traumatic stress disorder in children involved in road traffic accidents. *BMJ, 317*, 1619–1623.

Taylor S. & W. J. Koch. (1995). Anxiety disorders due to motor vehicle accidents: nature and treatment. *Clinical Psychology Review, 15*: 8, 721–738.

5

Brain Injury and the Mind: The Neuropsychology of Mild Traumatic Brain Injury

NIGEL H. WALTON, MA, PhD, AFBPsS

Consultant Neuropsychologist

Introduction

Mild traumatic brain injury (MTBI) accounts for approximately 70% of all head injury and represents a major, but largely unrecognised, healthcare problem (Mandel, 1989). Despite the term "mild", deleterious changes to family and occupational functioning frequently follow such injuries, yet the neuropsychological consequences of MTBI remain poorly understood and are all too frequently inadequately assessed. This can result in considerable distress for sufferers and their carers, as the changes that overtake an individual following MTBI are misunderstood and misinterpreted. The potential to overlook the neuropsychological consequences of MTBI has relevance in legal settings where personal injury victims may not receive the compensation they deserve.

There remains no universally accepted definition of MTBI. For the purposes of this chapter, I will regard as mild, head injuries that produce brief, or no loss of consciousness and a period of post traumatic amnesia (PTA) of less than 1 hour. This includes head injuries without direct head strike or whiplash injuries. Such injuries seem capable of causing persistent neuropsychological deficit in a subgroup of the population (Ettlin, Kischka,

Reichmann et al, 1992; Sweeney, 1992; Bohnen, Jolles & Verhey, 1993), though there exists some conflicting evidence (McLean, 1995). Moderate injuries with similar duration of loss of consciousness and PTA extending between 1–24 hours also meet many of the same problems in diagnosis and management.

Animal studies have shown that the mechanisms of MTBI are the same as those of more severe head injury. These include:

(i) Contusions due to differential motion between the brain and the skull
(ii) Stretching, tearing and shearing of neurones including small contusions and haemorrhages (diffuse axonal injury or DAI)
(iii) chemical abnormalities resulting from excessive neural depolarisation and abnormal agonist/receptor interactions

Dixon, Taft & Hayes (1993)

The nature of this damage is such that hard neurological signs are rare and even sophisticated neuroimaging techniques, such as high-powered MRI, may not show structural damage. However *absence of evidence is not evidence of absence*. For obvious reasons there are few post-mortem studies but one study has examined a group of MTBI victims who subsequently died of unrelated causes. All had damage to the fornices which are the major hippocampal projection pathways and are involved in the consolidation of new memories (Blumbergs, Scott, Manavis, Wainwright, Simpson & McLean, 1994).

There are no physiological markers that will predict severity of outcome better than Glasgow Coma Scale (GCS), duration of loss of consciousness and post traumatic amnesia (PTA) (Alexander, 1995). PTA refers to the period from the initial loss of consciousness or injury to the time when *continuous, ongoing* memories can be formed. It is best measured in the immediate aftermath of the injury and should be undertaken over several days to avoid the confounding effects of "islands" of memory. This is a phenomenon whereby an individual may appear to have regained ongoing memory for a while, only to lapse back into amnesia later. A single assessment can therefor erroneously suggest resolution of PTA. However, an estimate of the duration of PTA can generally be obtained by taking a careful history from the patient and a relative.

There is general agreement that the majority of individuals suffering MTBI improve markedly in the three to six months post injury. Whether or not this equates to *recovery* is a different matter (Lezak, 1995). Furthermore there are consistent reports of a significant minority (25–30%) who experience persisting neuropsychological and psychological difficulties at six months, one year or longer (Alexander, 1995; Bohnen, Jolles, Twijnstra, Mellink & Wijnen, 1995; Leininger, Gramling, Farrell, Kreutzer & Peck, 1990). Neuropsychologists have been influential in drawing attention to the subtle but nonetheless disruptive, cognitive sequelae of MTBI (Stuss, 1995). However given the relative paucity of our understanding of the mechanisms and nature of brain injury following MTBI, it remains a challenging area for the neuropsychologist, who is required to determine the presence or absence of brain damage. Neuropsychologists in legal and clinical settings, are also often asked to determine whether there is organic *or* psychological damage following head injury. The question is fundamentally flawed inasmuch as there is no clear dichotomy and the two probably never exist entirely independently. More likely the two co-exist in an extremely complex fashion, each confounding the other. This is arguably never more the case than when examining the consequences of MTBI.

Neuropsychological Assessment of MTBI

Neuropsychological assessment is a complex and sophisticated undertaking. This is particularly true in MTBI where deficits may be very subtle and measurable only in particular aspects of cognition. A neuropsychological assessment must involve an examination of pre-morbid and current intellectual functioning, attention/concentration, memory and executive skills. If a sound diagnosis is to be made, the neuropsychologist must take into account a variety of factors, in addition to the test scores. Clinical history, the nature of the complaints, the patient's presentation and attitude towards the examiner and the examination, the *way* in which they pass or fail particular tests and the degree to which complaints and deficits fit a given neuropsychological syndrome, must all be integrated into the final opinion. *The scores do not portray the results in full.*

In MTBI, neuropsychological deficits typically cluster around a range of abilities encompassing concentration, new learning and memory, sustained and focused attention and speed of information processing (Bohnen, Jolles & Verhey, 1993; Binder, 1986; Leininger, Gramling, Farrell, Kreutzer & Peck, 1990). Such deficits may exist against a background of essentially normal intellectual functioning and executive functioning, though subtle deficits may also be found in these areas. Information processing deficits may be apparent only under the most demanding test conditions, requiring specific neuropsychological assessment techniques if they are to become fully apparent (Gronwall, 1989).

The mainstay of neuropsychological assessment is the Wechsler Adult Intelligence Scale-Revised (WAIS-R). Alas the summary IQ scores derived from this test tell us little about subtle deficits in cognition. Recent research, however, suggests that an analysis of the factor structure of the WAIS-R, in particular the *Freedom from Distractibility* factor (Digit Span, Arithmetic and Digit Symbol Substitution) may provide greater predictive power than traditionally used methods of analysis such as VIQ:PIQ discrepancies and individual subtest score scatter (Crawford, Johnson, Mychalkiw & Moore, 1997).

A multitude of tests exist to test new learning and memory and executive functions. It is not the purpose of this chapter to provide detailed descriptions of them. However, it should be noted that the power and reliability of neuropsychological assessment is increased by the administration of multiple tests so that patterns of performance can be analysed. Good neuropsychological practice requires that aberrant performances on individual tests be interpreted with extreme caution (if at all) and sound diagnosis requires evidence of difficulty on a range of measures tapping a specific area of cognition (e.g. verbal memory) prior to diagnosis.

Two tests that have received particular attention in the assessment of MTBI have been the Paced Auditory Serial Additions Task (PASAT) and the Stroop Colour Word Test and its modifications (Bohnen, Jolles & Twijnstra, 1992). These tests are regarded as being sufficiently demanding to tease out the subtle effects of MTBI that can be missed by more traditional testing methods (Batchelor, Harvey & Bryant, 1995). Both require the individual to perform against strict time constraints, thereby testing the individual's capacity for speeded information processing. This appears to be a sensitive indicator of disrupted cognitive function. Both also require the individual to display sustained attention and flexibility of thinking and the latter test also requires the capacity for selective attention and the ability to avoid responding to salient but incorrect response tendencies.

Psychological Factors

Individuals who suffer a traumatic brain injury typically do so in very distressing circumstances. The event is usually regarded as a life crisis. They suffer pain and shock and are then faced with the frightening perception that they are not as cognitively able as they were. This is particularly the case for individuals working in cognitively demanding environments where even a minor diminution in cognitive ability is likely to make itself felt. They are apt then to develop symptoms of depression and anxiety as they attempt to cope with a return to work and the resumption of pre-accident activities and responsibilities. Persistent symptoms following MTBI may thus reflect both underlying organic brain damage *and* psychological factors. Recent research has focused on attribution theory as a possible explanation of maintenance of symptoms. Mittenberg, DiGiulio, Perrin & Bass (1992) suggest that the symptoms experienced by MTBI victims are sustained by the fact that they are anticipated or expected to follow head injury. They suggest that MTBI victims become hypervigilant to minor cognitive lapses and post-concussional symptoms, and attribute them to their injury. They argue that patients and clinicians alike underestimate the frequency with which these symptoms occur in the normal population. In contrast to these findings, Aubrey, Dobbs & Gail Rule (1989) reported that lay persons knowledge of the likely consequences of MTBI was dissimilar to the complaints of injury victims. This suggests that there may exist unique sequelae of MTBI. Clearly more work is required to disentangle this controversy.

Malingering vs Exaggeration

In legal settings there is understandably much interest in the presence of exaggeration and/or malingering. Given the possibility of financial compensation for injury there is obvious potential for secondary gain factors to influence performance during neuropsychological testing. Miller (1961) focused attention on malingerers when he suggested that most of his patient's symptoms resolved after settlement of litigation. He cited this as evidence that his patients were exaggerating their deficits in an effort to secure undue financial compensation. This assertion has though been frequently challenged. Thompson (1965) for example, showed that 75% of a large sample did not demonstrate resolution of symptoms following settlement of litigation. The issue of "malingering" thus remains poorly understood. In particular insufficient attention is paid to the difference between malingering and exaggeration. The two are not at all the same thing.

It is vital that health professionals and the courts are made aware of the differences between exaggeration and deliberate malingering (which is rare in my clinical experience). Exaggeration can occur for a variety of understandable and valid reasons. Typically individuals who have suffered MTBI face sceptical and sometimes hostile medical and legal fraternities who have little insight into the profound disruption that even minor decrements in concentration or speed of processing skills can exert on an individual's capacity to function socially and at work. Spouses, families and carers are also typically unsophisticated in their understanding of the sequelae of minor head injury and are often unsympathetic towards symptoms that result from seemingly inconsequential injuries. This can lead an individual to exaggerate symptoms (quite possibly unconsciously) in an effort to "demonstrate" to the world that they are suffering. In short, exaggeration may be a "cry for help". This is particularly true for individuals functioning at high levels where demands on rapid and accurate cognitions are great. Thus victims find themselves under pressure to *demonstrate* that they have suffered an injury to explain their inefficiencies or inability to cope in settings where they had done so previously. The situation is further complicated when there exists some secondary gain for the injured party to maintain illness behaviour. This is by no means always financial gain but may involve gratification from the increased attention they receive from family or friends or an excuse to cease an activity (e.g. work) that was previously unpleasant or stressful.

Malingering on the other hand might be regarded as a deliberate and fully conscious attempt to mislead for the purposes of financial compensation or obvious gain. Typically such patients are more overt in their actions and will frequently react aggressively if confronted by an examiner. There are numerous qualitative methods that may help in the detection of malingering. For example many individual's who are deliberate malingerers will be reluctant to talk in detail about their symptoms and will react in a hostile and evasive fashion to continued questioning. In contrast those with a more hysterical basis to their presentation will talk happily and in detail about the effects of their injury. In addition there are countless qualitative and quantitative neuropsychological observations and measurements that can alert the clinician to the presence of malingering. Malingerers are for example more likely to produce bizarre and profoundly impoverished results on testing and as mentioned above will frequently react aggressively if the notion of psychological or even deliberate manipulation is raised. Deficits far in excess of the nature and severity of the injury and complaints that make no neurological sense are also useful qualitative signs.

Despite the potential for an experienced neuropsychologist to expose deliberate under-performance, the objective measurement of exaggeration and malingering remains a challenge. Whilst diagnosis will always involve careful and skilled qualitative observation of the patient, standardised, scientific methods of differentiating between genuine and fraudulent performances continue to be sought.

Currently the most popular tools for this purpose are the Rey 15 Item Memory Test and tasks involving two-alternative, forced-choice paradigms, such as the Warrington Recognition Memory Test. The first of these involves giving the patient a task that is in fact very simple but that is presented as difficult. There exists the assumption that all but the most demented of patients can pass this test and poor performance therefore likely reflects exaggeration. The latter method involves presenting a large number of items that require a simple choice between two items, one of which is correct. Thus pure guessing will result in ~50% hit rate and scores below chance indicate a degree of deliberate under-performance.

The problem with the Rey 15 Item Memory Test is that it lacks both sensitivity and specificity. Thus if a patient performs poorly, one is alerted to the possibility that they may be exaggerating, but one cannot assume that their performance reflects a deliberate or fully conscious intention to deceive. There is, for example, some evidence to suggest that patients with severe memory or attentional problems may also do poorly on the test for entirely appropriate reasons. If on the other hand the patient performs normally, our own research suggests one cannot rule out malingering (see below). Additionally determining the cut-off point for impaired performance remains problematic. Lee, Loring & Martin (1992) have suggested 7/15 as an appropriate cut-off but there is no universal agreement. Furthermore there is no method of scoring intrusions. It is also feasible that a sophisticated patient will be able to determine that the task is simple and may be aware that they are being examined for exaggeration.

In an effort to provide redress to this situation, Rawling (1993) published the Simulation Index (SI) which attempted to provide a more sophisticated analysis of neuropsychological performance using the two most widely used clinical test batteries, the Wechsler Adult Intelligence Scale-Revised (WAIS-R) and the Wechsler Memory Scale-Revised (WMS-R). Errors made by severely brain damaged patients and those suspected of malingering were analysed to determine patterns of response that differentiated the two groups.

We are currently conducting our own study (Walton & McCarter, in preparation) to examine the use of neuropsychological assessment, SI, Rey 15 Item Memory Test and Warrington Recognition Memory Test in the detection of exaggeration in an MTBI population. We have thus far examined 18 patients with brief or no loss of consciousness and with some documented PTA not exceeding 24 hours. All were given a thorough neuropsychological assessment as part of litigation. Patients were classified by two experienced clinical neuropsychologists (RMcC & NHW) as having a) genuine MTBI profiles, b) profiles significantly confounded by psychological factors or c) malingerers. 17/18 were given the Rey 15 Item Memory Test and 6/18 were given the WRMT. All scores were subsequently independently and blindly rated by an assistant psychologist using the Simulation Index.

The neuropsychologists classified 8/18 as showing profiles inconsistent with brain injury. The Simulation Index rated 7/18. There were no patients rated by the neuropsychologists as genuine that were rated as simulators using the SI. The Rey 15 Item Memory Test failed to identify any of the simulators (using the recommended cut-off score of 7/15). Data for the Warrington Recognition Memory Test are insufficient at this stage, though qualitatively performance on this test did not prove useful, the test correctly classifying 2/6 but producing 3/6 false negative results.

Interestingly scores on the WAIS-R and Wechsler Memory Scale-Revised (WMS-R) were significantly lower in the simulating group. This suggests that unsophisticated neuropsychological analysis of these scores could easily lead to false assumptions of impaired neuropsychological performance following

MTBI. Whilst our preliminary results suggest that a large minority of patients with MTBI show reliable signs of simulation, there remains a majority who do not and in whom there is evidence of genuine neuropsychological deficit.

Conclusions

- MTBI may produce damage to the brain in the absence of loss of consciousness or even direct head strike. This may result from diffuse axonal injury or chemical changes within the brain or both. Whilst the mechanisms of MTBI remain poorly understood, this does not allow us to rule out their existence.
- There may be persistent neuropsychological deficits following MTBI that are likely to affect concentration, sustained and focused attention, speed of information processing and memory. The detection of these deficits requires careful and appropriate neuropsychological testing and experienced clinical evaluation of those test results.
- Such deficits are likely to exert a more marked impact on individuals who function in demanding occupational settings, where creative approaches are required for coping with multiple simultaneous demands under conditions of stress. In such settings even a mild deterioration in ability or reliability of performance may have profound consequences (e.g., what potential for lapses of concentration or minor errors would we tolerate in an airline pilot?).
- Evaluation of the consequences of MTBI requires sophisticated neuropsychological testing and interpretation, including reliable measures designed to differentiate genuine profiles from simulated ones.
- Differing patterns of performance may reveal deficits consistent with MTBI, psychological factors or malingering. These will have very different prognoses and potential to benefit from intervention.

References

Alexander, M. P. (1995). Mild traumatic brain injury: Pathophysiology, natural history, and clinical management. *Neurology*, *45*: 1253–1260.

Aubrey, J. B., Dobbs, A. R. & Rule, B. G. (1989). Laypersons' knowledge about the sequelae of minor head injury and whiplash. *Journal of Neurology, Neurosurgery, and Psychiatry*, *52*: 842–846.

Batchelor, J., Harvey, A. G. & Bryant, R. A. (1995). Stroop Colour Word Test as a measure of attentional deficits following mild head injury. *The Clinical Neuropsychologist. 9*(2): 180–186.

Binder, L. M. (1986). Persisting Symptoms After Mild Head Injury: A review of the Postconcussive Syndrome. *Journal of Clinical and Experimental Neuropsychology, 8*(4): 323–346.

Blumbergs, P. C., Scott, G., Manavis J., Wainwright H., Simpson D. A. & McLean A. J. (1994) Staining of amyloid precursor protein to study axonal damage in mild head injury. *The Lancet, 344,* 1055–1056.

Bohnen N, Jolles J. & Twijnstra A. (1992). Modification of the Stroop Colour Word Test improves differentiation between patients with mild head injury and matched controls. *The Clinical Neuropsychologist, 6*: 178–188

Bohnen, N., Jolles, J. & Verhey, F. R. J. (1993). Persistent neuropsychological deficits in cervical whiplash patients without direct headstrike. *Acta neurol. belg., 93*: 23–31.

Bohnen, N. I., Jolles, J., Twijnstra, A., Mellink, R. & Wijnen, G. (1995). Late neurobehavioural symptoms after mild head injury. *Brain Injury, 9*(1): 27–33.

Crawford, J. R. & Allan, K. M. (1997). Estimating Premorbid WAIS-R IQ with Demographic Variables: Regression Equations Derived from a UK Sample. *The Clinical Neuropsychologist, 11*(2): 192–197.

Crawford, J. R., Johnson, D. A., Mychalkiw, B. & Moore, J. W. (1997). WAIS-R Performance Following Closed-Head Injury: A Comparison of the Clinical Utility of Summary IQs, Factor Scores, and Subtest Scatter Indices. *The Clinical Neuropsychologist, 11*(4): 345–355.

Dixon, C. E., Taft, W. C. & Hayes, R. L. (1993). Mechanisms of mild traumatic brain injury. *Journal of Head Trauma Rehabilitation, 8*(3): 1–12.

Ettlin, T. M., Kischka, U., Reichmann, S., Radii, E. W., Heim, S., Wengen, D. & Benson, F. (1992). Cerebral symptoms after whiplash injury of the neck: prospective clinical and neuropsychological study of whiplash injury. *Journal of Neurology, Neurosurgery, and Psychiatry, 55*: 943–948.

Gronwall, D. (1989). Cumulative and persisting effects of concussion on attention and cognition. In H.S. Levin, H.M. Eisenberg & A.L. Benton (Eds) *Mild Head Injury.* Oxford University Press, New York.

Lee, G. P., Loring, D. W. & Martin, C. W. (1992). Rey's 15 item visual memory test for the detection of malingering: Normative observations on patients with neurological disorders. *Psychological Assessment, 4*: 43–46.

Leininger, B. E., Grambling, S. E., Farrell, A. D., Kreutzer, J. S. & Peck, E. A. (1990). Neuropsychological deficits in symptomatic minor head injury patients after concussion and mild concussion. *Journal of Neurology, Neurosurgery, and Psychiatry, 53*: 293–296.

Lezak, M. D. (1995) *Neuropsychological Assessment* (3rd Ed). Oxford University Press, New York USA.

Mandel, S. (1989). Minor head injury may not be 'minor'. *Head Injury, 85*(6): 213–225.

McCarter R. J. & Walton N. H. (in preparation) Concordance between the Simulation Index and neuropsychological diagnosis in mild traumatic brain injury.

McLean, A. J. (1995). Brain Injury without Head Impact? *Journal of Neurotrauma, 12*(4): 621–625.

Mild Traumatic Brain Injury Committee of the Head Injury Interdisciplinary Special Interest Group of the American Congress of Rehabilitation Medicine, (1993).

Miller, H. (1961). Accident neurosis. *British Medical Journal, 1*: 919–925.

Mittenberg, W., DiGiulio, D. V., Perrin, S. & Bass, A. E. (1992). Symptoms following mild head injury: expectation as aetiology. *Journal of Neurology, Neurosurgery, and Psychiatry*, *55*: 200–204.

Rawling, P. J. & Brooks, D. N. The Simulation Index: a method for detecting factitious errors on the WAIS-R and WMS. *Neuropsychology*, *4*: 223–238.

Stuss, D. T. (1995). A sensible approach to mild traumatic brain injury. *Neurology*, *45*: 1251–1252.

Sweeney, J. E. (1992). Nonimpact Brain Injury: Grounds for Clinical Study of the Neuropsychological Effects of Acceleration Forces. *The Clinical Neuropsychologist*, *6*(4): 443–457.

Thompson, M. R. (1965). *Post-traumatic psychoneurosis a statistical survey*. American Journal of Psychiatry, *121*: 1043–1048.

6

Injuries to the Brain

DANIEL SILVERMAN, M.D.

Capital Neurological Associates, Albany, New York, U.S.A.

TRISHUL DEVINENI, B.S., B.A.

Center for Stress & Anxiety Disorders, University at Albany, SUNY, Albany, New York, U.S.A.

Introduction

The aim of this chapter is to review general aspects of the pathology and physiology of mild closed head injury (CHI). While much is known about the pathophysiologic correlates of severe head injury, relatively little scientific knowledge has been gathered about the pathophysiologic processes involved in mild CHI. Recently, more systematic attention has been paid to mild CHI and the body of methodologically sound, empirical research has been steadily growing in this area. It is not the goal of this chapter to provide an exhaustive review of the biomedical literature pertaining to mild CHI. Rather, our goal is to introduce major topics relevant to a general understanding of current research findings on the pathophysiology of mild CHI. For a more detailed, technical discussion of each of these areas, refer to the corresponding primary literature cited throughout the chapter.

Each of the sections of this chapter correspond to some of the major research areas related to mild CHI. First, the definition of mild CHI is elaborated upon followed by presentation of data on the scope of the problem. Next, biomechanical models of closed head injury are discussed in some detail. This is followed by a brief review of some of the major pathologic processes proposed to account for the neurophysical underpinnings of mild CHI. Related to these pathophysiologic findings, evidence gathered from neuroradiologic imaging and electrophysiologic studies in mild CHI patients are discussed. Finally, we will review some of the potential pathophysiologic correlates of postconcussive syndrome, a stereotypic cluster of chronic subjective complaints that frequently follow CHI.

Epidemiology of Head Injury: Magnitude of the Problem

Motor vehicle accidents (MVAs) are the leading cause of death resulting from unintentional injuries in the United States. Of these unintentional injury deaths, more than one third are attributable to head injuries. Head injury is a prevalent and serious national health care problem in the United States. About 2 million Americans experience head injury traumas of varying severity each year. MVAs are the single leading cause of closed head injuries and are the most common cause of injury seen in hospital emergency departments and other acute care settings. Obtaining reliable estimates of the frequency of CHI is complicated by the lack of agreement on the clinical features of CHI and inconsistent use of terminology to refer to these conditions. Nonetheless, advances in assessment methods such as the development of sophisticated neuroradiologic procedures (e.g., CT, MRI, PET, SPECT) have resulted in an accumulation of evidence indicating that CHI is a major public health problem in most industrialized countries. The best current estimates show an U.S. annual incidence of 150 per 100,000 for mild CHI from all causes, accounting for over 75% of all reported head injuries (U.S. DHHS, 1989).

In terms of other injuries, so called whiplash injuries, where the neck and head are thrown back and forth from the accelerative-decelerative forces of impact, following MVAs are the most common cause of cervical injuries with an incidence of over 1 million per year in the U.S. Whiplash-related injuries have been associated in some studies with many of the symptoms characteristic of postconcussive syndrome (e.g., dizziness, headache, memory deficits, concentration difficulties) that are frequent complaints among mild CHI patients (Evans, 1992b).

With respect to mortality data, an average of 52,000 Americans die each year following head injury traumas from all causes. More than one third of these head injury-related deaths result from MVAs (Sosin et al., 1995). With an annual death rate of about 7 per 100,000 people, MVAs are the second leading cause, behind firearms, of head injury-related death in the United States (CDC, 1996a). In 1992, the death rate associated with traumatic head injuries from all causes was about 19.3 per 100,000 residents (Sosin et al., 1995). Overall, MVAs are the leading cause of injury-related mortality in the United States among people aged 1 to 64, accounting for about one third of all deaths resulting from injuries (CDC, 1996b). Clearly, head injuries serve as a frequent etiology for injury-related mortality resulting from MVAs. However, it should be noted that mild CHI, uncomplicated by other more severe concomitant primary or secondary injuries, is much more commonly associated with morbidity outcomes than mortality.

The human costs of head injury in terms of the emotional and physical burden borne by those who are injured and their family and friends are incalculable. Long-term physical and psychological disability is common, even in cases of "mild" head injury. The economic burden of head injury to U.S. society is also enormous. The limited data on estimated monetary costs of head injury (in 1985 dollars) totals a staggering $37.8 billion (Max et al., 1991). These financial costs represent direct medical care and rehabilitation expenditure as well as indirect costs associated with lost wages of the injured individual and work productivity losses to the nation.

Several large-scale community and national epidemiologic studies indicate that head injuries resulting in hospitalization and long term disability are a very common occurrence in the United States. The Federal Interagency Head Injury Task Force (U.S. DHHS, 1989) estimates that 70,000 to 90,000 persons each year experience serious long term disability as a result of brain injury. Rates in the United States of mild to moderate brain injury, defined as a closed head injury resulting in some degree of loss of consciousness, are estimated to run much higher. Based on data from the National Health Interview Survey, a representative probability sample of the non-institutionalized civilian U.S. population, 1.5 million individuals each year sustain a non-fatal brain injury that does not result in institutionalization or permanent disability, yielding an annual rate of 618 per 100,000 U.S. residents in 1991 (Sosin et al., 1996). MVAs are the single largest cause of non-fatal closed head injuries in the United States, accounting for about 28% of all mild to moderate brain injuries. Other authors estimate that as much as 50% of all head injury-related morbidity in the U.S. is accounted for by MVAs (Kraus & Sorenson, 1994). This figure represents about 186,500 or half of all head injuries resulting in hospitalization.

Annually, about 373,000 Americans are hospitalized as a result of head injuries from all causes (Kraus & Sorenson, 1994). The results of the National Health Interview Survey indicate that medical care-seeking is common among head injured persons: 75% of those with brain injury sought some form of medical attention; of these, 14% were treated in private or community clinics and offices, 35% were treated and released from hospital emergency departments, and 25% were hospitalized. Males, teenagers, and young adults were found to be at greatest risk of sustaining brain injury severe enough to require medical attention. Thus, it appears based on the national data that the incidence of MVA-related mild to moderate brain injury in the United States is substantial. Moreover, these data indicate that at least one fourth of individuals suffering from brain injury from any cause never seek formal medical attention, suggesting that these figures may significantly underestimate the true extent of the problem.

In terms of risk factors associated with sustaining brain injury, males are about twice as likely to incur a head injury due to all causes as females (Sosin et al., 1989). Teenagers and young adults in the age range of 15–24 are at the highest risk of incurring brain injuries. Consistent with the overall injury data, males are over twice as likely to experience MVA-related head injuries compared to females. About half of all Americans hospitalized for MVA-related head injuries are within the ages of 15–35 (Sosin et al., 1989). We may infer from these data that young adult males are the subgroup of the U.S. population at greatest risk of suffering MVA-related brain injuries.

The existing data indicate that closed head injuries resulting from MVAs are a common occurrence in the United States. CHIs of varying degrees of severity occur in about two-thirds of all MVAs in the United States. This situation prevails in spite of considerable measures taken by government agencies at the federal, state, and local levels over the past 30 years to promote safer roadways (e.g., by easing congestion), more crashworthy vehicles (e.g., mandatory airbags), better driver education (e.g., proper use of occupant restraint systems), and harsher penalties for drunk driving. These government initiatives have resulted in declining rates of head injury-related mortality in MVAs, although the inevitable consequence is that the rates of morbidity associated with debilitating mild to moderate head injuries have increased steadily over the past 30 years among this increasingly large group of MVA *survivors*. This mild to moderate brain injured group experiences significant long-term disability, impairment in basic bodily functions (e.g., vision, memory), and markedly decreased quality of life. This brain injured MVA survivor group represents a significant national public health care challenge to all levels of the medical treatment community, particularly the acute trauma care and rehabilitation systems.

Definitions of Mild Head Injury

For the purposes of our discussion only closed or blunt, nonpenetrating head injuries will be considered. It should be noted that in clinical practice

Table 1. Head Injury Classification

Head injury severity	Glasgow Coma Scale Score
Mild	13–15
Moderate	9–12
Severe	3–8

and among researchers, the terms *mild closed head injury* and *mild traumatic brain injury* are used interchangeably to refer to essentially the same condition. These terms are treated as synonymous in the present chapter. However, for the sake of clarity and consistency, the somewhat arbitrary decision was made to use variations on the term *mild closed head injury* throughout this chapter.

These conditions certainly represent a wide spectrum in terms of the qualitative degree of cerebral injury. Present classification systems divide closed head injury into three general categories: mild, moderate, and severe. Historically, these were defined by the Glasgow Coma Scale (GCS) score (see Table 1) at initial assessment. Nevertheless, it must be recognized that other initial assessment variables not accounted for by the GCS may significantly effect outcome. The GCS by itself does not take into account many confounding variables. For example, drug or alcohol intoxication may effect the primary assessment. Additional injuries need to be taken into account and other focal neurological deficits should be considered to increase diagnostic and prognostic accuracy. The presence of skull or facial fractures and intracerebral hematomas will certainly have major implications for subsequent morbidity.

Most present definitions of minor CHI classify individual as having mild head injuries based on a GCS score of 13 to 15 at initial assessment with no focal neurological deficits or breach of the cranial vault. An acute loss of consciousness is not required for a classification of mild head injury, and any loss of consciousness should be transient with total duration under 30 minutes. Perhaps the most comprehensive operational definition was recently developed by the Mild Traumatic Brain Injury Committee, Head Injury Interdisciplinary Special Interest Group of the American Congress of Rehabilitation Medicine (1993). According to these criteria, a person with mild traumatic brain injury (TBI) is one who has traumatically induced physiologic disruption of brain function, as manifested by at least *one* of the following:

1. Any period of loss of consciousness;
2. Any loss of memory for events immediately before or after the accident;

3. Any alteration in the mental state at the time of the injury (e.g., feeling dazed, disoriented, or confused);
4. Focal neurological deficits(s) that may or may not be transient (*Note*: Focal neurological signs, if permanent, are nonetheless often used as exclusionary criteria by researchers when defining mild head injury).

Excluded from the diagnosis of mild TBI are cases where *any* of the following are true:

1. Posttraumatic amnesia exceeds 24 hours;
2. Loss of consciousness is greater than 30 minutes;
3. Glasgow Coma Scale score is less than 13, beyond 30 minutes post-injury.

This definition does not exclude cases in which the head is struck by a blunt object, or where the brain undergoes an acceleration-deceleration movement without direct external trauma to the head or cervical region (e.g., whiplash). The issue of whether whiplash can actually produce minor head injury remains controversial. Clearly some biomechanical and pathophysiological differences exist between a direct, physical blow to the head versus the inertial forces of acceleration-deceleration injury. These differences are important to recognize when examining the sequelae of minor head injury. Nevertheless, these patients are often difficult to reliably characterize based on available signs and symptoms. Many descriptions rely on subjective self-reports of head injured patients. Archival data largely from case reports indicate that historical accounts by victims of minor head injuries, particularly MVA-related injuries, are notoriously inaccurate. Therefore distinguishing these two forms of injury etiology is a daunting task. The fairly common occurrence of combined injuries further complicates our understanding of the distinction. Experimental data with non-human primates has accumulated to support the view that whiplash injuries may indeed produce microscopically observable cerebral damage (Ommaya et al., 1968). This issue will be explored in greater detail in later parts of this chapter.

Often a GCS score of 13–14 (inclusive in the definition of mild head injury) reflects an acute period of confusion or disorientation. Yet in some cases, the presence of mild head trauma may not even become evident until the patient begins to manifest some of the chronic, long-term symptoms typically associated with this condition. Moreover, minor head injury may easily be overlooked in cases of multiple traumas. Therefore, the diagnosis in many cases may only be made retrospectively when certain characteristic posttraumatic symptoms develop. These symptoms include possible cognitive impairments. Most commonly observed are recent memory deficits, as well as disruption in concentration, judgment, and other executive functions. Impairments in movement abilities such as strength and coordination and

Table 2. Glasgow Coma Scale

Eyes open	Never	1
	To pain	2
	To verbal stimuli	3
	Spontaneously	4
Best Verbal Response	No response	1
	Incomprehensible sounds	2
	Inappropriate words	3
	Disoriented and converses	4
	Oriented and converses	5
Best Motor Response	No response	1
	Extension (decerebrate rigidity)	2
	Flexion abnormal (decorticate rigidity)	3
	Flexion withdrawal	4
	Localizes pain	5
	Obeys	6
Glasgow Coma Score	*Total*	*3–15*

Note. The scale is used by circling the appropriate number for each item. The total score is computed by summing the individual scores.

sensory systems such as tactile and visual sensation disturbance may also be manifested. Additionally, some behavioral changes may be evident including emotional lability and lassitude.

Another clinically troubling and unanswered question is whether a formal distinction should be made between individuals presenting with a GCS score of 13 or 14 and those with a perfectly "normal" score of 15. It becomes readily apparent when reviewing the scale items (see Table 2) that this may be a heterogeneous group. This heterogeneity was illustrated by a case review study of 3370 patient records performed by Culotta and colleagues (1996). In this review of head injury patients admitted to a trauma unit, the rate of abnormal CT scans and the need for neurosurgical intervention increased significantly as GCS scores dropped from 15 through 13.

Some researchers define mild head trauma to exclude patients with abnormal imaging studies. However, application of this criterion becomes a complex issue as a few cases of what appear to be mild head injury have demonstrated small petechial hemorrhages on MRI scans (Alexander, 1995).

Physics of Closed Head Injury

The brain has a gelatinous consistency and is suspended in cerebrospinal fluid. It is partially compartmentalized by flexible dural membranes that are anchored to the calvarium. The skull is a rigid structure with internally irregular contours. The brain itself, although quite soft, is not compressible. The mechanics of mild head injury in MVAs is a result of an initial, sudden acceleration of the cranium with the internal structures slightly lagging behind due to inertial forces. Immediately subsequent to application of this force, sudden deceleration of the cranial vault is followed by a slight lag in the deceleration of the brain. The result is that the brain tissue will be compressed at the site where physical force is applied, and will be pulled away from the opposite side (Elson et al., 1994). Surface contusions may result from impact of the brain as a whole against these irregular, internal calvarial surfaces and shear stresses may also develop as a result of this push-pull motion.

In an early study, Holbourn (1943) postulated that linear acceleration would produce little relative motion between parts of the brain; however, more rotational movements would produce shearing injury due to the torque produced from this angular momentum on compartmentalized regions of the brain. It has also been postulated that physical stresses applied by shearing forces may effect the brain stem, which becomes compressed when the neck is in extension and stretched in flexion (Elson et al., 1994). Such activity could occur in whiplash injury. Some analytical data obtained using modified human models suggest that the shear forces produce maximal injury in the corpus collosum. If the force is increased sufficiently, there is subsequent damage in the brainstem. It may be that the dural structures (the falx and tentorium cerebri) serve to concentrate the shear forces in these particular two brain regions (Nishimoto et al., 1998).

Holbourn's hypotheses have received considerable support by Gennarelli and colleagues (1982) using animal models. In experiments with primates, Gennarelli showed that deceleration forces produce diffuse axonal injury (DAI) in all animals with initial loss of consciousness for more than 15 minutes. Interestingly, the presence of DAI was much more likely when forces were applied in either a lateral or oblique direction and less likely in saggital (forward-backward) motion. In laterally-induced injuries, coma of greater than six hours occurred in 20 of 26 primates. Saggital or oblique-directed force did not produce coma lasting for greater than six hours in any of the test animals. It appeared that the magnitude of lateral motion was proportional to the degree of DAI. Additionally, this appeared to directly correlate with the induction of traumatic coma.

Unfortunately, the significant anatomical differences that exist between humans and other primate species limits our ability to extrapolate from these data. The inertial forces that are generated when kinetic energy is transferred to the brain are largely dependent on the relative masses of the cranium and its contents. For example, rhesus monkey cranium is only 8 percent of the human cranial weight, and even the chimpanzee brain is only 30 percent the weight of the human brain (Jennett & Teasdale, 1981). Also, the spatial configuration of internal structures differs somewhat across the primate species. Additional anatomical variables, including the angle of the brainstem to the cervical cord and cerebral hemispheres, will influence the force vectors and the resultant injury. It has been clearly demonstrated that many traumatic brain injury models developed and tested in lower animals do not reflect the same gross pathological abnormalities that have been found in humans (Cruz et al., 1998). Therefore, the biochemical and ultrastructural abnormalities demonstrated in small species (e.g., rodents) may not correspond to human pathophysiologic changes.

Pathology of Closed Head Injury

There is abundant clinical and experimental evidence documenting the manifold physical consequences of closed head injury. In addition to producing alterations on an ultrastructural level, closed head trauma may have profound effects on the cerebral vasculature and blood flow. Alterations may also occur on a biochemical level with the release of excitatory neurotransmitters and cytotoxic free radicals in response to tissue damage.

Diffuse Axonal Injury. Diffuse degeneration of the cerebral white matter as a consequence of closed head injury in humans had been recognized as early as 1956 by Strich who hypothesized that diffuse axonal injury (DAI) was caused by shearing stresses brought about by rotational forces occurring at the moment of impact. After studying postmortem brain tissue from 59 head injury victims, Oppenheimer (1968) postulated four mechanisms by which these shearing forces produce injury. The first mechanism is established by direct impact on hard structure, such as sudden pressure of the free edge of the tentorium abutting the brainstem. The second mechanism would be sudden stretching of small vessels resulting in small tears and resulting petechial hemorrhages. The third and fourth mechanisms speak specifically to DAI. Nerve fibers may be stretched or torn without hemorrhaging, or nerve fibers may be disrupted as they cross a blood vessel. By examining brains of head injury victims who died at different time intervals from the moment of injury, Oppenheimer was able to characterize a temporal sequence of pathological changes. By 24 hours post-trauma, reacting glial cells were noted to enlarge and appear in clusters. Axons were noted to form retraction balls in these regions. By three weeks, reactive astrocytes were evident in the regions around these clusters. By six weeks, diffuse microglial proliferation was evident in areas of axonal degeneration.

Most of the brains Oppenheimer studied were in victims of severe head injury, however, in five cases the cerebral injuries were very minimal. The cause of death in these cases was most often related to fat embolism or pneumonia. Nevertheless, microglial clusters and axonal injury were evident in these probable cases of minor head injury. In one example of these cases illustrated by Oppenheimer, there were only 10–15 minutes of posttraumatic amnesia and no loss of consciousness. In this particular case, histological studies revealed significant loss of myelin and numerous axonal retraction bulbs in the midbrain. Oppenheimer concluded that even a mild concussive injury could produce these microscopic changes.

Clear evidence for the presence of axonal injury in mild head trauma has recently been provided in a topographical analysis by Blumberg and colleagues (1995). In this study of 12 closed head injury victims, six patients had sustained mild head trauma, but succumbed to other injuries. By employing a sophisticated scoring technique to identify axonal damage, Blumberg documented axonal injury for all patients in this sample. The mild head injury patients showed evidence of axonal degeneration in the corpus collosum and fornices without indication of concomitant vascular injury.

Cerebral Autoregulation. Cerebral blood flow normally remains fairly constant despite variations in systemic blood pressure. This homestatic mechanism which is intrinsically and autonomously controlled by the cerebral vasculature, is known as cerebral autoregulation. This regulatory mechanism is in part managed by arteriolar muscular control of vascular resistance. In normotensive individuals, cerebral blood flow will remain constant even with large systemic mean arterial pressure variations between 50 and 150 mm Hg. The mechanism is as follows: as mean arterial pressure increases, cerebral vasculature will constrict to maintain cerebral blood volume; and conversely, as mean arterial pressure falls, cerebral arterioles will dilate to maintain blood flow. It is a well documented phenomenon that in moderate and severe closed head injury, cerebral autoregulation may be compromised (Ropper & Kennedy, 1988). This disruption can result in significant neuronal damage secondary to ischemia. If similar dysregulatory effects are demonstrable in the case of minor head injuries, this would suggest that such individuals may be at increased risk for ischemic neuronal injury. Such effects have been demonstrated recently in a study by Junger and colleagues (1997). Using transcranial Doppler (TCD), cerebral blood flow was monitored while systemic blood pressure was varied by the use of bilateral thigh cuffs. It was found that 8 of 29 (28 %) of the mild head injury patients had either severely impaired or completely absent cerebral autoregulation. These patients were all evaluated within 48 hours of their initial head injury. Furthermore, experimental rodent models of mild head injury suggest an increased vulnerability of hippocampal neurons to a subsequent hypoxic insult (Katoh et al., 1998). The immediate clinical implications of these results may relate to circumstances in which victims of minor head injuries are exposed to significant blood pressure variations. Such a scenario is quite common since these patients often have concomitant injuries that require urgent surgical intervention. In fact, Strebel et al. (1997) had the opportunity to test this hypothesis in a patient who had suffered a mild head injury in a MVA. This individual required an orthopedic procedure six days post-MVA. Autoregulation was tested after anesthesia induction using phenylephrine to raise systemic blood pressure and TCD to measure blood flow. An almost complete absence of cerebral autoregulation was demonstrated, both under anesthesia and after regaining consciousness. The possibility of such regulatory dysfunction jeopardizing the mild head injured patient's neurological outcome as a result of ischemic neuronal damage is therefore a real concern.

It has been postulated that long-term alterations in cerebral blood flow may have a role in the chronic symptoms of mild head injury. Although to date there are no conclusive reports of chronic autoregulatory dysfunction in patients with mild head injury, there is data supporting impairment in cerebral blood flow in these patients. Studies of cerebral blood flow using a Xenon (Xe)-133 inhalation technique have shown both regional and interhemispheric blood flow abnormalities in patients with chronic posttraumatic headache (a common result of mild head trauma; Gilkey et al., 1997). To date, no conclusive evidence is available linking these blood flow alterations to postconcussive symptomatology. However, these reports generally do support the theories of chronic organic abnormalities in victims of minor head injury.

Neurochemical Abnormalities. Free radicals, byproducts of both normal and abnormal metabolic processes, have been implicated in a multitude of neurodegenerative disorders. They have also been implicated as a confounding influence in ischemic stroke. The biochemically unstable structure of these molecules result in progressive tissue damage through lipid peroxidation producing increased vascular permeability and through the stimulation of excitatory neurotransmitters. Furthermore, there is growing evidence that oxygen-free radicals are linked to hypoperfusion, impaired energy metabolism, and ultimately axonal degeneration (Hall & Braugher, 1993). These neuropathologic changes result in localized edema and tissue necrosis. Studies using animal models have suggested a role for oxygen-free radicals in tissue damage resulting from head injury (Hall et al., 1994; Nishio et al., 1997). However, there is little evidence to date indicating a role for free radicals in the pathology of mild head injury among humans.

Several experimental studies with rats have demonstrated transient release of excitatory neurotransmitters including glutamate and aspartate following head injury. Acetylcholine levels have also shown high rates of transient turnover after head injury in both humans and experimental animal models (Hayes & Dixon, 1994). The release of these neurotransmitters may be the result of widespread neuronal depolarization in response to the mechanically induced stress of injury. Large extracellular increases of ionic potassium, a signature of widespread depolarization, have been shown in experimental models of head injury (Katayama et al., 1990). Further, these data indicate that a concussive event may lead to an indiscriminate release of excitatory neurotransmitters as a direct result of mechanically induced efflux of potassium.

In addition to free radicals and excitatory neurotransmitters, elevated levels of beta-endorphins have been found in the cerebrospinal fluid (CSF) of closed head trauma patients. This is the case even in those presenting with mild head trauma (Pasaogla et al., 1996). It has been suggested that release of these neuropeptides may in fact be destructive, as some opiate antagonists have shown to have a neuroprotective role in both spinal cord trauma and cerebral ischemia (Hayes & Dixon, 1994).

Neuroimaging Studies

For obvious reasons, pathological specimens are largely unavailable or difficult to acquire in victims of mild head injury. Therefore, great efforts have been made to assess neurological sequelae through the use of neuroradiologic imaging studies. One of the dilemmas that result from this research effort is that some radiologic abnormalities might exclude these cases from being considered mild head injuries based on some formal diagnostic criteria or standard clinical practice. If one is to exclude gross abnormalities such as large cerebral contusions and hematomas from consideration, the task is narrowed to identifying subtle abnormalities that could yield clues to the myriad symptoms seen in mild brain injury (e.g., postconcussion syndrome).

CT. The value of computerized tomography (CT) imaging in the assessment and management of closed head injury has been well established. French and Dublin (1977) reviewed 1000 consecutive head injury cases using CT. Sixty three percent were scanned within the first 72 hours of admission of which 51 percent were abnormal. Abnormalities ranged from cortical contusions to subdural and epidural hematomas. Among those patients initially classified as alert and neurologically intact, 13 percent manifested some abnormality on CT. It must be noted however, that these patients were not defined as neurologically "normal" at the time of scanning, but necessarily at their initial evaluation. Therefore the assessment utility of CT for "mild head trauma" was not established by this work. In a study comparing CT and magnetic resonance imaging (MRI) in the evaluation of head trauma, Kelly et al. (1988) found only one case in 36 patients with mild head trauma with an abnormality on CT and etiology linked to the initial injury.

The question regarding the specific value of CT scanning in evaluation of mild head trauma victims was addressed by Mohanty and colleagues (1991). In a total of 348 patients with an initial GCS score of 13 or better, only 12 showed abnormalities on CT imaging. These few patients with abnormal scans nevertheless exhibited no neurological defects or sequelae. Mohanty concluded that no clinical utility appeared to exist for CT scanning in patients with mild head trauma, except in cases where there was an indication of a basal skull fracture.

MRI. There is fairly conclusive evidence supporting the utility of magnetic resonance imaging (MRI) to demonstrate abnormalities in severe and moderate head injury that may not appear on a CT scan. In a study by Wilberger et al. (1987), frontal, temporal, and subcortical lesions were found in 24 head injury patients who had normal CT scans. Late MRI studies, performed between 4 to 24 months post-injury, have shown similar results (Grosswasser et al., 1987). It has been much more difficult to demonstrate abnormal MRI studies in patients with mild head trauma. In a retrospective review of 100 patients with clinically significant head trauma, Kelly et al. (1988) found no identifiable abnormalities on MRI in 33 of 36 patients who were categorized as sustaining minor head injuries. In only one of the remaining three patients was an abnormality (a chronic subdural hematoma) found that was clinically relevant to initial injury. However, in a smaller study of 20 consecutive hospital admissions for mild or moderate closed head trauma, Levin et al. (1987) revealed focal brain lesions attributable to the initial trauma in 90 percent of the patients. Mild head injury was represented in eight of these cases. Among the most impressive abnormalities for these cases were parenchymal lesions in the frontal and temporal lobes. Lesions were also identified in both the cortical and subcortical regions. Additionally, in a prospective analysis by Doezema et al. (1991), 6 of 58 patients with minor head injury had abnormal MRI scans. These abnormalities included three cortical contusions and three cases of small subdural hematomas. Two of these subdural hematomas were not evident on CT scanning. Mittl and colleagues (1994) found evidence of diffuse axonal injury in 6 of 20 patients with mild head injury using MRI. All of these patients had normal CT scans at initial evaluation. In a selective study of 17 head trauma cases, Maeder et al. (1991) performed volumetric analysis of MRI scans conducted more than one year post-injury. These patients were selected on the basis of having demonstrable frontal lesions. Despite these criteria, five of the seventeen patients had minor head trauma. Volumetric analysis revealed cortical volume loss in four of these patients. One of the four also showed subcortical volume loss.

PET and SPECT. Given the dearth of evidence of observable structural injury in patients with mild head injury, other techniques have been utilized to measure potential changes in physiologic parameters in these individuals. In particular, single-photon emission computerized tomography (SPECT) and positron emission tomography (PET) have recently been studied extensively since these techniques have value in assessment of functional changes. Ichise and colleagues (1994) compared the findings of Technetium-SPECT, MRI, and CT in 29 brain injured individuals with 17 patient controls. Fifteen of the 29 (52%) experimental cases were classified as having mild head injuries, with an average Glasgow Coma Scale score of 14. In this group, over 50 percent showed abnormalities on SPECT imaging compared to 25 and 15 percent on MRI and CT, respectively. SPECT abnormalities were found most commonly in the frontal and temporal lobes. Using a different isotope, Otte et al. (1996) found evidence of hypoperfusion in the parieto-occipital regions of whiplash victims who had persistent, subjective postconcussive complaints one to four years after their injury.

Although many studies such as these demonstrate a high sensitivity of SPECT in revealing abnormalities in mild head injury, it is probable that a significant number of these results are false positives. For example, in a study conducted by Jacobs et al. (1994), 24 percent of patients with positive SPECT scans at three months post-injury were completely free of symptoms. Because of this high rate of false positives, Jacobs and colleagues (1996) performed an additional evaluation of 136 patients with mild head injury at 3, 6, and 12 months post-injury. SPECT abnormalities were correlated with clinical symptoms in order to test the sensitivity and specificity of this technique. Three-month assessments again showed a high false positive rate, thus replicating their findings from the previous study. Notably, the false positives tended to drop considerably at 12 months. Conversely, false negative SPECT scans were low at three months, with sensitivity of 91%, and dropped to nil at 6 and 12 months, representing 100% sensitivity.

The above data suggests potential clinical utility for SPECT imaging in the objective evaluation of mild head injury. Moreover, since SPECT scans correlate with cerebral perfusion, it might be surmised that it is revealing neuropathologic changes not detectable by other imaging methods. However, identical perfusion abnormalities have been identified in patients suffering from major depression (Ito et al., 1996). This concern was recently examined by Bicik et al. (1998) in a study of whiplash patients using PET and SPECT imaging. In this study, abnormalities in the frontopolar areas on flourodeoxyglucose (FDG)-PET scans were correlated with clinically elevated scores on the Beck Depression Inventory among whiplash patients. Thus, the source of frontopolar hypometabolism in these patients remains ambiguous. Furthermore, defects observed in the parieto-occipital lobes were found in both controls and mild head injury patients. MRI data suggested these defects were artifactual, and related to cortical mass. It appears at this time that some healthy skepticism is advisable when weighing the evidence of SPECT and PET imaging as a reflection of pathologic changes in mild head trauma or whiplash injury.

Electrophysiologic Studies

Electrophysiologic measurement employing such techniques as electroencephalogram (EEG) and auditory evoked potentials has a possible advantage in the study of mild head injury due to its sensitivity in detecting subtle changes in physiology. Several studies have documented EEG abnormalities in mild head injury provided these recordings were taken soon after the injury. Rapid normalization of the EEG tracings has been observed with short time latencies post-injury (Young & Silberstein, 1994). Therefore, it does not appear that there is any clinical utility of EEG in verifying the presence of a mild head injury.

Short-latency brainstem evoked potentials measure computer averaged waveforms produced in response to a repetitive auditory stimulus. Five peaks are identified which represent neuronal responses from the caudal to rostral brainstem (Chiappa, 1983). Several studies have shown abnormalities on brainstem evoked responses persisting for several months after mild head injury in 10 to 27% of patients (Rowe & Carlson, 1980; Benna et al., 1982). These results indicate a potential brainstem pathology in these patients not detectable with neuroradiologic imaging techniques. Unfortunately, these reports failed to find any significant correlation between the presence of postconcussive symptoms and abnormal evoked responses. This negative result, coupled with the large percentage of normal evoked responses seen in mild head injury patients suggest little clinical utility for short-latency evoked potentials.

Pathophysiologic Correlates

A large descriptive literature exists supporting the existence of chronic symptomatology in mild head injury victims (the so called "postconcussive syndrome"). The most common postconcussive symptoms include headache, dizziness, cervical pain, impaired concentration, memory deficits, anxiety, and depression (Evans, 1992a). The pathogenesis of these symptoms, however, remains elusive. Are these symptoms based on a purely psychological response to the provoking traumatic incident? What role does compensation and liability claims play in symptom etiology and maintenance? While it is not within the scope of this review to address such questions, it nevertheless is apparent from the data available thus far that pathophysiologic changes do indeed occur as a result of mild head trauma. To reliably correlate these neuropathologic findings with the symptom complex of postconcussive syndrome remains a formidable challenge for investigators. Although the process of diffuse axonal injury has been documented, it is by no means clear that these findings are related to specific clinical symptoms. Moreover, the permanency of these findings is unclear. It well known that axons are capable of regenerating with the growth of both myelinated and unmyelinated sprouts (Povlishock & Becker, 1985). This phenomena has been demonstrated in mammalian models exposed to moderate head trauma. Remarkably, after 12 months virtually complete recovery was observed by both light and electron microscopic analysis (Erb & Povlishock, 1991). While this finding might help explain the frequently observed recovery of most mild to moderately injured patients in the first year, it does not inform us about the outliers who remain symptomatic for several years post-injury.

Despite experimental models suggesting remarkable regenerative potential of central nervous tissue and recovery of function in test animals, persistent neurologic symptoms are common and almost stereotypic in a significant minority of mild head injury victims. The neuropsychological sequelae of mild head injury will be discussed in a later chapter of this text.

Chronic tension and migraine headaches with posttraumatic onset have been well documented in mild head injury victims (Randolph, 1992). As noted previously, the release of excitatory neurotransmitters post-injury as well as the observed increase in levels of intracellular sodium, calcium, chloride, and extracellular potassium, bear striking resemblance to the neurochemical changes implicated in migraine headache. It has been suggested that these similar alterations may implicate a common pathway for both migraine and posttraumatic headache (Packard & Ham, 1997). However, the anatomic and biochemical substrates for these complaints remain speculative at this time.

Chronic dizziness is a vexing complaint for clinicians treating head injured patients and a very common postconcussive symptom. Despite the absence of true symptomatic vertigo in many of these patients, evidence from posturography and electronystagmography has linked these symptoms to vestibular impairment (Mallinson & Longridge, 1998).

Visual blurring may be accounted for by impaired accommodation. This condition, known as convergence insufficiency, has been reported in as much as 16 percent of acute head injury cases with 58 percent having persistent difficulties (Kowal, 1992). Additionally, diplopia has been found to occur as a result of oculomotor nerve palsies, particularly cranial nerve IV palsies, resulting from mild head trauma (Kwartz et al., 1990).

Conclusion

Mild closed head injury has received increasing research attention since the pioneering studies performed in the 1940's and 50's. Systematic research efforts have been underway attempting to elucidate the pathologic mechanisms underlying the symptomatology of postconcussive syndrome. The study of mild CHI poses numerous difficult problems, many of which have been highlighted throughout this chapter. Progress in the empirical evaluation of the neuropathology of mild head injury has been inevitably slowed by practical and ethical considerations and current methodological limitations. The study of mild head injury is further complicated by the necessity of detecting subtle anatomical or physiologic alterations, in contrast to the gross abnormalities characteristic of more severe forms of head injury. Nonetheless, promising results implicating potential pathophysiologic processes have been obtained with recent advances in radiologic imaging and other assessment technology. Theoretical advances in ever more sophisticated conceptual models of mild CHI have been made with ongoing testing of these models in animal and human studies offering compelling data to support a pathophysiologic basis of mild head injury. Progress in conducting *in vivo* histological assays of mild head injured patients also offers potential of developing a better understanding of the pathologic changes accompanying mild CHI and how these abnormalities account for the symptomatology of postconcussive syndrome. Systematic attempts to meaningfully tie together the results of functional assessment data (e.g., neuropsychological testing) with pathologic studies offers potential for better understanding the complex clinical manifestation of concussive injury. What seems clear at this time is that integration among the various diverse research efforts employing both functional and physiologic levels of analysis is needed. While the challenge to researchers is substantial, the steady progress being made offers hope that a more complete understanding of mild head injury is attainable in the foreseeable future.

References

Alexander, M. P. (1995). Mild traumatic brain injury: Pathophysiology, natural history, and clinical management. *Neurology*, *45*, 1253–1260.

American Congress of Rehabilitation Medicine: Report of the Mild Traumatic Brain Injury Committee, Head Injury Interdisciplinary Special Interest Group (1993). Definition of mild traumatic brain injury. *Journal of Head Trauma Rehabilitation*, *8*(3), 86–87.

Benna, P., Bergamasco, B., Bianco, C., Gilli, M., Ferrero, P. & Pinessi, L. (1982). Brainstem auditory potentials in postconcussion syndrome. *Italian Journal of Neurological Sciences*, *3*(4), 281–287.

Bicik, I., Radanov, B. P., Schafer, N., Dvorak, J., Blum, B., Weber, B., Burger, C., Van Schultess, G. K. & Buck, C. (1998). PET with ^{18}fluordeoxyglucose and hexamethylpropylene amine oxime SPECT in late whiplash syndrome. *Neurology*, *51*, 345–350.

Blumberg, P., Scott, G., Manavis, J., Wainwright, H., Simpson, D. A. & McLean, A. J. (1995). Topography of axonal injury as defined by amyloid precursor protein and the sector scoring method in mild and severe closed head injury. *Journal of Neurotrauma*, *12*(4), 565–572.

Centers for Disease Control and Prevention, National Center for Injury Prevention and Control. (November, 1996a). *National summary of injury mortality data, 1988–1994*. Atlanta, GA: Author.

Centers for Disease Control and Prevention, National Center for Injury Prevention and Control. (1996b). *Ten leading causes of death tables, 1994*. Atlanta, GA: Author.

Chiappa, K. H. (1983). *Evoked potentials in clinical medicine*. New York: Raven.

Cruz, J., Minoja, G., Mattioli, C., de Carvalho, W. B., Petitjean, M. E., Marginaud, E., Okuchi, K. & Massei, R. (1998). *Neurologic and Neurosurgical Emergencies*. Philadelphia: W. B. Saunders.

Culotta, V. P., Sementilli, M. E., Gerold, K. & Watts, C. C. (1996). Clinicopathological heterogeneity in the classification of mild head injury. *Neurosurgery*, *38*(2), 245–250.

Doezema, D., King, J., Tandberg, D., Espinosa, M. & Orrison, W. (1991). Magnetic resonance imaging in minor head injury. *Annals of Emergency Medicine*, *20*(12), 1281–1285.

Elson, L. M. & Carley, C. C. (1994, March). Mechanisms and pathophysiology of mild head injury. *Seminars in Neurology*, *14*(1), 8–18.

Erb, D. E. & Povlishock, J. T. (1991). Neuroplasticity following traumatic brain injury: A study of GABAergic terminal loss and recovery in the cat dorsal lateral vestibular nucleus. *Experimental Brain Research*, *83*(2), 253–267.

Evans, R. W. (1992a). The postconcussion syndrome and the sequelae of mild head injury. *Neurologic Clinics*, *10*(4), 815–844.

Evans, R. W. (1992b). Some observations on whiplash injuries. *Neurologic Clinics*, *10*(4), 975–997.

French, B. N. & Dublin, A. B. (1977). The value of computerized tomography in the management of 1000 consecutive head injuries. *Surgical Neurology*, *7*, 171–183.

Gennarelli, T. A., Thibault, L. E., Adams, J. H., Graham, D. I., Thompson, C. J. & Marcincin, R. P. (1982). Diffuse axonal injury and traumatic coma in the primate. *Annals of Neurology*, *12*, 564–574.

Gilkey, S. J., Ramadan, N. M., Aurora, T. K. & Welch, K. M. A. (1997). Cerebral blood flow in chronic posttraumatic headache. *Headache*, *37*(9), 583–587.

Grosswasser, Z., Reider-Grosswasser, I., Soroker, N. & Machtey, Y. (1987). Magnetic resonance imaging in head injury patients with normal late computerized tomography scans. *Surgical Neurology*, *27*, 331–337.

Hall, E. D. & Braugher, J. M. (1993). Free radicals in CNS injury. *Research Publications – Association for Research in Nervous and Mental Disease*, *71*, 81–105.

Hall, E. D., Andrus, P. K., Yonkers, P. A., Smith, S. Z., Zhang, J. R., Taylor, B. M. & Sun, F. F. (1994). Generation and detection of hydroxyl radicals following experimental head injury. *Annals of the New York Academy of Sciences*, *738*, 15–24.

Hayes, R. L. & Dixon, C. E. (1994). Neurochemical changes in mild head injury. *Seminars in Neurology*, *14*(1), 25–31.

Holbourn, A. H. S. (1943). Mechanics of head injury. *Lancet*, *2*, 438–441.

Ichise, M., Chung, D., Wang, P., Wortzman, G., Gray, B. G. & Franks, W. (1994). Technetium-99m-HMPAO SPECT, CT, and MRI in the evaluation of patients with chronic traumatic brain injury: A correlation with neuropsychological performance. *Journal of Nuclear Medicine*, *35*(2), 217–226.

Ito, H., Kawashima, R. & Awata, S. (1996). Hypoperfusion in the limbic system and prefrontal cortex in depression: SPECT with anatomic standardization technique. *Journal of Nuclear Medicine*, *37*, 410–414.

Jacobs, A., Put, E., Ingels, M. & Bossuyt, A. (1994). Prospective evaluation of technetium-99m-HMPAO SPECT in mild and moderate traumatic brain injury. *Journal of Nuclear Medicine*, *35*(6), 942–947.

Jacobs, A., Put, E., Ingels, M., Put, T. & Bossuyt, A. (1996). One year follow-up of technetium-99m-HMPAO SPECT in mild head injury. *Journal of Nuclear Medicine*, *37*, 1605–1609.

Jennett, B. & Teasdale, G. (1981). *Management of Head Injuries: Contemporary Neurology, no. 20.* Philadelphia: Davis.

Junger, E. C., Newell, D. W., Grant, G. A., Avellino, A. M., Ghatan, S., Douville, C. M., Lam, A. M., Aaslid, R. & Winn, H. R. (1997). Cerebral autoregulation following minor head injury. *Journal of Neurosurgery*, *86*(3), 425–432.

Katayama, Y., Becker, D. P., Tamura, T. & Hovda, D. A. (1990). Massive increases in extracellular potassium and the indiscriminate release of glutamate following concussive brain injury. *Journal of Neurosurgery*, *73*(6), 889–900.

Katoh, H., Shima, K., Nawashiro, H., Wada, K. & Chigasaki, H. (1998). Selective hippocampal damage to hypoxia after mild head injury in the rat. *Acta Neurochirurgica Supplementum*, *71*, 247–249.

Kelly, A. B., Zimmerman, R. D., Snow, R. B., Gandy, S. E., Heler, L. A. & Deck, M. D. F. (1988). Head trauma: Comparison of MRI and CT experience in 100 patients. *American Journal of Neuroradiology*, *9*, 699–708.

Kowal, L. (1992). Ophthalmic manifestations of head injury. *Australian and New Zealand Journal of Ophthalmology*, *20*(1), 35–40.

Kraus, J. F. & Sorenson, S. (1994). Epidemiology. In J. Silver, S. Yudofsky & R. Hales (Eds.) *Neuropsychiatry of Traumatic Brain Injury* (pp. 3–41). Washington, DC: American Psychiatric Press.

Kwartz, J., Leatherbarrow, B. & Davis, H. (1990). Diplopia following head injury. *Injury*, *21*, 351–352.

Levin, H. S., Amparo, E., Eisenberg, H. M., Willimas, D. H., High, W. M., Jr., McArdle, C. B. & Weiner, R. L. (1987). Magnetic resonance imaging and computerized tomography in relation to the neurobehavioral sequelae of mild and moderate head injuries. *Journal of Neurosurgery*, *66*, 706–713.

Maeder, P., Wirse, A., Bajc, M., Schalen, W., Sjoholm, H., Skeidsvoll, H., Cronqvist, S. & Ingvar, D. H. (1991). Volume of chronic traumatic frontal brain lesions measured by MR imaging and CBF tomography. *Acta Radiologica*, *32*, 271–278.

Mallinson, A. I. & Longridge, N. S. (1998). Dizziness from whiplash and head injury: Differences between whiplash and head injury. *American Journal of Otology*, *19*(6), 814–818.

Max, W., MacKenzie, E. J. & Rice, D. P. (1991). Head injuries: Costs and consequences. *Journal of Head Trauma Rehabilitation*, *6*(2), 76–91.

Mittl, R. L., Grossman, R. I., Hiehle, J. F., Hurst, R. F., Kauder, D. R., Gennarelli, T. A. & Alburger, G. W. (1994). Prevalence of MR evidence of diffuse axonal injury in patients with mild head injury and normal head CT findings. *American Journal of Neuroradiology*, *15*(8), 1583–1589.

Mohanty, S. K., Thompson, W. & Rakower, S. (1991). Are CT scans for head injury patients always necessary? *Journal of Trauma*, *31*(6), 801–804.

Nishimoto, T. & Murakami, S. (1998). Relationship between diffuse axonal injury and internal head structures on blunt impact. *Journal of Biomechanical Engineering*, *120*(1), 140–147.

Nishio, S., Yonoki, M., Noguchi, Y., Kawauchi, M., Asari, S. & Ohmoto, T. (1997). Detection of lipid peroxidation and hydroxyl radicals in brain contusion of rats. *Acta Neurochirurgica Supplementum*, *70*, 84–86.

Ommaya, A. K., Faas, F. & Yarnell, P. (1968). Whiplash injury and brain damage: An experimental study. *Journal of the American Medical Association*, *204*, 285–289.

Oppenheimer, D. R. (1968). Microscopic lesions of the brain following head trauma. *Journal of Neurology, Neurosurgery, and Psychiatry*, *31*, 299–306.

Otte, A., Ettlin, T., Fierz, L. & Mueller-Brand, J. (1996). Parieto-occipital hypoperfusion in the late whiplash syndrome: First quantitative SPECT study using technetium-99m bicisate (ECD). *European Journal of Nuclear Medicine*, *23*, 72–74.

Packard, R. C. & Ham, L. P. (1997). Pathogenesis of posttraumatic headache and migraine: A common headache pathway? *Headache*, *37*(3), 142–152.

Pasaoglu, H., Inci Karakucuk, E., Kurtsoy, A. & Pasaoglu, A. (1996). Endogenous neuropeptides in patients with acute traumatic head injury, I: Cerebrospinal fluid beta-endorphin levels are increased within 24 hours of trauma. *Neuropeptides*, *30*(1), 47–51.

Povlishock, J. T. & Becker, D. P. (1985). Fate of reactive axonal swellings induced by head injury. *Laboratory Investigation*, *52*(5), 540–542.

Ropper, A. H. & Kennedy, S. K. (1988). *Neurological and Neurosurgical Intensive Care* (2nd ed.). Rockville, MD: Aspen.

Rowe, M. J. & Carlson, C. (1980). Brainstem auditory evoked potentials in postconcussion dizziness. *Archives of Neurology*, *37*(11), 679–683.

Sosin, D. M., Sacks, J. J. & Smith, S. M. (1989). Head injury associated deaths in the United States from 1979–1986. *Journal of the American Medical Association*, *262*, 2251–2255.

Sosin, D. M., Sniezek, J. E. & Thurman, D. J. (1996). Incidence of mild and moderate brain injury in the United States. *Brain Injury*, *10*(1), 47–54.

Sosin, D. M., Sniezek, J. E. & Waxweiler, R. J. (1995). Trends in death associated with traumatic brain injury, 1979 through 1992: Success and failure. *Journal of the American Medical Association*, *273*(22), 1778–1780.

Strebel, S., Lam, A. M., Matta, B. F. & Newell, D. W. (1997). Impaired cerebral autoregulation after minor head injury. *Surgical Neurology*, *47*(2), 128–131.

Strich, S. J. (1956). Diffuse degeneration of the cerebral white matter in severe dementia following head injury. *Journal of Neurology, Neurosurgery, and Psychiatry*, *19*, 163–185.

U.S. Department of Health and Human Services. (1989). *Interagency head injury task force report*. Washington, DC: Author.

Wilberger, J. E., Deeb, Z. & Rothfus, W. (1987). Magnetic resonance imaging in cases of severe head injury. *Neurosurgery*, *20*, 571–576.

Young, W. B. & Silberstein, S. D. (1994). Imaging and electrophysiologic testing in mild head injury. *Seminars in Neurology*, *14*(1), 46–52.

7

Road Accidents and the Mind: The Post-Concussional Syndrome

DR R. R. JACOBSON MD, FRCPsych, MRCP

St. George's Hospital Medical School, Department of Psychiatry, Jenner Wing, Cranmer Terrace, London, SW17 0RE, United Kingdom

Abstract

Current models of post-concussional symptoms after mild head injury rest on the dichotomy between organic and psychogenic factors, which underpins Lishman's (1998) formulation; organic genesis and psychologically-driven persistence. Recent prospective studies of mild head injury and perspectives from cognitive behavioural and health psychology, are reviewed with a focus on patterns of recovery. It is argued that the organic-psychogenic conceptualisation inadequately explains persistent post-concussional symptoms. Psychosocial, cognitive-behavioural and motivational factors and the coping process may influence post-concussional symptoms over their entire time course, in particular the late phase.

A multifactorial model of chronic post-concussional symptoms is proposed which integrates biological (organic and psychophysiological stress response) processes with these factors. It is through the recognition and identification of separate processes that questions about outcome, the limits of the impact of organic and psychosocial factors, the nature of exaggeration, and appropriate therapy, may be resolved.

Introduction

The post-concussional syndrome refers to the emergence and variable persistence of a group of symptoms following head injury, particularly mild head injury (MHI). Most descriptions include somatic symptoms (headache, dizziness, fatiguability) accompanied by psychological symptoms both cognitive (poor memory and concentration) and affective (irritability, emotional lability, depression and anxiety). A third to a half of patients experience the syndrome over the first few weeks after mild head injury (Lishman 1988, Lidvall et al 1974, Levin et al 1987, Fenton et al 1993). Whilst most become asymptomatic in the ensuing months, a substantial minority experiences persistent symptoms 6 months to a year later (Alves et al 1986, Fenton et al 1993).

Much debate has surrounded the aetiology of post-concussional symptoms (PCS) after MHI (Miller 1961, Symonds 1962, Rutherford et al 1978, Binder 1986, Lishman 1988, Montgomery et al, 1991, Jacobson 1995). Most researchers accept that brain injury can occur with mild concussion and underly initial PCS, but argue over whether or not chronic or persistent PCS have an organic basis. Controversy still dances attendance on this putative syndrome, for which the American Psychiatric Association provides research criteria in DSM-IV (1994), in need of further study.

The simultaneous occurrence of physical and emotional trauma means that conventional models of the post-concussional syndrome tend to be dichotomous with symptoms viewed as of physiological (Lishman, 1988) or psychological aetiology (Newcombe et al, 1994). This division of opinion is most polarised after **mild head injury**, the focus of this review. The aim of this chapter is to provide a framework within which current research can be understood.

Lishman's (1988) careful review of the literature up to 1987 concluded that physiological factors contributed mainly to the onset of the post-concussional syndrome, while psychological factors contributed more to its long-term course. Recent research, in particular the Belfast studies (Montgomery et al 1991, Fenton et al 1993, McClelland et al 1994) and perspectives from cognitive-behavioural and health psychology will be reviewed to examine this division and to clarify patterns of recovery. It is argued that in terms of the formation and persistence of PCS, the traditional distinction between physiological disorder and psychological disturbance, is outmoded, and that:

(1) psychosocial and cognitive-behavioural factors (including social support and stresses, personal resources and the coping process) may influence the entire spectrum of the postconcussional syndrome, including its onset, but more often its course and prognosis;

(2) organic factors, whilst important in the genesis of post-concussional symptoms, may also influence their persistence (Montgomery et al, 1991; Kant et al, 1997); and
(3) psychophysiological and cognitive processes mediate the effects of stress on the patient at all stages (Steptoe, 1991; Salkovskis and Clark 1993)

The problem of individual differences in susceptibility or persistence of post-concussional symptoms is a central concern, but can be best discussed when the various aetiological factors have been reviewed.

Post-Concussional Symptoms After Mild Head Injury

The terms 'minor' or 'mild' are used to define a head injury in which the period of unconsciousness is short (under 15 minutes – Medical Disability Society, 1988) or post traumatic amnesia (PTA) is under one hour, there is no skull fracture or known intracranial mass lesion, and the Glasgow Coma Scale (GCS) scores are 13 or more at admission. Severity of head injury is not defined in terms of outcome (Jennett & Bond, 1975).

Although the post-concussional syndrome is contentious, symptoms show remarkable uniformity across most series worldwide. Early post-concussional symptoms include headache and dizziness; and vomiting, nausea, drowsiness and blurred vision, which are short-lived. Symptoms evident after 1–3 months include headache (44%), dizziness (28%), fatigue (26%), anxiety (22%), insomnia (21%), noise sensitivity (17%), poor concentration (15%) and memory (10%), irritability (12%), depression (6%), light sensitivity, alcohol intolerance, or any one in this list (52%) – figures pooled from 4 series (Levin et al 1987, Lishman, 1988).

Controversy persists concerning the nature of persistent PCS (PPCS) after mild head injury, with considerable variation reported in their prevalence at various times after injury. At 3 months the point prevalence varies between 24% (Lidvall et al, 1974) and 84% (Rimel et al, 1981), at 6 months is under 30% and at 1 year under 20% (Table 1). Methodological differences between these studies are reviewed by Jacobson (1995).

The Cognitive Deficits

In a prospective controlled study of 57 patients in three American centres with minor head injury (loss of consciousness, LOC < 20 minutes, GCS 13–15), uncomplicated by a neuropsychiatric history, past head injury or history of substance/alcohol abuse, Levin et al (1987) reported deficits in digit span, information processing efficiency on the paced auditory serial addition

Table 1. Frequency of Persistent Complaints after Minor Head Injury

At 6 weeks	–	51%	(Rutherford et al, 1977)
	–	42%	(Montgomery et al, 1991)
At 3 months	–	84% (Poor memory 79%)	(Rimel et al, 1981)
	–	47%	(Lidvall et al, 1974)
	–	≥ 1 symptom 65%	(Keshavan et al, 1981)
	–	≥ 1 symptom 25%	(Alves et al, 1986)
At 6 months	–	1 or 2 symptoms 21%	(Fenton et al, 1993)
	–	≥ 3 symptoms 28%	(Fenton et al, 1993)
	–	≥ 1 symptom 24%	(Alves et al, 1986)
At 1 year	–	14.5%	(Rutherford et al, 1978)
	–	≥ 1 symptom 18.3%	(Alves et al, 1986)

task (Gronwall 1977), verbal and visual memory and visuo-motor speed compared with controls at base line. At 3 months there was virtually full recovery. Thus cognitive complaints were objectively verified early after minor head injury, as subacute neuropsychological deficits. The authors concluded that a single uncomplicated minor head injury produces no permanent disabling neuro-behavioural impairment in most patients who are free of pre-existing neuropsychiatric disorder and substance abuse.

Most studies confirm this subacute disturbance of attention, memory, and information-processing efficiency during the first few days after head injury, and demonstrate recovery in most patients by 1 – 3 months (Gronwall & Wrightson 1974, Lidvall et al, 1974, Dikmen et al 1986, Levin et al 1987). Post-concussional symptoms frequently occur, however, **even** in patients with recovered cognitive functioning (Lidvall et al 1974, Levin et al, 1987). When neuropsychological deficits are present **from the start,** their aetiology is usually considered to be **organic.**

While a dose-response effect of severity of head injury and neuropsychological problems has been demonstrated (Russell 1971, Levin et al, 1990), not all studies reveal significant cognitive deficits after mild head injury. Dikmen et al (1986) reported very mild and clinically insignificant neuropsychological deficits 1 month after head injury (coma < 1 hour or PTA > 1 hour, GCS > or = 12), but disruption of daily activities was extensive, mainly due to multiple injuries. Newcombe et al (1994) tested mild head injury subjects (PTA < 1 hour in 85%) and controls, within 48 hours and again after one month. They found virtually **no** differences between groups in memory tasks or rates of information-processing. The authors concluded that post-concussional symptoms are of psychological not physiological origin, and owe much to secondary effects, including iatrogenic factors.

To examine how post-concussional symptoms are related to the *severity* of head injury, Van Zomeren and Van den Burg (1985) and Hinkeldey and Corrigan (1990) studied the residual complaints of mainly severely head-injured subjects, who were not involved in litigation, several years after injury. Two broad classes of complaints were identified: (1) those that were related to severity of head injury, which included slowness, poor concentration, difficulty doing two things at once and forgetfulness; and (2) those unrelated to severity but strongly associated with anxiety, including crying, dizziness, irritability, headache, fatigue, hypersensitivity to noise, bustle or light, and depression.

Both sets of authors suggested that the second group of complaints, might be secondary to chronic effort by the patient to compensate for their neuropsychological deficits – the 'coping hypothesis'. The stage was set therefore for anxiety, arising independently of brain injury, to contribute to the severity of PCS.

If emotional and organic factors are separately related to PCS, then a combination rather than a single measure should better predict outcome. King (1996) examined the predictors of the severity of PCS three months after mild or moderate HI. Outcome was assessed using the Rivermead Postconcussion Symptom Questionnaire (RPQ), a list of 16 PCS each on a 5-point scale of increasing severity (King et al, 1995). By 10 days post-injury, 36% (N=50) had low scores on the RPQ, as did 72% (N=45) at 3 months. Measures of mood and psychological distress (Impact of Event Scale), rather than neuropsychological tests were most highly associated with the RPQ at 3 months. A combination of measures accounted for 74% of the variance of outcome (RPQ score).

The Belfast Studies – patterns and predictors of recovery

Most studies have tended to rely on normal uninjured controls rather than directly comparing patients with and without post-concussional symptoms after mild head injury. Lishman (1988) warned against the dangers of confounding causal, concomitant and chance associations between independent observations and stressed the need for systematic prospective studies.

An important prospective investigation of minor head injury from Belfast has illuminated the factors causing the emergence and persistence of post-concussional symptoms (Montgomery et al 1994, Fenton et al, 1993, McClelland et al, 1994). The authors studied consecutively admitted patients with mild head injury and a PTA under 12 hours (46% < 1 hour), excluding those with alcohol consumption on the day of head injury, a history of head injury or brain disease, substance abuse or other injuries. Patients received a range of clinical (including the Present State Examination (PSE) for psychiatric disorder), social and laboratory investigations (EEG power spectra analysis, brainstem auditory evoked potential (BAEP) recordings, and a 4-choice reaction time measure of attention), during recovery and at follow-up at 6 weeks and at 6 months. The drop-out rate was under 5%.

All patients had symptoms initially; 42% at 6 weeks and 54% at 6 months. Initially, 44% of patients had more than one symptom, and 19% had abnormal neurological signs.

The psychiatric "case" rate (PSE) at 6 weeks was 36%, mostly anxiety and depression, with 29% borderline cases (level 4 on the PSE), compared with a 4% case rate in matched general practice controls. Both physiological and psychosocial factors were found to contribute to the emergence of post-concussional symptoms. There was clear evidence of early cortical and brain stem changes. The cortical changes (in EEG theta power spectra) were mostly transient, while brainstem conduction time delays found initially were largely unaltered at 6 weeks follow-up. In another study, the brainstem auditory evoked potentials were delayed in 27% of young males with PTAs mostly < 1 hour (McClelland et al, 1994). When the two studies were combined, brainstem conduction times were found to correlate with the duration of PTA and severity of PSE caseness (McClelland et al, 1994).

In the main study, choice reaction time was delayed initially and at 6 weeks, and improved over six months (Montgomery et al, 1991). Chronic social adversity, older age and female gender were associated with psychiatric caseness at 6 weeks. Neither life events, social support or premorbid social adjustment distinguished acute and chronic outcome groups (Fenton et al, 1993). Three patterns of recovery emerged (Table 2):

(i) *acute* (52%), with loss of symptoms at 6 weeks and symptom-free at 6 months;
(ii) *chronic* (15%), with persistent symptoms during the 6 months follow-up;
(iii) *symptom exacerbation,* over the 6 months, seen in a third.

Brainstem findings were related to outcome. In the acute group, a half had delayed brainstem auditory evoked potentials initially, reducing to 6% at 6 weeks. By contrast all the chronic group had delayed brainstem auditory evoked potentials (BAEPs) at day 0 and again at 6 weeks. In patients with symptom-exacerbation, only 1 out of 10 showed delayed brainstem auditory evoked potentials initially, and none at 6 weeks: emotional symptoms were worse in this group. As only 9% of patients were seeking compensation, this cannot therefore be the major mechanism of persisting post-concussional symptoms.

Table 2. Patterns of recovery and brainstem dysfunction in mild head injury Montgomery et al, 1991)

	Abnormal brainstem auditory evoked potentials	
	Day 0	6 Weeks
1. ACUTE GROUP – 52 %		
Recovery within 6 weeks	54%	6%
2. CHRONIC GROUP – 16%		
Symptoms persist over 6 months	100%	100%
3. SYMPTOM EXACERBATION GROUP 32%	12.5%	0%
Symptoms increase from 6 weeks to 6 months		

Table 3 sets out the findings which up to 1988 support, but since then, modify Lishman's (1988) conclusion that physiological factors contribute mainly to the emergence of post-concussional symptoms and psycho-social factors more to their persistence. The prospective Belfast studies soften this aetiological distinction by showing that, in addition, social adversity contributes to the emergence of post-concussional symptoms and brainstem dysfunction to their persistence.

Aetiological Factors

The factors relevant to psychiatric disability after head injury were fully reviewed by Lishman (1988), and only recent research on these factors is discussed here.

Pre-traumatic Factors: The Problem of Pre-existing Conditions

Civilian head injury occurs disproportionately in young males, unskilled and semi-skilled workers, substance abusers and those with past head injuries. Factors affecting differential road traffic accident risk, an indirect risk indicator of head injury, include inter alia transient influences (stress, alcohol and fatigue), demographic factors (male > female, youth and driving experience), cognitive skills (detection of embedded figures, attention switching and visual acuity) and three personality traits (Type A behaviour, antisocial attitudes and low thoroughness in decision-making) (Elander et

Table 3. Post-concussional symptoms

Risk Factors for Formation	Risk Factors for Persistence
Organic	*Organic*
Cerebral Blood Flow changes (1) SPECT Studies (3), (4)	Delay of 6 weeks in BAEPs (2) Cumulative PASAT impairment from repeated minor head injuries (5) and subconcussive injury in boxers (6), (7)
Reaction time & information processing (8), (9) EEG spectra (2) Brainstem conduction time – BAEPs (2), (10) BAEP delay correlation with PTA (12)	PTA, intellectual impairment (11) Possible anterior hypometabolism on PET (13) ? Apo E4 status (14)
MRI studies (15), (16) NMDA receptor changes (17), (18)	
Clinical	*Clinical*
Early headache, diplopia, CNS signs (19), (20)	'Caseness' at 6/52 predicts 6.5x risk of post-concussional chronicity at 6/12 (21) Emotional shock (19) Neuroticism (11) Past psychiatric illness (22) Type of accident
Psychosocial	*Psychosocial*
Age, Female sex, chronic social adversity (all associated with caseness at 6 weeks) (21)	Age, female sex, social class, – chronic social adversity at 6 months (21) Blame to employers (20)

Key

1. Taylor & Bell, 1966
2. Montgomery et al, 1991
3. Gray et al, 1992
4. Nedd et al, 1993
5. Gronwall & Wrightson, 1975
6. Barth et al, 1989
7. Casson et al, 1984
8. Gronwall, 1977
9. MacFlynn et al, 1984
10. Montgomery et al, 1984
11. Keshavan et al, 1981
12. McClelland et al, 1994
13. Ruff et al, 1994
14. Teasdale et al, 1997
15. Levin et al, 1987
16. Mitchener et al, 1997
17. Faden 1996
18. Koura et al, 1998
19. Lidvall et al, 1974
20. Rutherford et al, 1977
21. Fenton et al, 1993
22. Kay et al, 1971

al 1993). Together with a vulnerable personality, past psychiatric history and genetic liability (Dencker 1960), these factors influence the risk and course of post-concussional disability.

Alcohol abuse and the cumulative effects of multiple head injuries on information processing (Gronwall & Wrightson 1975) were likely to have elevated post-concussional symptom rates in Rimel et al's (1981) study, where these risk factors were reported in a third of subjects. Although at admission a third to a half of head-injured persons are intoxicated, the incidence of alcohol abuse often rises after head injury, the dual disability magnifying disinhibition, aggression, impaired judgement and cognitive deficits (Karol & Hallo-Poe, 1987).

Alcohol toxicity delays brain repair (West et al 1982, Lishman et al 1987). Recognition that alcoholism is the 'silent saboteur' in rehabilitation, has led to the development of specialised treatment programs in the USA (Langley et al 1990).

In the Belfast studies, head injured patients had twice as many adverse life events as controls in the year before injury, but as many chronic social difficulties and equivalent premorbid adjustment. By contrast, head injured patients with chronic post-concussional symptoms had more chronic social adversity but equivalent premorbid personality, social adjustment and life events compared with those whose post-concussional symptoms had remitted (Rimel et al, 1981).

Peri- and Post-Traumatic Factors

Pathology. The most consistent pathology after mild to moderate head injury is diffuse axonal injury. Damaged axons mount a recovery with sustained reactive sprouting and growth cone formation (Povlishock & Coburn 1989), but this is unlikely to be a complete or targeted regeneration.

Imaging Studies. Magnetic resonance imaging (MRI) has detected altered signal intensities ("lesions") within one week of head injury in 92% of patients scanned, almost twice as many as with computed tomography (CT). Most of the lesions detected by MRI but not by CT are found in the frontal and temporal regions (Eisenberg & Levin, 1989). In a small study of mild head injury, tentative structural-functional associations were reported (Eisenberg & Levin, 1989), but these are likely to be more complex after more severe head injury (Wilson et al, 1988, 1992).

Single photon emission computed tomography (SPECT) scans reveal more frequent and more extensive changes in regional cerebral blood flow than lesions on CT scans, and more areas of diametrically opposite change than

CT (Gray et al, 1992, Nedd et al, 1993). SPECT changes may account for a clinical deficit when MRI and CT brain scans fail to do so (Newton et al 1992, Jacobs et al, 1994, Varney et al, 1995, Kant et al, 1997).

Recent studies suggest that SPECT abnormalities may be present in patients with persistent post-concussional symptoms (PPCS) when structural imaging is normal. Jacobs et al (1996) carried out SPECT and CT on 136 subjects with mild head injury within 4 weeks of injury and noted PCS. In cases with acutely abnormal SPECT, it was repeated at 3,6 and 12 months follow-up. SPECT was abnormal acutely in 73 (54%), of whom 38 also reported PCS. By 12 months 7% had abnormal SPECT and PCS, 2% abnormal SPECT and none PCS only. In those with initially normal SPECT, no PCS were found at 12 months. Patients with no abnormality clinically and on SPECT at any follow-up were, however, rarely followed-up again. This omission ruled out the possibility of symptom exacerbation or late onset PCS. The authors concluded that SPECT powerfully predicts PPCS.

In a study of 43 patients on average 15 months after mild head injury, SPECT was abnormal in 53%, while MRI and CT were abnormal in 9% and 4.6% respectively (Kant et al, 1997). SPECT appeared to be more sensitive in detecting functional abnormalities after mild head injury especially in those with PPCS than either CT or MRI. SPECT abnormalities were found in the frontal (54%) and temporal (24%) lobes, revealing areas of hypoperfusion which were discrete rather than diffuse as seen in depression (Goodwin et al, 1993). Interestingly, no relationship was found between SPECT and cognitive performance or Beck Depression Inventory Scores.

One small positron emission tomography study reported patchy fronto-temporal hypometabolism in 9 patients with persisting neuropsychological deficits in the absence of CT and MRI abnormalities after mild head injury, even in 4 patients without reported loss of consciousness (Ruff et al 1994). The authors' deduction of evidence for "neuropathology" is, however, open to interpretation. The base rate of regional hypometabolism in recovered head injured patients was not assessed. Furthermore, primary depression with or without depression-related cognitive impairment could also account for the imaging changes (Bench et al, 1992, 1993). Very careful replication of putative functional imaging abnormalities is required before claiming an "organic" basis for persistent post-concussional symptoms after mild head injury or recommending such scanning for medico-legal assessment.

Genetic, Cellular and Neurochemical Factors

The outcome of severe HI has been linked to Apoliprotein E4 allele status, a genetic risk factor for late-onset Alzheimer's disease (Stritmatter & Roses,

1995). Teasdale et al (1997) found the 6 month outcome of severe HI was twice as bad in those with a high frequency of Apo E4 alleles after adjustment for other prognostic factors. Whether this extends to recovery after MHI is not known.

Recent research on the pathology of head injury has focused on the changes occurring at biochemical and cellular levels in the first few hours after head injury (Hayes et al, 1989). Trauma is hypothesized to produce widespread depolarization of neurons and excessive release of excitatory neuro-transmitters, including glutamate (Faden 1996, Koura et al, 1998) and acetylcholine (Murdoch et al, 1998), which cause excitotoxic effects on postsynaptic neurons (Hayes et al, 1989). Excitoxicity contributes to structural pathology depending on the severity of head injury. Mild head injury may also produce enduring excitotoxic changes in neural function and memory deficits not accompanied by light or electron microscopic tissue damage (Lyeth et al, 1990).

The demonstration of early organic symptoms and pathology suggests their aetiological involvement in the emergence of post-concussional symptoms. It is the partial resolution of organic changes after mild head injury yet persistence of post-concussional symptoms which limits the utility of the organic model.

Psychophysiological Stress Response

The most researched physiological process linking stress and illness is psychophysiological hyperreactivity, the tendency to respond to behavioural stress with abnormally large autonomic, endocrine or neuro-physiological reactions, or to display delayed habituation or recovery after stress ceases (Steptoe 1991). Hyperreactivity may arise on a constitutional or learned basis; or it may be restricted to specific organ systems. It may perpetuate "dizziness" after vestibular damage recovers (Flor & Turk, 1989, Clark et al, 1994, Eagger et al, 1992), and cause pain-site-specific muscular arousal, such as greater EMG responses from neck muscles during mental stress in patients with tension headache (Flor et al, 1990). The EMG stress response is symptom-specific (Flor & Turk 1989). Thus hyperreactivity may maintain the stability of certain post-concussional symptoms, particularly under chronic stress. Subjects with recovered headache may experience tension headache under stress, which will reinforce illness beliefs and attribution of symptom to injury, thereby impairing coping skills.

Emotional Impact and Cognitive Appraisal

Anxiety and depression are the most frequent psychiatric disorders after mild head injury, influenced by age, social adversity, past psychiatric history and brain-stem dysfunction (McClelland et al, 1994). Irritability, aggression and enhanced sensitivity to distress may also occur (Jacobson et al, 1994). Pre-injury psychopathology is frequent and often overlooked (Whetsell et al, 1989).

In the Oxford study, one-fifth of motor vehicle (MVA) accident victims, with whiplash or multiple injuries, reported severe initial distress characterised by mood disturbance and horrific memories (Mayou et al, 1993). This acute stress reaction was associated with neuroticism and not being unconscious. A quarter developed three overlapping types of chronic disorder: mood disorder, post-traumatic stress disorder (PTSD), and travel anxiety. PTSD and travel anxiety were associated with initial horrific memories, but unlike mood disorders not with past neurotic disposition. This indicates probable different aetiologies for the mood and post-traumatic disorders. In a one year prospective follow-up of MVA survivors, 65% of drivers and 44% of passengers reported lingering effects on their driving behaviour, including phobic avoidance in a fifth (Mayou and Bryant, 1994). This co-morbidity is an obvious contributor to persistent post-concussional symptoms.

Can PTSD Result from Minor Head Injury?

Rates of PTSD found in unselected samples of MVA victims are on average 26% and in American epidemiological surveys about 9% (Blanchard & Hickling, 1997). In Oxford, UK, the rate was 8% at 3 months and 11% within a year (Mayou et al, 1993). According to DSM-IV (1994), PTSD cannot arise after concussive head injury as the patient has not experienced the traumatic event because of loss of consciousness and post-traumatic amnesia – a view supported by several studies (Mayou et al, 1993; Sbordone 1992; Sbordone & Liter, 1996). The issue, however, is a source of controversy and debate (McMillan, 1996, 1997). Although Mayou et al (1993) found that PTSD did not occur in MVA survivors with unconsciousness, case reports have been published more recently of minor and severe HI patients with PTSD (McMillan 1996, King 1997). McMillan (1996) reported 10 cases of PTSD after a range of severity in HI, in whom "windows" of experience during PTA allowed emotional trauma to occur. These "windows" were recall of events near to the impact before brief retrograde amnesia, eg a lorry approaching and thinking that death was imminent; recall of distressing events after the end of a short PTA or during 'islands' of memory within PTA; and later "windows" – waking disabled in hospital without recall of the accident; distressing recollections based on self-generated accounts and pictures or the reports of others – "vicarious traumatization".

In recent group studies, acute stress disorder has been reported in 14–27% and PTSD in 17–33% of patients with MHI (Ohry et al, 1996, Bryant & Harvey, 1995, 1998).

Concussion and Acute Dissociation

Received wisdom states that traumatic brain injury arises only after concussive injury ie where there has been loss of consciousness even if only brief (Pearce, 1995). If loss of consciousness (LOC) and PTA are brief and there is no reliable witness, then it may be uncertain whether amnesia ever occurred at the time of the accident or whether "unawareness" reflected head injury or emotional shock. The validity of patients' reports of whether or not they lost consciousness at the time of the accident is unknown, especially if LOC is claimed yet not confirmed in Casualty records. These issues confound interpretation of occasional studies which report CT or SPECT abnormalities in patients who do not report LOC (Jenkins et al, 1986, Varney et al, 1995). The symptoms of acute stress disorder and PTSD, especially if accompanied by tension headache, closely resemble PCS. Acute stress disorder includes the dissociative symptoms of reduced awareness, depersonalisation, derealisation and amnesia, which are commonly reported during PTA in subjects with MHI (Grigsby & Kaye, 1993).

A reduction in awareness of one's surroundings or "being in a daze" may therefore reflect either brief loss of consciousness or a dissociative symptom during acute stress (APA, 1994) in the absence of concussion. If unconsciousness or registration failure are very brief, memories of part of the trauma may still be formed. Horrific memories may then evoke acute stress reactions or post-traumatic stress disorder, whose symptoms overlap with post-concussional symptoms. This suggests a dual aetiology for selected "post-concussional symptoms".

Cognitive complaints are frequently found in 'pure' anxiety disorders. Experimental cognitive psychology has established that patients suffering from anxiety disorders, including post-traumatic stress disorder, exhibit a cognitive bias that selectively favours the processing of threat material (Thrasher et al, 1994) . Attention is preferentially allocated to threat-related cues, decreased to neutral cues, and may be generally impaired in some anxious subjects (Eysenck 1993). Thus anxiety can generate cognitive complaints after

Table 4. Post concussional-type symptoms without head injury

Uncomplicated whiplash (Radanov et al 1994a, 1994b; Bicik et al 1998)
Chronic Pain (Shapiro et al 1993, Crombez et al 1997, Iverson and McCracken, 1997)
Minor medical problems (Lees-Haley & Brown, 1993)
PTSD (San Francisco Bay earthquake 1989 - Cardena & Spiegel, 1993)
Depression (APA, 1994)
Anxiety states (Fox et al, 1995; Wells & Matthews, 1996)
Expectation (Mittenberg et al, 1992)

head injury with minimal or no unconsciousness, and could potentially maintain these symptoms beyond neuropsychological recovery from mild concussive head injury.

What Conditions other than Head Injury Cause Post-concussional-type Symptoms?

Many MVA survivors have multiple injuries, which often give rise to chronic pain. Chronic pain patients may report cognitive and affective symptoms similar to PCS in the absence of head injury. Cognitive complaints related to forgetfulness (29%), difficulty maintaining attention (18%) and impaired concentration and thinking (16.5%) were reported in pain patients, of whom 81% met Category C of the DSM-IV research criteria for post concussional disorder (Iverson & McCracken, 1997). PCS-type symptoms may therefore occur in the absence of a concussive head injury; examples are given in Table 4.

Expectation as an Aetiological Factor

The high frequency and universality of post-concussional symptoms after head injury has implied that a common denominator, cerebral insult, is the principal cause. These very post-concussional symptoms may, however, occur as often in **uninjured** subjects (McLean et al, 1983, 1984, Dikmen et al, 1986, Gouvier et al, 1988) , including twins discordant for head injury (Dencker 1960). Imaginary concussion can reveal expectations in subjects with no personal knowledge or experience of head injury of a coherent cluster of symptoms identical to the post-concussional symptoms reported by head injury patients (Mittenburg et al, 1992). In this study, head injury patients underestimated the premorbid prevalence of these symptoms compared to the base rate in controls, suggesting a causal role for symptom expectation in the post-concussional syndrome. Expectations about post-concussional symptoms may result in re-attribution of benign symptoms to the head injury, selective attention to them and anxiety, which together increase their subjective intensity, reinforcing expectation and avoidant behaviours (Warwick & Salkovskis, 1989).

These attributional and cognitive factors may explain why post-concussional symptoms can persist in certain patients after mild head injury even in the absence of (Newcombe et al, 1994), or beyond the recovery of neuropsychological deficits (Levin et al, 1987). The risk of persistence may be influenced by symptom attributional style (Robbins & Kirkmayer 1991).

Iatrogenic effects

Expectations are especially important when the patient lacks an obvious explanation for his symptoms (Barsky & Klerman, 1983). This may explain why education and reassurance benefit post-concussional symptoms (Kelly 1975, Minderhoud et al, 1980). Kelly (1975) suggested that post-concussional symptoms originate in minor brain damage, but are then perpetuated mainly by the failure of doctors to validate them and to provide information and reassurance about their favourable prognosis.

Secondary emotional distress after mild head injury aggravates post-concussional symptoms and time off work (Binder 1986, Wrightson & Gronwall 1981). Early clinical intervention reduces disability as follows: It provides information and support on managing post-concussional symptoms; coping with slower information processing; likely prognosis and recovery times; advice how to reduce the effects of stress on symptoms and vice versa, and on graded resumption of activities after discharge (Wade et al 1997, 1998). A randomised controlled trial suggested that early specialist intervention significantly reduced social morbidity and post-concussional symptoms 6 months after HI. The benefit appeared in the mild and moderate but not severe HI groups (Wade et al, 1998). Nonetheless significant numbers of patients revealed persistent difficulties. In selected cases cognitive restructuring, counselling, and antidepressant medication are beneficial (Levin et al 1987, Mittenburg & Burton, 1994).

Accident Circumstances and Blame

Disability tends to differ between types of accident (Lishman, 1988), whose setting may lead to persisting fear, anger and resentment. Blame is an important factor in predicting post-concussional symptoms and time off work after accidents. More post-concussional symptoms were reported at 6 weeks where an employer or impersonal organisation were to blame, rather than oneself, another person or an "Act of God" (Rutherford 1989).

Attribution research distinguishes between two dimensions of blame – causal responsibility and culpability (Brewin, 1984). A person feels causally responsible if he or she has acted in such a way as to produce the outcome. Culpability, on the other hand, implies a moral evaluation of "deservingness of blame" for the outcome. In a study of industrial accidents, measures of culpability at follow-up were strongly related to time off work and recovery, indicating that the patient who felt that his accident was due to his own carelessness or negligence returned to work more quickly, as noted in patients with mild head injury (Rutherford 1989). Brewin (1984) argues that future studies should attempt to assess independently the influences of culpability and causal responsibility on return to work and compensation-seeking.

Clinical observation suggests that the perceived adequacy of justice and retribution also influences resentment and motivation for compensation. Resentment may fuel the "scapegoat motive," whereby the patient pins the blame for pre-morbid and subsequent life difficulties on the head injury. The power of resentment to perpetuate symptoms has been little researched.

Social Sequelae

Rates of unemployment, depression and social isolation are raised in patients with mild head injury and in family members (Florian et al, 1989). While marital dissatisfaction and parenting difficulties are frequently reported, their premorbid frequencies are unknown. Disability may be prolonged by the family response which, initially adaptive, may become entrenched and reinforce the patient's sick role (Kreutzer et al, 1992). This operant factor includes overprotection, resulting in child-like dependence and altered family roles (Tarsh & Royston, 1985), including caregiver depression (Kreutzer et al, 1994).

The Effects of Litigation

In a follow-up study by Rutherford and Fee (1988), 39% of litigants had symptoms at settlement on average 22 months after head injury, and 34% still had symptoms one year later. Litigation resulted in more than doubling of the long-term symptom rate. Do patients with worse post-concussional symptoms engage in litigation, or is the different outcome due to the medico-legal process? The stresses of litigation include "medical limbo" – that is having a condition that eludes diagnostic and prognostic consistency.

The patient's exposure to doubt, sceptical appraisal and conflicting medical advice biases his/her beliefs about the controllability of the "illness" and affects coping responses and treatment adherence (Leventhal et al, 1992, Pincus et al 1994). The patient may sense that he must nurture his suffering, which serves as his main weapon in blaming those who are to compensate him.

Compensation Neurosis

The term compensation neurosis refers to symptoms, psychological reactions or disability which occur after an injury and which are thought to be produced or maintained by a compensation claim (Weighill 1983, Mendelson 1995). In practice, disability persists long after expected recovery, or subjective symptoms exceed objective findings, or both occur.

Miller (1961) coined the term "accident neurosis" for post-concussional symptoms and attributed them entirely to compensation-seeking. A large body of authoritative research has challenged such an extreme position, derived from a highly selective medico-legal perspective. Thus, while Miller contended that post-concussional symptoms are rarely observed after severe head injury, McKinley et al (1983) found post-concussional symptoms in over half their patients six months after injury. Miller stated that the syndrome was only seen in compensation situations, yet many studies around the world have demonstrated post-concussional symptoms with similar rank order in head injury patients in whom compensation-seeking was infrequent.

Mayou (1995) has suggested that if compensation is a major determinant of outcome, then the following predictions can be made: the clinical picture is consistent with "compensation neurosis", claims suggest exaggeration, the outcome is worse than for subjects not seeking compensation, there is evidence of disputes about the extent of disability and loss, and symptoms improve on settlement. In the Oxford prospective study of legal and compensation proceedings after motor vehicle accidents, in which concussion was uncommon, compensation-seekers wanted compensation for losses and acknowledgement of their distress. Some were outraged by the unwillingness of others to admit responsibility. Outcome appeared similar in those who sought compensation and those who did not (Mayou 1995).

Resolution of post-concussional symptoms after settlement is uncommon (Thompson 1965, Kelly & Smith 1981, Mendelson 1981, Tarsh & Royston 1985, Rutherford & Fee 1988). Moreover, when treatment was applied early and efficiently, compensation and non-compensation patients did not differ in recovery time (Kelly, 1975). In their reviews of the subject, Weighill (1983) and Mendelson (1985) considered that the term compensation neurosis has no validity, and should be replaced by accepted DSM-III-R classifications such as: malingering, factitious disorder, or somatization/conversion disorder.

Malingering is defined as the intentional production of false or grossly exaggerated physical or psychological symptoms motivated by external incentives, such as financial gain (APA, 1994). **Factitious disorders** involve the intentional production of symptoms or signs to assume the sick role in the absence of external incentives (APA, 1994). The distinction between **somatization/conversion disorders** and malingering can be difficult (Resnick, 1989, Cunnien 1989, APA 1994). A diagnosis of conversion disorder does not imply an absence of organic disease (Merskey & Trimble, 1979).

Exaggeration of somatic complaints may be understood in terms of: (a) psychological factors (psychosocial stress, operant factors, anxiety, depression) affecting post-concussional symptoms, (b) motivational factors (factitious disorders and malingering), and (c) somatoform disorders (somatization, conversion and pain disorders, and hypochondriasis) – Table 5. DSM-IV (APA, 1994) provides a useful decision tree for somatoform disorders, which may present with subtle or shifting combinations.

Recent research on the detection of malingering is reviewed by Cunnien (1989), Rogers (1997), and Mendelson (1995).

Standardised approaches to the assessment of dissimulation have been developed (Rogers et al, 1992), which may hold considerable promise in the medico-legal evaluation of post-concussional symptoms, alongside

Table 5. Typology of exaggeration of disability

1. Unintentional	–	stress > coping resources
	–	psychiatric disorder – anxiety, depression, somatoform disorders (pain disorder, conversion reaction, hypochondriasis).
	–	operant conditioning – pain or postconcussional behaviours maintained by reinforcement, even in the absence of stimulation.
2. Intentional	–	internal incentive, to assume sick role – factitious disorder
	–	external incentive, financial gain – malingering
3. Combinations of 1 + 2		

specialised interview techniques (feedback, clarification of ambiguity, confrontation), neuropsychological tests (Leng & Parkin 1995), corroborative records, collateral and repeat interviews, and ultimately covert surveillance.

While compensation-seeking cannot be considered a necessary or sufficient cause of post-concussional symptoms in most head injury patients, amongst litigants, malingering is a real issue, particularly in those in whom the presence or extent of injury is in doubt, but who nevertheless claim significant disability. Assessing the various roles of genuine psychiatric disorder, secondary gain, the sick role, and malingering in the exaggeration of symptoms is especially difficult.

A Multifactorial Model of Chronic Post-Concussional Symptoms

What general model is appropriate to the complicated evidence about chronic post-concussional symptoms? The heterogeneity of outcome after mild head injury seems to require an integration of biological with social, cognitive, affective and behavioural factors. Jacobson (1995) has proposed a multifactorial model which is similar to current models of persistent pain (Turk & Rudy, 1992)

Table 6. A Model of persistent post-concussional symptoms

1. Organic factors.
2. Psychogenic perspective.
3. Motivational view – intentional exaggeration
   internal – factitious – the sick role
   Incentive → internal / external
   external – malingering – compensation
4. Operant conditioning – unintentional exaggeration
   – PC behaviours MAINTAINED by reinforcement
5. Psychophysiological stress response – e.g. hyperreactivity of vulnerable organs.
6. Cognitive – Behavioural perspective
   – information processing model which integrates 1 – 5 into beliefs, appraisals, expectations, self-perceptions and coping responses **over time.**

The variability of patient responses to a mild head injury is more understandable and more predictable, if the multiple influences on post-concussional symptoms and their changing combinations over time are jointly considered. Organic forces contend with a rubric of psychological factors, including attention, anxiety (stress responses and personality traits), prior learning history, the meaning of the situation, blame, and environmental responses.

Although organic factors precipitate the initial report of post-concussional symptoms in most cases, psychological, social and behavioural factors may maintain and exacerbate levels of complaint and disability over time. This aetiological divide has, however, been narrowed by the prospective bio-social studies from Belfast. Therefore, post-concussional symptoms that persist over time should not be viewed as either solely physiological or purely psychological. Rather, persistent symptoms are maintained by an interdependent set of organic, psychosocial and behavioural factors. A model that focuses on only one of these central sets of factors will inevitably be incomplete.

The application of the cognitive-behavioural perspective, which stands in contrast to the purely organic or psychological view, focuses on the patient, rather than on symptoms or pathophysiology. Emphasis is laid on the patient's beliefs, appraisals and coping responses as direct influences on the severity and disability of post-concussional symptoms (Turk & Rudy, 1992). Thus, symptom exacerbation in certain head injured patients (Montgomery et al, 1991) can only be understood if psychological, operant, and motivational factors are considered and integrated into the patients' coping responses. Headache that is interpreted as signifying ongoing tissue damage is likely to produce more suffering than when viewed as the result of a minor injury, although the amount of nociceptive input in the two cases may be equivalent. Both cognitive-behavioural and psychophysiological factors mediate the coping response which impacts on post-concussional symptom severity and disability. Table 7 summarises the cognitive factors likely to be involved in persistent PCS. Symptom-specific psychophysiological stress responses, which have been described for pain, poor concentration and dizziness (Flor & Turk, 1989, Brandt 1990), may maintain the stability of certain post-concussional symptoms.

The proposed model, discussed more fully elsewhere (Jacobson 1995), attempts to account for patterns of recovery (Table 2), the known aetiological factors of persistent symptoms (Table 3), the views of neuropsychologists on causation (Mittenburg & Burton, 1994), and also to serve as a guide to comprehensive treatment.

Table 7. Cognitive Factors in the PCS

Expectation	–	imaginary concussion → "PCS"
Attribution	–	benign symptoms re-attributed to HI → vicious circle of anxiety/avoidance
Symptom attributional style		
Emotional impact	–	acute stress reaction
	–	PTSD, adjustment reaction
	–	depression, sensitivity to stress
Attention altered to threat-related cues		
Blame – causal responsibility		
– culpability varies with time off work		
Perceived adequacy of justice and retribution		
Resentment		
"Illness beliefs" – controllability, coping responses, treatment adherence, catastrophizing cognitions		
Lack of education, reassurance → 2° emotional distress		
Stress of litigation – medical limbo, scepticism, and conflicting advice bias illness beliefs		
– doubles the long-term symptom rate (Rutherford & Fee, 1988)		

Conclusion

Concepts about the post-concussional syndrome and disability will influence its assessment, views on causation and methods of treatment. Recent research in neuropsychiatry, and cognitive and health psychology distinguishes processes with characteristic properties which combine to explain persistent post-concussional symptoms. It is constructed around the scaffold of Lishman's (1988) model of organic genesis and psychosocial/neurotic persistence of post-concussional symptoms. Most neuropsychologists believe that cerebral dysfunction is the chief mechanism underlying post-concussional symptoms after mild head injury, followed by anxiety and depression, and that selective attention to post-concussional symptoms and secondary gain are the more important maintenance factors. The principal influences on persistent post-concussional symptoms have been reviewed and fit with neuropsychologists' views on causation and the wide variety of currently effective treatments, including education (Wade et al, 1998), antidepressant medication, and cognitive restructuring. Future studies should evaluate this tentative model for its ability to clarify causation, match patients to treatment and predict outcome.

References

Alves, W. M., Colohan, A. R., O'Leary, T. J., Rimel, R. W. & Jane, J. A. (1986). Understanding post-traumatic symptoms after minor head injury. *Journal Head Trauma Rehabilitation, 1*: 1–12.

American Psychiatric Association (1994). *Diagnostic and Statistical Manual of Mental Disorders.* DSM-IV, 4th Edn. Revised. Washington DC:.

Barsky, A. J. & Klerman, G. L. (1983) Overview: hypochondriasis, bodily complaints, and somatic styles. *American Journal of Psychiatry, 140*: 273–283.

Barth, J. T., Alves, W. M., Ryan, T. V., Macciocchi, S. N., Rimel, R. W., Jane, J. A. & Nelson, W. E. (1989). In *Mild Head Injury. Mild head injury in sports: neuropsychological sequelae and recovery of function.* (Ed. Levin, H.S., Eisenberg, H. M., Benton, A. L.) pp. 257–275. Oxford University Press, Oxford.

Bench, C. J., Friston, K. J., Brown, R. G., Scott, L. C., Frackowiak, R. S. J. & Dolan, R. J. (1992). The anatomy of melancholia – focal abnormalities of cerebral blood flow in major depression. *Psychological Medicine, 22*: 607–615.

Bench, C. J., Friston, K. J., Brown, R. G., Frackowiak, R. S. J. & Dolan, R. J. (1993). Regional cerebral blood flow in depression measured by positron emission tomography: the relationship with clinical dimensions. *Psychological Medicine, 23*: 579–590.

Bicik, I., Radanov, B. P., Shafer, N., Dvorak, J., Blum, B., Weber, B., Burger, C., Von Shulthess, G. K. & Buck, A. (1998). PET with 18 fluorodeoxyglucose and hexamethylpropylene amine oxime SPECT in late whiplash syndrome. *Neurology, 51* (2): 336–40.

Binder, L. M. (1986). Persisting symptoms after mild head injury: A review of the postconcussive syndrome. *Journal Clinical Experimental Neuropsychology, 8*: 323–346.

Blanchard, E. G. & Hicking, E. J. (1997). After the Crash. Assessment and Treatment of Motor Vehicle Accident Survivors. *American Psychological Association,*Washington DC

Brandt, T. (1990). Vertigo – a systematic approach. In *Recent advances in Neurology.* (Kennard, C. Ed.) Vol. 6, Ch. 3, pp. 59–84. Churchill Livingstone, London.

Brewin, C. R. (1984). Attributions for industrial accidents: Their relationship to rehabilitation outcome. *Journal Social and Clinical Psychology, 2*: 156–164.

Bryant, R. A. & Harvey, A. G. (1995). Acute stress response: a comparison of head injured and non-head injured patients. *Psychological Medicine, 25*: 869–874

Bryant, R. A. & Harvey, A. G. (1998). Relationship between acute stress disorder and post traumatic stress disorder following mild traumatic brain injury. *American Journal of Psychiatry, 155*; 625–629.

Cardena, E. & Spiegel, D. (1993). Dissociative reactions to the San Francisco Bay Area earthquake of 1989. *Americal Journal of Psychiatry, 150*: 474–478

Casson, I. R., Siegel, O., Campbell, E. A., Tarlan, M., Di Domenico (1984). A. Brain damage in modern boxers. *Journal of American Medical Association, 251*: 2663–2667.

Clark, M. R., Sullivan, M. D., Fischl, M., Katon, W. J., Russo, J. E., Dobie, R. A. & Voorhees, R. (1994). Symptoms as a clue to otologic and psychiatric diagnosis in patients with dizziness. *Journal Psychosomatic Research, 38*: 461–470.

Cunnien, A. J. (1989). Psychiatric and medical syndromes associated with deception. pp 13–64 (Rogers R. editor) *Clinical Aspects of Malingering and Deception.* Guildford Press: New York.

Crombez, G, Eccleston, C., Baeyens, F. & Eelen, P. (1997). Habitation and the interference of pain with task performance. *Pain, 70* (2–3): 149–154

Dencker, S. J. (1960). Closed head injury in twins. *Archives of General Psychiatry, 2*: 569–575.

Dikmen, S., McLean A, & Temkin, N. (1986). Neuropsychological and psychosocial consequences of minor head injury. *Journal Neurology, Neurosurgery and Psychiatry*, *49*: 1227–1232.

Eagger, S, Luxon, L. M., Davies, R. A., Coelho, A. & Ron M. A. (1992). Psychiatric morbidity in patients with peripheral vestibular disorders: a clinical and neuro-otological study. *Journal of Neurology, Neurosurgery and Psychiatry*; *55* (5): 383–7

Eisenberg, H. M. & Levin, H. S. (1989). Computer tomography and magnetic resonance imaging in mild to moderate head injury. Ch. 8, pp. 133–141 (Eisenberg HM, Levin HS, Benton AL, editors) *Mild Head Injury*, Oxford University Press, Oxford.

Elander, J., West, R. French, D. (1993). Behavioural correlates of individual differences in road traffic crash risk: an examination of methods and findings. *Psychological Bulletin*, *113*: 274–294.

Eysenck, M. W. (1993). *Anxiety – the Cognitive Perspective*. Lawrence Erlbaum, Hove, England

Faden, A. I. (1996). Pharmacological treatment of central nervous system trauma. *Pharmacology and Toxicology*, *78*, 12–17.

Fenton, G., McClelland, R., Montgomery, A., MacFlynn, G. & Rutherford, W. (1993). The postconcussional syndrome : social antecedents and psychological sequelae. *British Journal of Psychiatry*, *162*: 493–497.

Fernandez, E. & Turk, D. C. (1989). The utility of cognitive coping strategies for altering pain perception: A meta-analysis. *Pain*, *38*: 123–135.

Flor, H., & Turk, D. C. (1989). The psychophysiology of chronic pain: Do chronic pain patients exhibit symptom-specific psychophysiological responses? *Psychological Bulletin*, *105*: 215–259.

Flor, H., Birbaumer, N. & Turk, D. C. (1990). The psychobiology of chronic pain. *Advances in Behavioural Research and Therapy*, *12*: 47–84.

Florian, V., Katz, S. & Lahav, V. (1989). Impact of traumatic brain damage on family dynamics and functioning: a review. *Brain Injury*, *3*: 219–233.

Fox, D. D., Lees-Haley, P. R., Earnest, K. & Dolzeal-Wood, S. (1995). Post-concussive symptoms: base rates and etiology in psychiatric patients. *Clinical Neuropsychologist*, *9*(1): 89–92.

Goodwin, G. M., Austin, M.-P., Dougall, M., Ross, C., Murray, C., O'Carroll, R. E., Moffoot, A, Prentice, N. & Ebmeier, K P. (1993). State changes in brain activity shown by the uptake of 99MTc-exametazime with single photon emission tomography in major depression before and after treatment. *Journal of Affective Disorders*, *29*; 243–253

Gouvier, W. D., Uddo-Crane, M. & Brown, L. M. (1988). Base rates of post-concussional symptoms. *Archives of Clinical Neuropsychology*, *3*: 273–278.

Gray, B. G., Ichise, M. & Chung, D. G. et al. (1992). Tc-99m-HMPAO SPECT in the evaluation of patients with a remote history of traumatic brain injury: a comparison with X-ray computed tomography. *Journal Nuclear Medicine*, 33: 52–58.

Grigsby, J. Kaye, K. (1993). Incidence and correlates of depersonalisation following head trauma. *Brain Injury*, *7*: 507–513

Gronwall, D. (1977). Paced auditory serial addition task: a measure of recovery from concussion. *Perceptual & Motor Skills*, *44*: 367–373.

Gronwall, D. & Wrightson, P. (1974). Delayed recovery of intellectual function after minor head injury. *Lancet*, *ii*: 605–9.

Gronwall, D. & Wrightson, P. (1975). Cumulative effects of concussion. *Lancet*, *2*: 995–997.

Hayes, R. L., Lyeth, B. G., Jenkins, L. W., Zimmerman, R., McIntosh, T. K., Clifton, G. L. & Young, H. F. (1989). Neurochemical mechanisms of moderate head injury: implications for treatment. pp 54–79. (Levin, H. S., Eisenberg, H. M., Benton, A. L. Eds.). *Mild Head Injury*, Oxford University Press, Oxford.

Hinkeldey, N. S. & Corrigan, J. D. (1990). The structure of head-injured patients' neurobehavioural complaints: a preliminary study. *Brain Injury*, *4*: 115–133.

ICD-10. The ICD-10 Classification of Mental and Behavioural Disorders. *Clinical descriptions and diagnostic guidelines*. (1992) World Health Organisation, Geneva.

Iverson, G. L. McCracken, L. M. (1997). 'Postconcussive' symptoms in persons with chronic pain. *Brain Injury*, *11*; 783–790.

Jacobs, A., Put, E. & Ingels, M. et al. (1994). Prospective evaluation of technetium-99m-HMPAO SPECT in mild and moderate traumatic brain injury. *Journal of Nuclear Medicine*, *35*: 942–947.

Jacobs, A, Put, E., Ingels, M., Put, T. & Bossuyt, A. (1996). One year follow-up of Technetium-99m HMPAO SPECT in Mild Head Injury. *Journal of Nuclear Medicine*, *37*: 1605–1609.

Jacobson, R. R., White, R. E. B. (1991). The neuropsychiatry of head injury. *Current Opinion in Psychiatry*, *4*: 116–122.

Jacobson, R. R., Kent, A. & White, R. E. B. (1994). Head injury and affective disorders. *Focus on Depression*, *2*: 1–4.

Jacobson, R. R. (1995). The Post-Concussional Syndrome: physiogenesis; psychogenesis and malingering. An integrative model. *Journal of Psychosomatic Research*, *39*, 675–693.

Jacobson, R. R. & Kopelman, M. D. K. (1998). Cardinal features of Organic Psychiatric Disorder. (Stein, G. S., Wilkinson, G., Ed.). *Seminars in General Adult Psychiatry*. Gaskell Press, London, pp. 954–1026.

Jenkins, A., Teasdale, G., Hadley, M. D. M., MacPherson, P. & Rowan, J. O. (1986). Brain lesions detected by magnetic resonance imaging in mild and severe head injuries. *Lancet*, *ii*: 445–446.

Jennett, B. & Bond, M. R. (1975). Assessment of outcome after severe brain damage: A practical scale. *Lancet*, *i*: 480–487.

Kant, R., Smith-Seemiller, L., Isaac, G. & Duffy, J. (1997). Tc-HMPAO SPECT in persistent post-concussion syndrome after mild head injury: comparison with MRI/CT. *Brain Injury*, *11*: 115–124.

Karol, R. L. & Hallo-Poe D. (1987). *Brain injury and alcohol: a workbook for making decisions after injury*. Thompson & Co, Minneapolis.

Kay, D. W. K., Kerr, T. A. & Lassman, L. P. (1971). Brain trauma and the post-concussional syndrome. *Lancet*, *2*: 1052–1055.

Kelly, R. E. (1975). The post-traumatic syndrome: an iatrogenic disease. *Forensic Science*, *6*: 17–24.

Kelly, R. & Smith, B. N. (1981). Post-traumatic syndrome: another myth discredited. *Journal Royal Society Medicine*, *74*: 275–277.

Keshavan, M. S., Channabassavanna, S. M. & Reddy, G. N. (1981). Post-traumatic psychiatric disturbances: patterns and predictors of outcome. *British Journal of Psychiatry*, *138*: 157–160.

King, N. S., Crawford, S., Wenden, F. J., Moss, N. E. G. & Wade, D. T. (1995). The Rivermead post-concussion symptoms questionnaire: a measure of symptoms commonly experienced after head injury and its reliability. *Journal Neurology*, *42*; 587–592.

King, N. S. (1996). Emotional, neuropsychological, and organic factors: their use in the prediction of persisting post concussion symptoms after moderate and mild head injuries. *Journal Neurology, Neurosurgery and Psychiatry*, *61*; 75–81

King, N. S. (1997) .Post traumatic stress disorder and head injury as a dual diagnosis: "islands" of memory as a mechanism. *Journal of Neurology, Neurosurgery and Psychiatry*, *62*: 82–84

Kirmayer, L. J., Robbins, J. M. & Paris, J. (1994). Somatoform disorders: personality and the social matrix of somatic distress. *Journal of Abnormal Psychology*, *103*: 125–136.

Koura, S. S., Doppenberg, E. M., Marmarou, A., Choi, S., Young, H. F. Bullock, R. (1998). Relationship between excitatory amino acid release and outcome after severe head injury. *Acta Neurochirurgica suppl*, *71*, 244–246, Vienna.

Kreutzer, J. S., Marwitz, H. H. & Kepler, K. (1992). Traumatic brain injury: Family response and outcome. *Archives of Physical Medicine & Rehabilitation*, *73*: 771–778.

Kreutzer, J. S., Gervasio, A. H. & Complair, P. S. (1994). Primary caregivers' psychological status and family functioning after traumatic brain injury. *Brain Injury*, *8*(3): 197–210.

Langley, M. J., Lindsay, W. O., Lam, C. S. & Priddy, D. A. (1990). A comprehensive alcohol abuse treatment programme for persons with traumatic brain injury. *Brain Injury*, *3*: 235–246.

Leng, N. R. C. & Parkin, A. J. (1995). Exaggerated or simulated memory disorder by neuropsychological methods. *Journal of Psychosomatic Research*, *39*: 767–776.

Lees-Haley, P. R. & Brown, R. S. (1993). Neurological complaint base rates of 170 personal injury claimants. *Archives of Clinical Neuropsychology*, *8*: 203–209.

Lees-Haley, P. R., Williams, C. W., Zasler, N. D., Marguilies, S., English, L. & Stevens, K. B. (1997). Response bias in plaintiff's histories. *Brain Injury*, *11*, 791–795.

Levin, H. S., Gray, H. E., Eisenberg, H. M. & Ruff, R. M. (1990). Neurobehavioural outcome 1 year after severe head injury: experience of the traumatic coma data bank. *Journal Neurosurgery*, *73*: 699–709.

Levin, H. S., Amparo, E. G., Eisenberg, H. M., Williams, D. H., High, W. M., McArdle, C. B. & Weiner, R. L. (1987). Magnetic resonance imaging and computerized tomography in relation to the neurobehavioural sequelae of mild and moderate head injuries. *Journal Neurosurgery*, *66*: 706–713.

Leventhal, H., Diefenbach, M. & Leventhal, E. A. (1992). Illness cognition: using common sense to understand treatment adherence and affect cognition interactions. *Cognitive Therapy Research*, *16*: 143–163.

Lidvall, H. F., Lindroth, B. & Norlin, B. (1974). Causes of the post-concussional syndrome. *Acta Neurologica Scandinavica Suppl*, *56*: 1–144.

Lishman, W. A. (1998). *Organic Psychiatry*, Third Edn. Blackwell, Oxford.

Lishman, W. A., Jacobson, R. R. & Acker, C. (1987). Brain damage in alcoholism: current concepts. *Acta Medica Scandinavica Suppl,D 717*: 5–17.

Lishman, W. A. (1988). Physiogenesis and psychogenesis in the "Post-concussional Syndrome". *British Journal of Psychiatry*, *153*: 460–469.

Lyeth, B. G., Jenkins, L. W., Hamm, R. J., Dixon, C. E., Phillips, L. L., Clifton, G. L., Young, H. F. & Hayes, R. L. (1990). Prolonged memory impairment in the absence of hippocampal cell death following traumatic brain injury in the rat. *Brain Research*, *526*: 249–258.

McClelland, R. J., Fenton, G. W. & Rutherford, W. (1994). The post-concussional syndrome revisited. *Journal Royal Society Medicine*, *87*: 508–510.

MacFlynn, G, Montgomery, E., Fenton, G. W. & Rutherford, W. (1984). Measurement of reaction time following minor head injury. *Journal of Neurology, Neurosurgery and Psychiatry*, *47*: 1326–1331.

McKinlay, W. W., Brooks, D. N. & Bond, M. R. (1983). Post-concussional symptoms, financial compensation and outcome of severe blunt head injury. *Journal Neurology, Neurosurgery and Psychiatry*, *46*: 1084–1091.

McLean, A., Temkin, N. R., Dikmens, S. & Wyler, A. R. (1983). The behavioural sequelae of head injury. *Journal Clinical Neuropsychology*, *5*: 361–376.

McMillan, T. M. (1991). Post-traumatic stress disorder and severe head injury. *British Journal of Psychiatry*, *159*: 431–433.

Mayou, R., Bryant, B. & Duthie, R. (1993). Psychiatric consequences of road traffic accidents. *British Medical Journal*, *307*: 647–651.

Mayou, R. A. & Bryant, B. M. (1994). Effects of road traffic accidents on driving behaviour. *Injury*, *25*: 457–460.

Medical Disability Society (1988). *The management of traumatic brain injury*. The Medical Disability Society: Royal College of Physicians, London.

Mendelson, G. (1985). Compensation neurosis. An invalid diagnosis. *Medical Journal Australia*, *142*: 562–564.

Mendelson, G. (1995). Compensation neurosis revisited: Outcome studies of the effects of litigation. *Journal of Psychosomatic Medicine*, *39*; 695–706.

Mendelson, G. (1981). Persistent work disability following settlement of compensation claims. *Law Institute Journal* (Melbourne), *55*: 342–345.

Merskey, H., Trimble, M. (1979). Personality, sexual adjustment, and brain lesions in patients with conversion symptoms. *American Journal of Psychiatry*, *136*: 179–182.

Miller, H. (1961). Accident neurosis. *British Medical Journal*. *1*: 919–925, 992–998.

Minderhoud, J. M., Boelens, M. E. M., Huizenga, J. & Saan, R. J. (1980). Treatment of minor head injuries. *Clinical Neurology & Neurosurgery*, *82*: 127–140.

Mitchener, A. Wyper, D. J., Patterson, J., Hadley, D. M.. Wilson, J. T., Scott, L. C., Jones, M. & Teasdale, G. M. (1997). SPECT, CT, and MRI in head injury: acute abnormalities followed up at six months. *Journal of Neurology, Neurosurgery and Psychiatry*, *62*(6): 633–6.

Mittenberg, W., DiGuilio, D. V., Perrin, S. & Bass, A. E. (1992). Symptoms following mild head injury: expectation as aetiology. *Journal of Neurology, Neurosurgery and Psychiatry*, *55*: 200–204.

Mittenberg, W. & Burton, D. B. (1994). A survey of treatments for post-concussion syndrome. *Brain Injury*, *8*(5): 429–437.

Mobayed, M. & Dinan, T. G. (1990). Buspirone/prolactin response in post head injury depression. *Journal of Affective Disorders*, *19*: 237–241.

Montgomery, A, Fenton, G. W. & McClelland, R. J. (1984). Delayed brainstem conduction time in post-concussion syndrome. *Lancet*, *i*: 1011.

Montgomery, E. A., Fenton, G. W., McClelland, R. J., MacFlynn, G. & Rutherford, W. H. (1991). The psychobiology of minor head injury. *Psychological Medicine*, *21*: 375–384.

Murdoch, I., Perry, E. K., Court, J. A., Graham, D. I. & Deward, D. (1998). Cortical cholinergic dysfunction after human head injury. *Journal of Neurotrauma*, *15*: 295–305.

Nedd, K., Sfakianakis, G. & Ganz, W. (1993). 99m Tc-HMPAO SPECT of the brain in mild to moderate traumatic brain injury patients: compared with CT – a prospective study. *Brain Injury*, *7*: 469–479.

Newcombe, F., Rabbitt, P. & Briggs, M. (1994). Minor head injury: pathophysiological or iatrogenic sequelae? *Journal of Neurology, Neurosurgery and Psychiatry*, *57*: 709–716.

Newton, M. R., Greenwood, R. J., Britton, K. E., Charlesworth, M., Nimmon, C. C., Carroll, M. J. & Dolke, G. (1992). A study comparing SPECT with CT and MRI after closed head injury. *Journal of Neurology, Neurosurgery and Psychiatry*, *55*: 92–94.

Ohry, A., Solomon, Z. & Rattock, J. (1996). Post traumatic stress disorder in traumatic brain injury. *Brain Injury, 10*: 687–695

Pearce, J. M. S. (1995). Post traumatic syndrome and whiplash injuries. In *Clinical Neurology*. Ed. Kennard, C. Churchill Livingstone. Edinburgh.

Pincus, T., Peane, S., McClelland, A., Farley, S. & Vogel, S. (1994). Interpretation bias in responses to ambiguous cues in pain patients. *Journal of Psychosomatic Research*, 38: 347–353.

Povlishock J. T. & Coburn, T. H. (1989). Morphopathological change associated with mild head injury. In Levin, H. S., Eisenberg, H. M., Benson, A. L. (Ed.), *Mild Head Injury*, pp 37–53. Oxford University Press: Oxford.

Radanov, B. P., Stefano, D. I. & Schindrig, G. (1994). A relationship between early somatic, radiological, cognitive and psychosocial findings and outcome during a one-year follow-up in 117 patients suffering from common whiplash. *British Journal of Rheumatology, 33*: 442–448

Radanov, B. P., Stefano, D. I., Schindrig, G. & Sturzenegger, M (1994). Common whiplash: psychosomatic or somatopsychic? *Journal Neurology, Neurosurgery and Psychiatry*, 57: 486–490

Resnick, P. J. (1989). Malingering of post-traumatic disorders. In: Rogers, R. (Ed.), *Clinical Aspects of Malingering and Deception* (Ch. 6, pp. 84–103). Guildford Press, New York

Rimel, R. W., Giordani, B., Barth, J. T., Boll, T. J. & Jane, J. A. (1981). Disability caused by minor head injury. *Neurosurgery, 9*: 221–228.

Robbins, J. M., Kirmayer, L. J. (1991). Attributions of common somatic symptoms. *Psychological Medicine, 21*: 1029–1045.

Rogers, R., Bagby, R. M., Dickens, S. E. (1992). *Professional manual for the SIRS*. Psychological Assessment Resources, Tampa, Florida:

Rogers, R. (1997). *Clinical Assessment of Malingering and Deception* (2nd Edition) Guildford Press, New York.

Ruff, R. M., Crouch, J. A., Tröster, A. I., Marshall, L. F., Buchsbaum, M. S., Lottenberg, S. & Somers, L. M. (1994). Selected cases of poor outcome following a minor brain trauma: comparing neuropsychological and positron emission tomography assessment. *Brain Injury*, 8(4): 297–308.

Russell, W. R. (1971). *The traumatic amnesias*. Oxford University Press, London.

Rutherford, W. H. (1989). Postconcussion symptoms: Relationship to acute neurological indices, individual differences, and circumstances of injury. In: Levin, H. D., Eisenberg, H. M., Benton, A. L. (Ed.), *Mild Head Injury*, pp 217–228. Oxford Press, New York.

Rutherford, W. H. & Fee, C. R. (1988). A study of the effect of legal settlement on post-concussion symptoms. *Archives of Emergency Medicine, 5*: 12–17.

Rutherford, W. H., Merrett, J. D. & McDonald, J. R. (1977). Sequelae of concussion caused by minor head injuries. *Lancet, 1*: 1–4.

Rutherford, W. H., Merrett, J. D. & McDonald, J. R. (1978). Symptoms at one year following concussion from minor head injury. *Injury*, 10: 225–230.

Salkovskis, P. M., Clark, D. M. (1993). Panic disorder and hypochondriasis. *Advances in Behaviour Research and Therapy*, 15: 23–48.

Sbordone, R. J. (1992). Distinguishing traumatic brain injury from post-traumatic stress disorder. *Letter. Neurolaw, 1*: 3.

Sbordone, R. J. & Liter, J. C. (1995). Mild traumatic brain injury does not produce post-traumatic stress disorder. *Brain Injury, 9*: 405–412.

Steptoe, A. (1991) The links between stress and illness. *Journal of Psychosomatic Research, 35*: 633–644.

Stritmatter, W. J. & Roses, A. D. (1995). *Apoliprotein E and Alzheimer's disease*. Procedures of the National Academy of Science, USA, *92*: 4725–4727.

Symonds, C. P. (1962). Concussion and its sequelae. *Lancet, 1*: 1–5.

Tarsh, M. H. & Royston, C. (1985). A follow-up study of accident neurosis. *British Journal Psychiatry, 146*: 18–25.

Taylor, A. R. & Bell, T. K. (1966). Slowing of cerebral circulation after concussional head injury. *Lancet, ii*: 178–180.

Teasdale, G. M., Nicholl, J. A., Murray, G. & Fiddes, M. (1997). Association of apoliprotein polymorphism with outcome after head injury. *Lancet, 350*: 1069–1071.

Thompson, M. R. (1965). Post-traumatic psychoneurosis - a statistical survey. *American Journal Psychiatry, 121*: 1043–1048.

Thrasher, S. M., Dalgleish, T. & Yule, W. (1994). Information processing in post-traumatic disorder. *Behavioural Research Therapy, 32*(2): 247–254.

Turk, D. C. & Rudy, T. E. (1992). Cognitive factors and persistent pain: a glimpse into Pandora's box. *Cognitive Therapy Research, 16*: 99–112.

Van Zomeren, A. H. & Van Den Burg, W. (1985). Residual complaints of patients 2 years after severe head injury. *Journal of Neurology, Neurosurgery and Psychiatry, 48*: 21–28.

Varney, N. R., Bushnell, D. L. & Nathan, M. E. (1995). NeuroSPECT correlates of disabling mild head injury: preliminary findings. *Journal of Head Trauma Rehabilitation, 10*: 18–28.

Wade, D. T., Crawford, S. & Wenden, F. J. (1997). Does routine follow up after head injury help? A randomised controlled trial. *Journal of Neurology, Neurosurgery and Psychiatry, 62*: 478–84.

Wade, D. T., Crawford, S., Wenden, F. J., Crawford, S. & Caldwell, F. E. (1998). Routine follow up after head injury: a second randomised controlled trial. *Journal of Neurology, Neurosurgery and Psychiatry, 65*: 177–183.

Warwick, H. M. C., Salkovskis, P. M. (1989). Hypochondriasis. In: Scott, J. Williams, J. M. G. Beck, A. T. (ed.) *Cognitive Therapy in Clinical Practice*, pp. 78–102, Gower, London.

Weighill, V. E. (1983). "Compensation neurosis". A review of the literature. *Journal of Psychosomatic Research, 27*(2): 97–104.

Wells, A., Matthews, G. (1996). Anxiety and cognition. *Current Opinion in Psychiatry*, 9: 422–426.

West, J. R., Lind, M. D., Demuth, R. M., Parker, E. S., Alkana, R. L., Cassell, M. Black, A. C. (1982). Lesion-induced sprouting in the rat dentate gyrus is inhibited by repeated ethanol administration. *Science, 218*: 808–810.

Whetsell, K. A., Patterson, C. M., Young, D. H. & Schiller, W. R. (1989). Pre-injury psychopathology in trauma patients. *Journal of Trauma, 29*: 1158–1161.

Wilson, J. T. L., Hadley, D. M., Wiedmann, K. D. & Teasdale, G. M. (1992). Intercorrelation of lesions detected by magnetic resonance imaging after closed head injury. *Brain Injury, 6*: 391–399.

Wilson, J. T. L., Wiedman, K. D., Hadley, D. M., Condon, B., Teasdale, G. & Brooks, D. N. (1988). Early and late magnetic resonance imaging and neuropsychological outcome after head injury. *Journal of Neurology, Neurosurgery and Psychiatry, 51*: 391–396.

Wrightson, P., Gronwall, D. (1981). Time off work and symptoms after minor head injury. *Injury, 12*: 445–454.

8

Children and Young People: The Neglected Victims of Road Traffic Accidents

PAUL STALLARD

Consultant Clinical Psychologist, Department of Child and Family Psychiatry, Royal United Hospital, Combe Park, Bath, BA1 3NG, England

It is only comparatively recently that researchers have started to systematically investigate the psychological effects of traumas upon children (Yule 1994). The reasons for this are many and complex although an overriding factor has been the failure of parents and professionals to acknowledge that children, like adults, are significantly affected by traumatic events. Parents are understandably protective of their children and are often reluctant to acknowledge or may deny that their child has been significantly affected by a traumatic experience.

Within the professional literature there has been a debate as to whether children are significantly affected by traumatic events and whether a specific diagnosis of Post Traumatic Stress Disorder (PTSD) for children was required (Garmezy & Rutter 1985: Yule 1989). The basis of this argument centred upon the premise that the effects of trauma on the majority of children are short-lived and that their symptoms are different from those displayed by adults. This argument was, however, flawed being based upon insensitive psychometric assessment scales often completed by adults who have been found to fail to recognise the severity of the psychological effects experienced by their children (Yule 1999: McFarlane 1987).

There is now recognition that children are significantly affected by traumas and the psychological effects arising from single traumatic events have been detailed (Vogel & Vernberg 1993; Yule 1989, 1999). The psychological consequences of a range of disasters including bushfires (McFarlane 1987) earthquakes (Pynoos et al 1993), shipping accidents (Yule & Williams 1990), bombings (Curran et al 1990) and sniper attacks (Pynoos et al 1987) have now been documented. However, it has only been in the past few years that researchers have begun to investigate the psychological effects of more frequent and everyday traumas such as road traffic accidents.

Road Traffic Accidents

The earliest reports have taken the form of descriptive case studies in which researchers have highlighted the psychological changes arising from individual accidents. Jones & Peterson (1993) reported a case of a three year old girl who developed post traumatic stress disorder (PTSD) following a minor road traffic accident. The girl presented with regular nightmares, trauma related anxiety, attempted to avoid travelling in vehicles and became more aggressive in her play. Similarly, Thompson, McArdle & Dunne (1993) described three children aged 4, 11 and 13 who, following traffic accidents, experienced nightmares, separation anxiety, sleep disturbance, and were reluctant to travel by car.

A few studies have provided descriptive accounts of the psychological effects of road traffic accidents involving groups of children. Stallard & Law (1993) assessed 7 adolescents involved in a school minibus accident. Although the young people sustained comparatively minor physical injuries, most were suffering significant psychological distress when assessed six months after their accident. All experienced regular intrusive accident related thoughts, described feelings of acute anxiety, panic attacks and a heightened awareness of danger when travelling in vehicles. Difficulties talking with parents and concentrating on schoolwork were also reported. Casswell (1997) described an accident in which a bus driver and one pupil died when a school bus was struck by an articulated lorry. Assessments completed on 34 children in respect of compensation claims 9–15 months after the accident suggested that one in six children were at high risk of developing severe PTSD. Finally, Winje & Ulvik (1998) assessed the psychological effects reported by 28 children involved in a fatal bus crash 1 and 3 years after the accident. At one year, three-quarters of the children reported specific symptoms of post-traumatic stress, three-quarters were assessed to have a marked anxiety reaction and almost half a marked depressive reaction. Psychosomatic problems were common with approximately 60% reporting headaches and 20–40% sleeping difficulties, tiredness, pain and appetite problems. No clinically significant symptoms were observed when assessed three years post accident.

Despite the growing interest in child RTA survivors larger scale studies have been comparatively slow to emerge. The led Di Gallo & Parry Jones as recently as 1996 to conclude "there is a lack of systematic research into the range and management of the psychological sequelae of road traffic accidents in children and young people".

One of the earlier attempts at assessing the psychological consequences of more everyday road traffic accidents was reported by Canterbury & Yule (1997). Postal self-report questionnaires designed to assess the presence of a significant trauma reaction, anxiety and depressive reactions were sent to children who attended an accident and emergency department. Completed assessments obtained for 28 children involved in road traffic accidents indicated that approximately 10 months after their accident, one in six children had scores that would suggest the presence of PTSD. More comprehensive questionnaire data for 45 school aged children 4–7 months after their attendance at an accident and emergency department were obtained by Ellis, Stores & Mayou (1998). The data indicated that 33% of children were judged to be significantly affected by their accidents, 39% reported travel anxiety, 23% were depressed, 14% highly anxious and 17% reported nighttime difficulties.

The first prospective study utilising diagnostic interviews to assess the psychological consequences of RTA's was reported by Di Gallo, Barton & Parry-Jones (1997). They assessed 57 children aged 5–18 years of age 2–16 days and again at 12–15 weeks post accident. Symptoms reduced over time although at Time 2, 14% suffered from post traumatic stress disorder and 17% reported serious traffic-related fears. In a larger study, Mirza et al (1998) assessed 119 children aged 8–16 years four to seven weeks and six months after a road traffic accident. At six weeks 53 (45%) children presented with PTSD symptoms but by six months this had reduced to 19 (17%). Diagnostic interviews with 44 of the 53 children who had significant PTSD symptoms at six weeks revealed that 33 (75%) fulfilled the DSM-IV criteria for this condition.

Methodological Problems

This overview highlights the limited research that has investigated the psychological effects of road traffic accidents upon children. Whilst the current knowledge base is limited, methodological problems further restrict the conclusion that can be drawn. Sample sizes have generally tended to be small and variable rates of recruitment raise questions as to whether those children assessed are representative of the general population of child accident survivors. Similarly, whilst acknowledging the practical difficulties, the absence of appropriate control groups prohibits any conclusions that psychological problems in child RTA survivors are different from those found in the general population. Studies have investigated differing psychopathology with some focusing only on PTSD (Di Gallo, Barton & Parry-Jones 1997) whereas others have adopted a broader definition of psychological distress (Ellis, Stores, Mayou 1998). The presence of other significant psychiatric disorders such as anxiety and depression has rarely been formally assessed (Mirza et al 1998). Methods of assessment have ranged from children and/or parents completing postal questionnaires (Canterbury & Yule 1997: Ellis, Stores & Mayou 1998) to more comprehensive interviews undertaken with both children and their parents (Di Gallo, Barton & Parry Jones 1997: Mirza et al 1998). The presence of significant psychological distress has been determined on the basis of fulfilling stringent diagnostic criteria (Di Gallo, Barton & Parry-Jones) whereas others have used questionnaire scores to suggest possible psychiatric diagnosis (Stallard & Law 1993). Finally, the time at which the assessment was undertaken has ranged from less than 4 weeks (Di Gallo, Barton & Parry-Jones 1997), between 4–7 months (Ellis Stores & Mayou 1998: Mirza et al 1998: Stallard & Law 1993), 9–15 months (Canterbury & Yule 1997; Casswell 1997) and 3 years (Winje & Ulvik 1998) post trauma. Temporal variations in the reported frequency of symptoms prevent comparisons between studies.

The Bath Road Traffic Accident Project

In 1996 a prospective study was undertaken to systematically assess via semi-structured interviews the psychological effects of RTA's upon children. The findings of the Bath Road Traffic Accident Project have been reported in more detail elsewhere and so this paper will be limited to providing an overview of the project and a summary of key findings. (Stallard, Velleman & Baldwin 1998).

Over a 12-month period all children aged 5–18 who attended the accident and emergency department at the Royal United Hospital in Bath following involvement in a RTA were identified. A total of 278 children attended the department of which 119 (43%) were successfully assessed approximately 6 weeks post accident. In order to provide a comparison group, 66 children who attended hospital following sporting accidents were also assessed using the same protocol.

The assessment protocol incorporated the Clinician Administered PTSD Scale for Children (CAPS-C) (Nader et al 1994). This scale systematically assesses both the frequency and intensity of each of the 17 identified features of DSM-IV (Diagnostic and Statistical Manual of Mental Disorders) that contribute to the diagnosis of PTSD (APA 1994). In addition to assessing the diagnostic criteria for PTSD a semi-structured interview explored the effects of the accident upon various aspects of the child's everyday life including social life, friendships and relationships. Finally, children aged over 7 completed the self assessment PTSD screening battery suggested by Yule & Udwin (1991), namely the Impact of Event Scale (IES) (Horrowitz, Wilner & Alvarez 1979), Birleson Depression Inventory (Birleson 1981) and Revised Children Manifest Anxiety Scale (Reynolds and Richmond 1978).

Post Traumatic Stress Disorder. The average age of the children assessed was 13.9 years with over half being in the older, 15–18 age group. Car crashes were the largest accident type with approximately one quarter being pedestrians hit by vehicles, and one fifth involved in cycle accidents. The majority were discharged home after assessment although one in four were admitted to hospital for observation or treatment.

On the basis of the semi-structured assessment, 41 children (34.45%), 13 boys and 28 girls fulfilled the diagnostic criteria for PTSD when assessed six weeks post trauma. Of those involved in sporting accidents, only 2 (3%) were found to have PTSD. It would therefore appear that RTA's generate significantly more psychological distress than other forms of unexpected trauma such as sporting accidents.

The type of accident (i.e. car crash, cycle or pedestrian accident), accident status of the child (passenger, driver, pedestrian), and presence and severity of physical injuries (i.e. fractured bones, blows to the head, triage priority scores, hospital admission) were not predictive of significant psychological distress. Similarly children of all ages were affected by their accident although girls were significantly more at risk of developing PTSD than boys.

Effects upon everyday life. In addition to PTSD some children developed other trauma reactions. Psychometric scores suggest that approximately one in seven suffered from clinically significant anxiety and depressive disorders. The suggestion that children suffer from a range of trauma reactions other than PTSD has been highlighted and the rates obtained in this study are comparable to those reported by other researchers (Di Gallo, Barton & parry-Jones 1997: Ellis, Stores & Mayou 1998).

The accident resulted in a number of effects upon the child's everyday life with 40% reporting changes in their sleeping pattern with accident related dreams and difficulty falling asleep being the most common. Emotional changes were often reported with almost a quarter (23.5%) of children becoming more tearful. However the dominant feeling was that of anger with almost half feeling angry and intolerant of others (47.1%). A quarter (26.9%) reported travel related anxiety and half (50.4%) were regularly troubled by recurrent accident related thoughts. Some children reported that they kept themselves busy in order to avoid being troubled by these distressing images.

In terms of friendships, although the accident effected the social groupings of 1 in 7 children, significant changes in relationships were reported by one third. This was not however always a negative change and a number reported that they had become closer to their friends particularly if they were involved in the accident. However for a quarter of the children the accident resulted in them feeling distanced or estranged from others.

Conclusion

The results of this study suggest that at least in the short term, approximately one third of child RTA survivors suffer from PTSD. Our findings are however limited since assessment was undertaken only once, six weeks post trauma. The study by Di Gallo, Barton & Parry Jones (1997) suggests that PTSD varies over time and that fewer children will go on to develop chronic PTSD. Our preliminary follow-up data supports this finding and indicates that of a sub-group of 40 children followed-up 8 months post accident, almost half of those initially diagnosed with PTSD still fulfilled the diagnostic criteria. None of the 19 children who did not have PTSD at the initial assessment went on to develop this condition.

It is however important to recognise that whilst PTSD is seen by many as the "gold standard" against which trauma reactions are assessed PTSD refers only to a defined cluster of symptoms. RTA survivors present with other reactions, particularly anxiety and depressive symptoms and although these were not independently clinically assessed during our study, anecdotally we would suggest that these reactions are regularly experienced by children. Similarly the effects of the RTA upon the child's everyday life proved extensive with significant changes in social activity, friendships and emotional liability being reported. The importance of these changes should not be underestimated since, although they may not necessarily indicate any specific medical diagnosis, they nonetheless highlight the considerable re-adjustment the children are required to make.

Neither accident characteristics nor the nature or severity of personal injuries were related to the degree of psychological distress. This finding is consistent with research on adult RTA survivors and with other studies focusing upon children (Mayou, Bryant & Duthie 1993; Ellis, Stores & Mayou 1998). The objective severity of the accident was not therefore predictive of PTSD. Children involved in comparatively minor shunts suffered significant psychological distress. However, the way the individual perceives and cognitively appraises the accident does appear important. In our study we found a positive association between those children who perceived their accident as life threatening and poor psychological adjustment.

Finally, although this study has focused upon school aged children there is little doubt that pre-school children are equally affected by road traffic accidents. The presentation of symptoms in younger children may however vary and in particular, behaviour problems, toileting, clinginess, and accident-related play are commonly reported features (Street & Sibert 1998).

By way of an example, a two-year-old girl was referred to the author to assess the psychological consequences of a car accident that occurred 8 months previously. The girl was travelling home one evening with her older sister and mother when their car was hit by another that sped out of a side turning. Their car span around and was pushed across the road through a garden wall. Although the site of the impact was less than a metre from the girl's seat nobody was physically injured nor taken to hospital. However a number of changes were noted in the girl's behaviour over the coming weeks.

The girl had developed a good sleeping pattern but on the day after the accident became fearful of going to bed. She now sleeps with the light on and wakes two or three times each night. She displays more frequent temper tantrums, appears very alert whilst travelling in cars and is very startled and upset by loud unexpected noises. She has become extremely fussy with her eating and regularly wet herself for six weeks after the accident.

The accident was subsequently re-experienced in two main ways. Firstly the girl copied the noise of the impact by loudly banging her hand on the furniture. Her language was limited to two and three word sentences and she would accompany this by saying "man bang". Loud noises similar to those during the accident such as hot water pipes knocking and fireworks caused her intense distress resulting in her clinging tightly to her mother. Secondly the accident was acted out in play. Cars were banged into each other and little figures placed around them as she re-enacted the accident.

The girl became very distressed when travelling in cars and had to be physically manhandled into her seat for her next four journeys. Thereafter she remained reluctant to get into a car and would regularly say during journeys "man bang". In terms of responsiveness she became withdrawn at toddler group and would not play with the other children preferring instead to sit quietly beside her mother.

Clinical Implications

Increased awareness. The research to date would clearly indicate a need to increase awareness and recognition amongst professionals, parents and young people as to the possible psychological consequences of RTA's. Professionals in hospitals and GP surgeries need to be sensitive to the emotional needs of child accident survivors and provide parents and young people with age appropriate information about the possible psychological effects. The Child Accident Prevention Trust have developed a series of booklets designed to help children and parents understand the range of reactions and emotions they may experience after an accident and how they can learn to cope and feel better (Child Accident Prevention Trust 1998). The routine provision of such information to child RTA survivors would undoubtedly be of benefit and help them understand and normalise their reactions.

The greater availability of educational materials would also help parents and teachers understand that although RTA's are comparatively common children can be significantly affected and for some this may persist for a number of months. Behaviour problems, poor academic performance, irritability and moodiness may need to be seen as indications of unresolved trauma rather than willful naughtiness, defiance or laziness. Increased recognition may therefore facilitate more effective help seeking since at present specialist psychological services for children involved in RTA's are not routinely provided.

Early identification. In our study, at the end of the assessment interview, families were given an information leaflet including the telephone number of a psychologist to contact if they would like further help. By the end of the study only two parents had contacted the psychologist seeking assistance for their child suggesting that the vast majority of the psychological distress experienced by child RTA survivors is unrecognised and remains untreated.

A more proactive approach to the early identification of children at risk of developing significant psychological reactions would appear indicated. However children likely to be psychologically affected by their accident can not be predicted at the first point of emergency care on the basis of accident or physical injury characteristics. This has led some researchers to suggest that all child RTA survivors should be screened for psychological complications (Ellis, Stores & Mayou 1998). Whether non-mental health professionals could undertake this screening needs careful assessment. As reported by Di Gallo, Barton & Parry-Jones (1998) "the decision as to whether symptoms represent a normal psychological reaction following a distressing event and are likely to subside spontaneously, or reflect a disorder of function requiring psychological intervention, has to be taken very carefully".

Similarly, although the routine psychological screening of RTA survivors would ensure that children suffering significant distress as a result of their accident were identified this would have enormous implications for mental health services. The results of this study would suggest that at six weeks post trauma approximately 20,000 child RTA survivors in the UK each year would be diagnosed as experiencing PTSD. Furthermore, of these, approximately half will recover without any specialist intervention. Any screening programme therefore needs to be able to accurately identify those at risk of developing chronic symptoms rather than those experiencing significant although more transient reactions.

Preventative Interventions. An alternative approach is to provide RTA survivors with interventions designed to prevent the development of significant psychological reactions. Interventions such as critical incident stress debriefing have gained much popularity over recent years (Mitchell 1983) and the technique has been adapted for use with children either in a group setting or individually (Dyregov 1991: Pynoos & Eth 1986). However the value of psychological debriefing has been questioned since research with adults has found little evidence to suggest that it is effective in preventing future psychopathology (Bisson & Deahl 1994: Raphael, Meldrum & McFarlane 1995). Studies utilising this technique with children have rarely been reported although there are some suggestions that it maybe helpful and some promising results have been reported (Stallard 1999: Stallard & Law 1994). Randomised controlled trials using standardised interventions are required in order to determine whether routinely debriefing child RTA survivors is an effective way to reduce the development of significant psychological reactions.

References.

American Psychiatric Association. (1994). *Diagnostic and Statistical Manual of Mental Disorders.* (Fourth edition).Washington DC.

Birleson, P. (1981). The validity of depressive disorder in childhood and the development of a self-rating scale: A research report. *Journal of Child Psychology and Psychiatry, 22*, 73–88.

Bisson, J. I. & Deahl, M. P. (1994). Psychological debriefing and prevention of post-traumatic stress. More research is needed. *British Journal of Psychiatry, 165*, 717–720.

Canterbury, R. & Yule, W. (1997). The effects in children of road accidents. In M. Mitchel (Ed.), *The aftermath of road accidents. Psychological, social and legal consequences of an everyday trauma.* Routledge. London.

Casswell, G. (1997). Learning from the aftermath: The response of mental health workers to a school-bus crash. *Clinical Child Psychology and Psychiatry, 2*(4), 517–523.

Child Accident Prevention Trust (1998). *Getting over an accident.* Child Accident Prevention Trust. London.

Curran, P. S., Bell, P., Murray, A., Loughrey, G., Roddy, R. & Rocke, L. G. (1990). Psychological consequences of the Enniskillen bombing. *British Journal of Psychiatry, 156*, 479–482.

Di Gallo, A., Barton, J. & Parry-Jones, W. L. I. (1997). Road traffic accidents: early psychological consequences in children and adolescents. *British Journal of Psychiatry, 170*, 358–362.

Di Gallo, A. & Parry-Jones, W. L. I. (1996). Psychological sequelae of road traffic accidents: an inadequately addressed problem. *British Journal of Psychiatry, 169*, 405–407.

Dyregov, A. (1991). *Grief in children: A handbook for adults.* Jessica Kingsley, London.

Ellis, A., Stores, G. & Mayou, R. (1998). Psychological consequences of road traffic accidents in children. *European Child and Adolescent Psychiatry, 7*, 61–68.

Garmezy, N. & Rutter, M. (1985). Acute reactions to stress. In M. Rutter & L. Hersov (Ed.), *Child & Adolescent Psychiatry: Modern Approaches* (2nd edition). Oxford. Blackwell.

Horowitz, M. J. Wilner, N. & Alvarez, W. (1979). Impact of Event Scale: A measure of subjective stress. *Psychosomatic Medicine, 41*, 209–218.

Jones, R. W. & Peterson, L. W. (1993). Post traumatic stress disorder in a child following an automobile accident. *Journal of Family Practice, 36*, 223–225.

Mayou, R., Bryant, B. & Duthie, R. (1993). Psychiatric consequences of road traffic accidents. *British Medical Journal, 307*, 647–651.

McFarlane, A. C., Policansky, S. & Irwin, C. P. (1987). A longitudinal study of the psychological morbidity in children due to a natural disaster. *Psychological Medicine, 17*, 727–738.

Mirza, K. A. H., Bhadrinath, B. R., Goodyer, I. M. &Gilmour, C. (1998). Post-traumatic stress disorder in children and adolescents following road traffic accidents. *British Journal of Psychiatry, 172*, 443–447.

Nader, K. O., Kriegler, J. A., Blake, D. D. & Pynoos, R. S. (1994). *Clinician Administered PTSD Scale for Children (CAPS-C).* National Centre for PTSD. Boston.

Pynoos, R. S. & Eth, S. (1986). Witness to violence : the child interview. *Journal of the American Academy of Child Psychiatry, 25*, 306–319.

Pynoos, R. S., Fredrick, C., Nader, K., Arroyo, W., Steinberg, A., Eth, S., Nunez, F. & Fairbanks, L. (1987). Life threat and post traumatic stress in school-age children. *Archives of General Psychiatry, 44*, 1057–1063.

Pynoos, R. S., Goenjian, A., Tashjian, M., Karakashian, M., Manjikian, R., Manoukian, G., Steinberg, A. M. & Fairbanks, L. A. (1993). Post-traumatic stress reactions in children after the 1988 Armenian earthquake. *British Journal of Psychiatry, 163*, 239–247.

Raphael, B., Meldrum, L. & McFarlane, A. C. (1995). Does debriefing after psychological trauma work. *British Medical Journal, 310*, 1479–1480.

Reynolds, C. R. & Richmond, B. O. (1978). What I think and feel : A revised measure of children's manifest anxiety. *Journal of Abnormal Child Psychology, 6*, 271–280.

Stallard (1999). Debriefing adolescents after critical life events. In Raphael, B. (Ed.), *Stress debriefing: a critical appraisal of practice, evidence and clinical outcomes.* Cambridge University Press. Cambridge.

Stallard, P. & Law, F. (1993). Screening and psychological debriefing of adolescent survivors of life-threatening events. *British Journal of Psychiatry, 163*, 660–665.

Stallard, P., Velleman, R. & Baldwin, S. (1998). Prospective study of post- traumatic stress disorder in children involved in road traffic accidents. *British Medical Journal, 317*, 1619–1623.

Street, E. & Sibert, J. (1998) Post-traumatic Stress Reactions in Children. *Clinical Child Psychology and Psychiatry, 3*(4), 553–560.

Thompson, A., McArdle, P. & Dunne, F. (1993). Psychiatric consequences of road traffic accidents. Children may be seriously affected . *British Medical Journal, 307*, 1282–1283.

Vogel, J. M., & Vernberg, E. M. (1993). Task Force Report Part 1: Children's psychological responses to disasters. *Journal of Clinical Child Psychology. 22*(4), 464–484.

Winje, D. & Ulvik, A. (1998). Long-term outcome of trauma in children: the psychological consequences of a bus accident. *Journal of Child Psychology and Psychiatry, 39*(5), 635–642.

Yule, W. (1989). The effects of disasters on children. *Association for Child Psychology and Psychiatry Newsletter, 11*(6), 3–6.

Yule, W. (1994). Posttraumatic Stress Disorders. In Rutter, M., Taylor, E. & Hersov, L. (Eds). *Child and Adolescent Psychiatry: Modern Approaches* (3rd Edition). Blackwell Scientific Publication. Oxford.

Yule, W. (1999) Post-traumatic stress disorder. *Archives of Disease in Childhood,* 80(2), 107–110.

Yule, W. & Williams, R. (1990). Posttraumatic stress reactions in children. Journal of Traumatic Stress, *3*, 279–295.

Yule, W. & Udwin, O. (1991). Screening child survivors for post-traumatic stress disorder : experiences from the Jupiter sinking. British Journal of Clinical Psychology, *30*, 131–138.

9

Psychological Distress in Police Officers Attending Serious and Fatal Road Traffic Accidents

MARGARET MITCHELL, Ph.D.

Police Research Unit, Department of Psychology, Glasgow Caledonian University

The effects of road traffic accidents on "primary victims" is the main topic of this volume. UK statistics on death and injury on the roads indicate that over three thousand people die each year in road accidents, providing compelling evidence that dealing with road accidents is a frequent, and potentially very difficult task for the emergency services working at the accident scene. Substantial research exists on the impact of disasters and large scale accidents on emergency workers, although rather less exists on the effect of more "everyday" incidents such as road traffic accidents (RTAs). The purpose of this chapter is to describe the consequences of RTAs from the perspective of the professional "helpers" at the scene.

Ambulance workers, paramedics and firefighters have an obvious life saving role at a road accident, while the role of the police may be rather less well acknowledged and understood. The description of their tasks found in police training manuals – the control of other traffic, obtaining information from witnesses and survivors, and collecting sufficient facts to complete an accident report – is a dry and procedural account of what they do. It does not reflect the considerable assistance they give to very distressed people.

Nor does it reflect the fact that they themselves are witness to distressing serious or fatal injuries at the scene. Often they will be required to inform relatives of the death or serious injury of a loved person, and accompany the relative to hospital, or to identify victims. Police officers are exposed more frequently simply because they also attend less serious accidents, and those causing disturbance of traffic flow.

The possible effect on the health and welfare of individual officers of exposure to more serious accidents is of concern, naturally. But in turn, distress in the officers may affect how they deal with survivors and witnesses at the scene of an accident (Hetherington, Munro & Mitchell, 1997). Protecting the psychological well-being of police officers, therefore, has a very practical effect. The police, and the fire and ambulance services are an integral part of any accident scene. How they act, and care for those involved in accidents has the potential to ameliorate or exacerbate an already very bad situation. An approach to the people affected which concentrates only the procedure to be followed can appear cold or harsh. And such an approach may be the result of the officers' attempts to protect his or her own emotional status. Equally to be too emotionally involved or affected by others' distress is not helpful in getting the job done.

Police training does, however, tend to emphasise the procedural aspects of the work – the form filling, the preparation of accident reports – with rather less emphasis on how to manage the emotions of others and, indeed, their own emotional reactions. In our previous work it was found that police probationers learn how to deal with sudden death, and especially the management of emotions under the relatively informal guidance of supervisors and colleagues (Mitchell 1997a; 1997b). The work of the police at an accident scene is a difficult role, as will be seen.

Reported here is the experience of the police as represented by a sample from a large Scottish police service. The data were collected as part of a study of how police officers and police organisations manage critical incident reactions (Mitchell, Stevenson & Poole, 1999). In this chapter, the impact on individual officers is described, as are the implications for police organisations in the best ways of supporting staff.

The Study

Design. An age stratified sample of officers above the rank of probationer, and up to and including chief inspector was obtained from different occupational groups within the police (officers in traffic; mobile and foot patrol; firearms; the female and child unit; scenes of crime officers; the CID; and the support unit). Questionnaires covering many aspects of the experience of critical incidents, and aspects of occupational stress, were distributed and returned anonymously. Through this, the nature of critical incidents the officers had experienced and what was memorable or problematic about them were obtained.

The instrument. Respondents were asked if they could describe a single critical incident which was most memorable for them from any time during their police career. The section of the questionnaire was introduced as: "*In contrast to more routine police work, this final section is about serious work incidents you have attended which are memorable or significant for you. Sometimes these incidents are called traumatic. In asking you to recount one of these which may still bother you, we apologise in advance for any upset this may cause you. Bringing memories like this to mind can sometimes be quite upsetting for a short while, but perhaps you will also find the opportunity to write about it useful. You are reminded of the organisation's welfare support which is available for you to use should you wish*".

It was thought important to leave it open to the officers to describe which incidents they found memorable and significant and to not restrict their choice, for example, by asking if they had experienced any from a list of "typical" critical incidents. The question was asked in two different ways (fifty per cent of the sample each). In one form, post trauma symptoms were described in order to help the officer identify what types of incidents were being asked about, as follows: ". . . *even although it might have happened a while ago, you might find that thoughts about it, or quite clear images of it, can come to mind easily, at times spontaneously, or when you come across reminders of it. You might also find that you feel slightly disturbed for some reason when you do think about it.*".

In the second question format, respondents were simply asked to think of one incident which 'stood out' for them, as follows: ". . . *one particular incident at work which stands out most for you, regardless of how long ago or recently it happened*". It was found that those who were given the first question (which described typical post trauma reactions) reported a slightly higher mean number of total symptoms compared with those who were given the second question (which did not describe symptoms), but both forms of the question produced similar types and numbers of incidents. Importantly, the difference was not statistically significant. This is interesting in itself in terms of whether one can suggest symptoms to those completing questionnaires. It would appear that the effect is slight.

It is recognised that asking respondents to do this could prove distressing. Throughout the questionnaire and in covering letters, officers were encouraged to contact the Police Occupational Health and Welfare Unit should they experience any distress and were generally reminded of the support available for them. It is worth mentioning that research on disclosure suggests that writing about a significant experience can be distressing temporarily, although helpful and stress alleviating in the longer term (Duncan, Thomson & Sheffield, 1997).

The level of post trauma symptoms was measured using two instruments. The Revised Impact of Event Scale was used for the first two occupational groups sampled, and the Modified PTSD Symptom Scale (MPSS, Coffey, Dansky, Falsetti, Saladin & Brady, 1998) was used for all other groups. The use of the second type of instrument was in order to co-ordinate data collection with that being undertaken in another collaborating police organisation and also to obtain a measure of the frequency *and* the severity of symptoms, as the MPSS provides.

The sample. In total 1245 questionnaires were distributed and 612 completed responses were returned (49.1%). All 612 completed most of the questionnaire, 458 of the sample provided some comment on critical incidents, and 426 described incidents which could be content analysed (see Table 1). Thirty stated that "none stand out" or "none have caused any difficulty".

Twenty nine (n = 29) gave no description of the incident but provided other information – whether a description of the memorable aspects, when it occurred, and/or a rating of the post trauma symptoms associated with this incident. The reasons for this vary. It must be acknowledged that some would find it upsetting to describe particular incidents, and some respondents made this comment in their responses. Some also stated that they wished to ensure anonymity and which may have been compromised by their description of a particularly unusual incident.

Almost three quarters of the incidents described, unsurprisingly, were various forms and causes of death (including murder, accidental death, the death of a child or baby, or a suicide). It is of particular interest for present purposes that almost a third of the deaths described were the result of a road traffic accident (RTA), rendering RTAs as the largest single category of memorable critical incident. The multiple casualties resulting from the Lockerbie Disaster of December 1988 (causing 270 fatalities), and from the crash of the RAF Chinook helicopter on the Mull of Kintyre in June 1994 (causing 29 fatalities) were also frequently described.

With the information in Table 1 as background, the data for the present chapter is drawn from the sub-set of 96 who described a RTA. In this group, ten were female and 86 male; and a quarter (n = 23) were of supervisory rank. The mean length of service is 17 years (range 1.5 to 32 years) and the mean age was 38.4 years (25 to 54 years). The length of service and age of those describing RTAs was no different than the overall sample from which this sub-group was drawn. It is conceivable that repeated exposure

Table 1. What types of incidents did the respondents describe as memorable?

nature of incident	n
death	305 (71.5%)
various	129
road traffic accident	96
Lockerbie	60
Kintyre	20
threat	87 (20.4%)
personal threat	77
firearms	6
prolonged danger	4
abuse or cruelty	19 (4.4%)
direct	14
secondary sources (e.g. interview)	5
workplace morale issues	12 (2.8%)
complaint from public or supervisor	11
perceived workplace harassment	1
Total	426* (100%)

*This includes 3 others not categorised to protect the anonymity of respondent.

to the human sequelae of road accidents might "toughen" officers assigned to the traffic department, and hence they may not report them as significant, but 60% of the RTAs were described by traffic officers. While this is not surprising given their relatively high exposure, it does tend to argue against the idea that higher exposure "toughens" officers and reduces the impact.

How Memorable were the Incidents?

The fact that officers were asked about incidents that had taken place at any time during their career meant that respondents described accidents which had happened from two weeks to, in one example, twenty-five years previously. The mean length of time since the accident was 5.6 years. No significant relationship with post trauma symptoms was found between the length of service, or the age of the respondents. The fact that road accidents were recalled from all times during the length of service indicates that the passage of time does not necessarily reduce how memorable it is, or potentially its impact.

This would suggest that many other aspects of the incident or the person, and his or her circumstances, influence the degree to which an incident is associated with higher symptoms. Of the set of 96 accidents which were described, almost all respondents acknowledged that the incident was very easily brought to mind (74, 97%) and that it was recalled vividly (73, 95%). Three quarters (57, 74%) recalled experiencing a high degree of distress *at the time* of the incident.

It would appear, then, that significant incidents, such as these are not easily forgotten, and indeed one officer stated they recalled, "*the full incident . . . every aspect is very vivid, and always will be.*" Some appear to have this vivid recall and, one could say that the officers are "carrying" these memories around with them as they attend further accidents. This may pose the question of a possible interaction between previous experiences and current exposure to new or similar incidents. When considering that all these 96 incidents were remembered quite clearly, it is surprising that more are not associated with higher levels of post trauma symptoms. Indeed, 34 of the 96 respondents (35%) reported no symptoms at all.

What was Particularly Significant About the Memorable RTAs?

In order not to make assumptions about what was problematic about the incidents or why they were particularly memorable, respondents were specifically asked about that. Frequently this concerned the officer relating to the victims because of their similarity to their own personal circumstances, for example, ". . . the personal circumstances of the couple were so close to my own that I could easily see myself in their position." The personal meaning of an incident is no more acute than when a fellow officer is involved. It is inevitable that police officers will attend a fatal or serious accident involving a colleague who may be well known to them. This particular circumstance presents great difficulty for them and also poses a direct threat to the sense of invulnerability which the officer may feel in his or her role. In one instance the sight of the police uniform on the body was deeply problematic for the respondent. The nature and the extent of injuries were also easily recalled, for example, ". . . the sensation of a broken skull and the worry of what you will find when undressing the dead body." Further memorable aspects were the reactions of the people involved, for example, the reaction of a family when told of the death, or the bravery of the survivors and the youth or innocence of the deceased. Feelings of uselessness or guilt were also expressed when resuscitation failed at the scene, or the injured person died soon after the officer's arrival.

Which Incidents Were Associated With High Post Trauma Symptoms?

Eleven of the 96 incidents were associated with particularly high levels of post trauma symptoms, and they occurred between four months and twenty five years previously. Six were associated with scores above the clinical cut-off suggesting the existence of PTSD, and a further five were associated with 'high' scores (that is those within the quartile just below the cut-off level). The following is a description of the memorable characteristics of these particular incidents.

In one incident, the occupant of a car died while still being spoken to by the emergency services. This produced feelings in the officer that something more could have been done to save him. Two others involved the death of children: in one, two children were killed by a truck, resulting in the officer feeling extremely upset and shocked and then guilty about their own "inadequacy" at not being "in control" of their own emotions. In another, the officer was first on the scene of two children who were killed in a bus accident. Back up from other services was felt by him to be slow, resulting in feelings of anger and a sense of being let down by colleagues.

Included in this group is one involving a near accident in which the officer felt he was going to be killed. In this instance it was not only the shock of the near accident which made the incident memorable and problematic, but also the reaction of the other emergency workers at the scene who treated the situation as a joke.

Lengthy exposure to an extremely unpleasant scene was also, as might be expected, associated with higher symptoms. In one, the officer had to remain at the accident site while the accident investigation team completed their work, and also accompany the body to the mortuary and attend the post mortem.

It is well known that the untimely death of a child is problematic for all emergency workers, as it was for this group. In these eleven particularly difficult incidents, three were the deaths of children.

Protracted contact with a very damaged body was problematic, as was handling it, for example, to carry out an identification. In Scotland, not only do the police accompany the body to the mortuary, but in some jurisdictions will have to strip the body to prepare it for the post-mortem. Often they are required to take notes during the post-mortem. It is not necessary, procedurally, to have the same officers carry out all these tasks, although it is preferable for reasons of continuity. Rotation or relief of officers might go some way to reducing exposure to these particularly horrific incidents. Care needs to be taken here, however. Completing a task and seeing it through from start to finish is often helpful psychologically, so the way an officer is relieved from a duty and the explanation given to him or her is important if the officer is to understand that it is not a criticism of their performance.

Other incidents were associated with high scores. In one, a very young child slipped and fell under a vehicle having let go of his mother's hand. Another was a multiple fatality, which also required the officer to accompany the bodies to the mortuary. In another the car had burst into flames after hitting a lamp post burning the young occupant who, in a highly disfigured state, had to be searched in order to identify him. In yet another highly memorable incident, which clearly had significance to the organisation as a whole, a police officer was killed in an RTA.

Is the Occupational Context Important?

It is evident from this that simple exposure to horrific scenes is not the sole contributor to making an incident memorable and its being associated with symptoms of post trauma. Rather the personal meaning the officer attributes to the incident is important. Of particular interest when considering the wider context is that a sense of being let down or unsupported by colleagues or the organisation appears to be particularly difficult.

Other measures obtained through the questionnaire were coping measures and sources of occupational stress. Two should be mentioned here. Amongst other ways of coping, respondents were asked to rate how helpful they found "acknowledgement by a supervisor that it was a significant incident" in their coming to terms with the incident. The need to have the significance of the incident recognised by supervisors was found to be particularly important, and receiving such recognition bore an inverse relationship to the level of post trauma symptoms. As confirmation of the value placed on good management and support, a sense in day to day work that support and good communication was not forthcoming from supervisors, was also significantly associated with higher post trauma symptoms. Both of these measures correlated significantly with post trauma symptoms ($r = .-26, p < .01$, n = 82; and $r = .24, p < .01$, n = 81 respectively). The sample sizes are accounted for by the different measures of post trauma symptoms used, as explained above.

These relationships with occupational variables underline the importance of the *context* within which the incidents happen and the importance of support and recognition during and after an incident. A casual, harsh or off-hand approach from supervisors following a significant incident appears to be related to poorer long term psychological management of the incident in officers.

The Provision of Critical Incident Stress Debriefing (CISD) and Other Forms of Post Incident Care

Particular aspects of incidents seem to strike officers, and these seem to be important to the maintenance of emotionally charged recollections. While there are consistent and meaningful themes, it is certainly the case that even highly similar incidents do not strike all officers in exactly the same way, with the same health outcomes. This, of course, presents the challenge for the appropriate planning of post incident care for individuals. It would be simpler if reactions were predictable.

Considerable debate exists currently about the efficacy or even advisability of providing Critical Incident Stress Debriefing (CISD) following potentially traumatic incidents. It should be noted that the practice of CISD started in this police organisation in May 1994, so only 61 of the incidents described would have occurred within this time frame. Of these 61, ten reported having participated in a CISD following the incident they described, and 45 had not (13 missing data). This means that a relatively low number participated in a CISD since this form of support would have been available. When asked if they would have wanted to participate in a CISD had it been offered, 70 answered this question. It is interesting that 73% (51) said they would not.

Many of the comments of those who participated are positive, reflecting that they found it helpful to be able to express feelings and recognise that others feel the same. The following are typical statements: *"It was useful for officers to discuss feelings, to find out that I was not alone"*; *"Talking about an incident of this nature to anybody is useful"*; *"To learn that others felt as I did and sometimes worse"; and "It was good to hear different feelings and responses from the other personnel at the incident"*. As an interesting reflection of the police occupational culture, one said, *"I was able to discuss the incident and express my feeling without having to worry what was been said behind my back"*. Other comments were less positive, for example that debriefing was less useful if *"no-one volunteered their feelings first"*; and another said: *"It doesn't help you forget"*.

Whatever effect CISD may have on the level of psychological distress, if any, it does allow sharing of feelings and perceptions, which some clearly find helpful. It also allows education about the possible short and longer term effects of attending critical incidents, and dissemination of information about further psychological assistance. Within the police context both of these are positive features.

The problem of how to provide psychological and social support services which are acceptable to employees is particularly acute within the police service. When asked about their willingness to use such services, 57 (of the sub-sample of 96) provided answers. Although eleven said they would be quite happy to if necessary, 30 said they feared a lack of confidentiality and the possible effect that help-seeking might have on promotion and their image within the organisation.

Conclusion

Road traffic accidents clearly have the potential to give rise to significant levels of post trauma symptoms and the fact of their "everyday" nature should not suggest that they are managed easily. It would appear, however, that the majority of officers manage the work well without long term psychological harm. No information is available, however, from these data, on the number of officers who have not overcome the impact of critical incidents and who may temporarily be off work, or even retired from the service on grounds of psychological ill health. All the respondents in this sample were currently working, and even the eleven per cent who were experiencing considerable post trauma symptoms were at work. Officers demonstrably carry out acts of bravery, and manifest tremendous personal resilience to quite horrifying duties. The effects of very demanding work are, in some instances, never forgotten but may become part of the person's psychic constitution, while not preventing their ability to work. The effect of this on day to day functioning is an important question and its answer depends on a longitudinal analysis of the longer term impact on psychological well-being and work practices.

The support of officers needs to be part of the fabric of the organisation through the provision of health and welfare services, and support should also be provided informally and mutually through day to day interactions. The appreciation and support conveyed to the officer by an immediate supervisor is of the greatest importance in how the incident is dealt with psychologically, a fact which has been found in much of our other work (Mitchell, Munro, Thomson & Jackson, 1997; Mitchell, Cowan, Hamilton, Jackson & Speed, 1998; Mitchell, Stevenson & Poole, 1999).

Police officers' efforts to deal with this work should not, and cannot go unrecognised and perhaps a good supportive managerial structure is the best protection that can be offered to them. While such strategies as CISD demonstrate that the organisation "cares", a good manager provides evidence of this implicitly, every day.

Acknowledgements

Sincere thanks are due to the police officers who took part and to the Chief Constable for allowing the project to be carried out. The data were collected for a Health and Safety Executive project 3715/R54.069, *Managing post incident reactions in the police service* (Mitchell et al. 1999). The research assistance of Dr Kathryn Young and Rona Hamilton in this project is acknowledged.

References

Coffey, S. F., Dansky, B. S., Falsetti, S. A., Saladin, M. E. & Brady, K. T. (1998) Screening for PTSD in a substance abuse sample: Psychometric properties of a modified version of PTSD Symptom Scale Self-Report. *Journal of Traumatic Stress, 11(2), 393–399.*

Duncan, E., Thomson, K. & Sheffield, D. (1997) *Short-term health effects from written disclosure of real versus imagined traumatic events.* Fifth European Congress of Psychology. ISBN 0950457094

Hetherington, Munro, A. & Mitchell, M. (1997) At the Scene: Road accidents and the police. In Mitchell, M. (Ed.) *The Aftermath of Road Accidents: Psychological, Social and Legal consequences.* Routledge: London.

Mitchell, M., Munro, A., Thomson, D. & Jackson, J. (1997) *Exposing police probationers to sudden death.* Home Office Police Policy Directorate: London.

Mitchell, M., Cowan, M., Hamilton, R., Jackson, J. & Speed, E. (1998) *Facing Violence: Assessing the support and training requirements for police constables in Scotland.* Central Research Unit. Scottish Office: Edinburgh. ISBN 0 748 6936 4

Mitchell, M., Stevenson, K. & Poole, D. (1999) *Managing post incident reactions in the police service.* Health and Safety Executive Contract Research Report: London.

10

The Hidden Victims of Disasters and Vehicular Accidents: The Problem and Recommended Solutions

JEFFREY T. MITCHELL, Ph.D., CTS

University of Maryland and President, International Critical Incident Stress Foundation (ICISF)

GEORGE S. EVERLY, JR., PhD., CTS

Johns Hopkins University and Loyola College, Maryland

DOUGLAS J. MITCHELL, MPA

Lt. Retired Fire Department, New York, Certified Instructor for ICISF

The Problem

Case 1: In the mid 1970's a young firefighter /paramedic, who was on his way home from work late one night, came upon a horrific auto accident. The driver of a small car had crashed into the rear of a truck carrying pipes to a construction site. One of the pipes slid across the hood of the car, punctured the windshield and impaled a young woman in the passenger seat. When he approached the accident to assess the injured woman, he was shocked to find a twenty year old girl dressed in a brilliant white wedding gown. The gown was covered with blood and the victim was obviously dead. The pipe had gone through the woman's heart. The girl's new husband was in a drunken state and added to the chaos of the moment by punching the off duty rescuer in his left ear. The scene ended with police officers arresting the out of control husband as the extrication crew removed the body of his new wife from the car. For many months the firefighter could not get the image of the young woman in the wedding dress out of his mind. Every time he saw a wedding gown on display in a store, his mind replayed the image of the dead young woman impaled on a pipe in the small car.

Case 2: In New York City several years ago. Fire fighters were called to the scene of a motor vehicle fire on a busy highway. Upon arrival, a hose line was placed in operation to extinguish the fire. As the fire was extinguished, a drunk driver struck the rear of the fire apparatus where a fire fighter had been standing directing traffic. The impact severed the firefighters two legs and forced his body under the fire apparatus. He died at the scene in the arms of his fellow firefighters. They suffered powerful grief reactions and traumatic stress symptoms. No one present that day has been able to forget the details of the incident. Their grief and trauma was intensified when the drunk driver was so vigorously defended in a court of law. It was hard for them to understand why their friend had to die while doing something to help someone else.

The young firefighter's experience described in Case 1 and the reactions of the firefighters in Case 2 are not isolated nor are they unique. Many thousands of police officers, firefighters, paramedics and other first response and disaster personnel have experienced similar and even more severe psychological reactions to the traumatic events they encounter in the normal course of their everyday emergency services work.

Exposure to human tragedies of all types including small and large disasters, violence, auto accidents, terrorism, hurricanes, tornadoes, cyclones, earthquakes, floods, injuries and disease produces havoc in the lives of many of those who respond to help others. The effects of the forces of nature or of human beings raging out of control has been widely chronicled in both print and electronic media.

Numerous studies demonstrate that emergency personnel and disaster workers are vulnerable to work stress. For example, 42 rescuers were studied for a year after the San Diego air crash in 1978. Only 5 of the 42 personnel had any previous counseling before the disaster. One year after the disaster 13 (31 percent) were in counseling (Colen, 1979). In the United Kingdom, a researcher and ambulance officer, Tristan Ravenscroft, studied 1420 personnel in the London Ambulance Service (LAS) and concluded that job stress was the main reason for sickness in LAS staff. He reports that 97% of surveyed staff felt that stress was their main problem. He concluded that "… no less than 15% of LAS front-line staff self reported symptoms which crossed the threshold for acute Post Traumatic Stress Disorder (PTSD).

In addition, the inclusion for control purposes, of the 60 question version of the General Health Questionnaire showed that no less than 52% of the LAS staff were suffering from recent mental disturbance (or high levels of stress)." (Ravenscroft 1994, p. 35).

One study of LAS, concluded that "51% could not "switch off" and took work problems home with them. 34% said they often felt anxious or depressed at work. A quarter found their sleep disturbed by work pressures. 26% said that things were getting on top of them and 29% suffered from high blood pressure or frequent headaches. All these are generally recognized stress symptoms." (NUPE Briefing, 1991, p. 3).

Another group of LAS researchers randomly selected 40 personnel to determine if they were stressed by the types of calls they handled. An impressive 60% could be classified as having stress responses and 17% of the personnel were in the severe category of symptoms on the General Health Questionnaire and on the Impact of Event Scale (Thompson & Suzuki, 1991).

Similar findings have been noted in the United States and in Australia. Mitchell (1985) found 86.9% of 360 emergency workers stated that "they had been emotionally and physically affected by their work at one or more emergency events." Robinson (1994) performed an extensive study of 1380 ambulance officers and 1223 of their significant others. Robinson (1994, p.3) concluded, "A disturbing finding is that 65% of Officers report that they currently experience trauma reactions as a result of prior ambulance jobs [calls]. Seventeen percent report pervasive, strong response. Though this study does not define staff with Post-Traumatic Stress Disorder, the findings suggest that a high incidence exists."

Similar studies on clinical health care workers in hospitals are in concert with the findings for fire fighters, paramedics and police officers. Clinical health care staff in one study discussed their level of exposure to traumatizing events. 62% said that they had been exposed to a significant traumatic stress in their workplace.

In a study of Post Traumatic Stress Disorder (PTSD) in urban firefighters, Corneil (1993) confirmed a dose-response effect of exposure to a traumatic event and the prediction of PTSD. The PTSD rate among 641 Toronto firefighters was 16.2%. This prevalence rate is similar to the prevalence rate in Vietnam veterans and much higher than the prevalence of PTSD in the general population, about 1.97% (Helzer and others, 1987).

A recent feature which appeared on the popular MSNBC American television show indicated that after the Oklahoma City bombing there has been a drastic increase in domestic violence involving Oklahoma City police officers. The report also cited a 300% increase in divorce rate among member of the Oklahoma City Fire Department (Williams, 1998).

In 1983, line-of-duty deaths, serious line-of-duty injuries to emergency workers, death of children, deaths of adults, gory sights and sounds, violence against children, multi-casualty/mass casualty incidents, victims known to the rescuers, incidents involving severe personal threat to the emergency worker and prolonged operational events which end in a loss of life or a mission failure were considered to be the most highly stressful experiences for emergency personnel (Mitchell, 1983). A recent study of the duty related stressors, in firefighters and paramedics confirms this list of highly stressful experiences for emergency workers and adds insight into the factors which may intensify negative experiences for these front line workers. For example, the age of the victims being treated by rescue personnel has much to do with the intensity of the emotional response of emergency personnel (Beaton, et al., 1998)

The huge quantity of disastrous auto accidents throughout the world makes it virtually impossible for emergency response personnel to avoid exposure to items on the above lists such as gory sights and sounds, injury, death, sorrow, loss grief and pain. The potential for disruption to the lives of emergency operations personnel is demonstrated by fatal highway statistics alone. For example, in 1996 the US Department of Transportation's National Highway Traffic Safety Administration reported that police statistics indicate that almost 7 million motor vehicle accidents occurred in the United States. These accidents took a staggering toll of roughly 42,000 killed and produced 3.5 million injuries. The statistics also indicate that for 1996 one hundred and fifteen people died each day, which translates into one death for every 13 minutes of each day! Additionally, motor vehicle accidents were found to be the leading cause of death for every age group from six years of age through twenty-seven years of age.

In the Mind of the Rescuer

The psychological and physical impact of a traumatic event for emergency services personnel and other disaster workers is often intensified by a number of important factors. For example the rescuer's age, experience, status in the group and success or failure of activity in a specific mission can be crucial in lowering, or intensifying stress reactions. The mental view of the world which is held by the rescuer before, during and after the traumatic experience can alter the course of recovery from the trauma. For instance, if rescuers believe that they managed the job according to their training and skill level, they will recover faster psychologically than if they believe (even if their perception is inaccurate) that they made a mistake in managing the job. This is especially so if someone has been injured during the mission.

We will explore some other factors which might influence the impact of a traumatic stress on the emergency personnel. For people in the emergency services professions, accidents which produce personal injuries that require long term physical therapy and rehabilitation work can sometimes be viewed as indicators of personal incompetence, inefficiency or stupidity. They can be unusually harsh in their self evaluations and may develop depression as a result. This obviously complicates their recovery and ability to resume their work. Emergency personnel also experience a heightened sense of personal vulnerability when they see one of their own seriously injured at the scene. They might then hesitate to use a certain piece of equipment or to perform certain tasks.

Caregivers such as paramedics can occasionally become emotionally affected by seeing the suffering of others. Frequently strong bonds are developed between victims of motor vehicle accidents or disasters and their rescuers during prolonged extrication operations to free the trapped occupants from the mangled wreckage. When a victim expires, there is a deep sense of failure and loss on the part of the emergency service workers. They blame themselves for the failure. This, at times, results in excessive, uncontrollable anger. They may compare or contrast the plight of others to their own experiences. They may feel sympathy, survivor guilt, discomfort, anxiety, fear for the safety of their own loved ones and a host of other emotions. Court testimony may stir these emotions further and cause the emergency services worker to be adversely affected in court or later at work or home.

In the United States, outside the major metropolitan areas, the majority of rescue personnel render their services in volunteer fire and rescue departments. Many, therefore, work in their own communities and neighborhoods. They are frequently called on to assist people who are known to them. Sometimes it is a neighbor or friend who requires assistance. In some instances, the fire service is called to scenes in which their family members are involved. There are many stories told of fire fighters, paramedics and police officers responding to accidents that involve alcohol or drugs and their own children.

Distressing events involving pediatrics are routinely faced by the emergency forces. These can be among the most stress producing incidents for the emergency responders. Emergency responders relate these events to their own children or to important children in their lives. As a direct result they may become over-protective and hyper-vigilant of their children and other family members.

When multiple casualties are encountered during vehicular accidents or disasters, some emergency personnel have reported flashbacks and intrusive images for several weeks. The pressures associated with a multiple casualty incident are extreme. Later when they respond to other accidents involving groups of people they often report vivid memories of the previous event. More recent accident situations may serve as a trigger to make them feel that they are back at the original accident.

Other factors which play a role in the intensity of stress encountered by emergency personnel are their personality, their training, administrative support, level of supervision, group cohesion, views held by the media and the public about their work, gratitude from their communities, a sense of job satisfaction and accomplishment and a feeling of job mastery. Specific or unusual circumstances connected with the event may also be very distressing. One fire fighter paramedic, for instance, found a deceased eight year old child victim of a mass shooting incident who was wearing the exact same T-shirt that his son had on when the firefighter left for work that morning. He was quickly overcome by emotion at the scene since he had personalized the victim and thought of the dead child as if he were his own son.

Not all emergency services events are likely to produce strong reactions in emergency personnel. Only those which are "critical incidents" are likely to disturb and distress. A critical incident is one that has unusual emotional intensity associated with it. The emotional content can be so strong in a critical incident that it overwhelms the usual coping mechanisms and causes the personnel to dysfunction at the scene or later at home or work.

Routine events almost never cause intense distress among emergency workers. A typical list of disturbing significant critical incidents would include line-of-duty deaths, line-of-duty serious injuries, suicides of emergency personnel, mass casualty disasters or multiple casualty events, the killing or wounding of an innocent person in the performance of one's routine duties, police shootings, significant events involving children, events with considerable threat to the responders, prolonged incidents with negative outcomes, and any other severe distressing incident.

The Symptoms

Emergency responders can be effected physically, cognitively, behaviorally, and emotionally by the traumatic events they encounter. If the physical stress is strong enough, it may result in the death of a fire fighter. Statistics indicate that the primary cause of line of duty death for fire fighters is heart attack, secondary to stress. If the stress does not kill the individual, then other physical ailments may occur. Some of these may be ulcers, stomach digestive disorders, high blood pressure, and other psychologically generated illnesses.

A rescue person must be capable of making split second decisions that affect life and death situations. Stress may inhibit these individuals in their decision making process. There can also be an impairment of their mental capabilities especially higher cognitive functions. Diminished cognitive functions may, on occasion, adversely affect the entire field operation.

Emergency Services personnel may experience a change in behavior after a stressful event. Any major change in behavior should be a signal that something may be wrong. Supervisors should know their personnel well enough to identify when a significant change in behavior has occurred. Someone, who was normally quiet and reserved prior to a critical incident and is somewhat boisterous after the incident, should be seen as a person who may be exhibiting signals of distress in the aftermath of a critical incident.

Crying spells, intensifying depression, sleeplessness, mood, swings, angry outbursts, frustration with small tasks, a sense of helplessness, feelings of hopelessness and other signs of emotional distress may develop after emergency service responders engage rescue operations.

It should be noted that the symptoms discussed in the preceding paragraphs are a dramatically shortened list for the purpose of citing examples alone. Practically any cognitive, physical, emotional and behavioral symptom is possible after a traumatic event and the list could literally be pages long, Certainly the classic signs and symptoms of Post Traumatic Stress Disorder (PTSD), intrusion, avoidance and arousal, are not uncommon among emergency personnel.

The four main effects of stress (cognitive, physical, emotional and behavioral) on the emergency service personnel can occur immediately, may be delayed, or can become cumulative over time. In the event that they occur immediately, they may result in a great deal of embarrassment to the emergency worker, especially if emotional reactions occur in the presence of their co-workers. They fear that they will be perceived as weak or crazy and, therefore, they attempt to hide the symptoms of distress. Such covering behavior often leads to delays in the initiation of appropriate crisis intervention tactics that can be helpful in mitigating or resolving stress reactions before they take hold.

Emergency workers may experience delayed reactions to stressful events. The need to complete the operations causes many to deliberately suppress their immediate feelings. Suppressed feelings often come to the surface at inopportune and unexpected times. There may be enough time between the actual event and the reaction that the worker cannot understand the relationship between the two experiences. This may result in a feeling of uniqueness or a feeling of being out of control. "Why is this happening to me?" "Why aren't the others feeling this way also?" "Why is it happening now after so much time has passed?"

Finally, the stress reactions may accumulate over time. There may be a considerable pile-up effect of the emergency service worker's stressful work environment. Some personnel get an unusual number of stressful responses within a very short period of time, or several bad experiences in a row. Cumulated stress can explode into obvious and painful symptoms or its symptoms may grow gradually as time passes. The effects of cumulative stress show up then as gradual deterioration in health and performance and changes in relationship and personality.

For hundreds of years, there had been very little thought given to how emergency responders dealt with these stressful events. It was commonly thought that their technical training was enough to carry them through the tough times. It was falsely believed that they were invulnerable to the effects of stress. More and more, the recent literature indicates that emergency personnel are, in fact, vulnerable to the normal stress reactions, encountered by all other people. And, if appropriate steps are not taken to manage distress early enough, emergency personnel may develop PTSD. There seems to be a growing acceptance that traumatic stress reactions, called "critical incident stress" and the pathological condition of PTSD exists and that there are many prevention strategies and treatments available under the care and direction of professional mental health practitioners (Mitchell, 1985; Mitchell & Bray, 1990; Everly & Mitchell, 1997).

The Recommended Solutions

Crisis Intervention for Emergency Personnel

The previous pages of this chapter have attempted to provide the reader with an overview of the psychological toll that is extracted upon emergency personnel and disaster workers as a result of their work at repeated motor vehicle accidents and other tragedies. Given that it appears clear that rescuers work in a "high risk environment for psychological distress and disability, the issue of intervention becomes relevant. What steps are being taken to prevent and mitigate the adverse impact of activities at first response situations upon rescue personnel? A structured, organized and comprehensive approach to crisis intervention is emerging from the "high risk" occupational groups such as emergency personnel. This approach is called Critical Incident Stress Management (CISM) (Everly & Mitchell, 1997; Flannery, 1998) and is a result of the early work of Mitchell (1983). But the CISM approach is conceptually grounded in the pioneering formulations of Caplan (1964) as they pertain to prevention.

Critical Incident Stress Management (CISM) represents a powerful, yet cost effective approach to crisis response (Everly, Boyle, & Lating, in press; Everly, Flannery, & Mitchell, in press; Flannery, 1998; Everly & Mitchell, 1997) which unfortunately is often misrepresented and misunderstood. There exists numerous "debriefing models and other esoteric crisis interventions with which CISM is often confused. Let us attempt to clarify the CISM approach."

What is CISM? CISM is a comprehensive, integrative, multi-component crisis intervention system. CISM is considered comprehensive because it consists of multiple crisis intervention components which functionally span the entire temporal spectrum of a crisis. CISM interventions range from the pre-crisis phase through the acute crisis phase and into the post-crisis phase. CISM is also considered comprehensive in that it consists of interventions which may be applied to individuals, small functional groups, large groups, families, organizations, and even communities. The 7 core components of CISM are defined below and summarized in Table 1.

1. Pre-crisis preparation. This includes stress management education, stress resistance, mental preparedness and crisis mitigation training for both individuals and organizations.
2. Disaster services. These support services have been developed for large scale incidents' and they include school and community support programs demobilizations services, informational briefings, "town meetings", and staff advisement services.
3. Defusing. This is a 3-phase, structured small group discussion provided within hours of a crisis for purposes of assessment triaging, and acute symptom mitigation.
4. Critical Incident Stress Debriefing (CISD) refers to the "Mitchell model" or "ICISF model" (Mitchell & Everly, 1996) which is a 7-phase, structured group discussion, usually provided 1 to 10 days post-crisis (although in mass disasters may be used 3 weeks or more post-incident). The CISD is designed to mitigate acute symptoms, assess the need for follow-up, and if possible, provide a sense of post-crisis psychological closure.
5. One-on-one crisis intervention/counseling or psychological support throughout the full range of the crisis spectrum. This is the most frequently used of CISM interventions. Typically, this form of intervention consists of 1 to 3 contacts with an individual who is in crisis. Each contact may last 15 minutes to more than 2 hours, depending upon the nature and severity of the crisis.

Table 1. Critical Inident Stress Management (CISM): The Seven Core Components

Intervention	Timing	Activation	Goals	Format
1. Pre-crisis preparation	Pre-crisis phase	Anticipation of crisis	Set expectations. Improve coping.	Groups/Orgs.
2. Individual crisis intervention (1: 1)	Anytime. Anywhere	Symptom driven	Symptom mitigation Return to function, if possible. Referral, if needed Stress management	Individuals
Large Groups: 3a. Demobilizations & Staff Consult. (rescuers); 3b. Group Info. Briefing for schools, businesses and large civilian	Shift disengagement; or Anytime post crisis	Event driven	To inform, and consult To allow for psychological decompression Stress management Symptom mitigation	Large groups Organizations
4. Defusing	Post-crisis (within 12hrs.)	Usually symptoms driven	Possible closure. Triage	Small groups.
5. Critical Incident Stress Debriefing (CISD)	Post-crisis 1 to 10 days; At 3–4 weeks for mass disasters.	Usually symptom driven Can be event driven.	Facilitate psychological closure. Symptom mitigation Triage	Small groups
Systems: 6a. Family CISM; 6b. Organizational Consultation.	Anytime.	Either symptom driven or event driven	Foster support, communications. Symptom mitigation. Closure, if possible Referral, if needed.	Families Organizations
Family. 7. Follow-up; Referral	Anytime	Usually symptom driven	Assess mental status. Access higher level of care	Individual

6. Family crisis intervention, as well as organizational consultation.
7. Follow-up and referral mechanisms for assessment and treatment if necessary.

Specific guidelines for these interventions may be found in Mitchell & Everly (1996) and Everly & Mitchell (1997). While originally designed for the needs of emergency response personnel, the reader will note the general applicability to crisis and disaster situations for all individuals, not just emergency personnel. Indeed, CISM has been adopted by school systems, employee assistance organizations, many airlines, hospitals, the military, as well as, many fire departments, police departments, the Federal Bureau of Investigation, the United States Marshals Service, the United States Secret Service, the Bureau of Alcohol, Tobacco & Firearms, to name just a few. The comprehensive CISM program is summarized in Table 1.

As one would never attempt to play a round of golf with only one golf club, one would not attempt the complex task of intervention within a crisis or disaster with only one crisis intervention technology. As crisis intervention, generically, and CISM, specifically, represent a sub-specialty within behavioral health, one should not attempt application without adequate and specific training. CISM is not psychotherapy, nor a substitute for psychotherapy. CISM is a form of psychological "first aid".

As noted earlier, CISM represents an integrated, multi-component crisis intervention system. This system's approach underscores the importance of using multiple interventions combined in such a manner as to yield maximum impact to achieve the goal of crisis stabilization and symptom mitigation. Although in evidence since 1983 (Mitchell, 1983), this concept is commonly misunderstood as evidenced by a recent article by Snellgrove (1998) who argues that the CISD group intervention should not be a stand alone intervention. This point has, frankly, never been in contention. The CISD intervention has always been conceived of as one component within a larger functional intervention framework. Admittedly, some of the confusion surrounding this point was engendered by virtue of the fact that in earlier expositions, the term CISD was used to denote the generic and overarching umbrella program/system, while the term "formal CISD" was used to denote the specific 7 phase group discussion process. The term CISM was later used to replace the generic CISD and serve as the overarching umbrella program/system as noted in Table 1 (see Everly & Mitchell, 1997).

The effectiveness of CISM programs has been empirically validated through thoughtful qualitative analyses, as well as through controlled investigations, and even meta-analyses (Everly, Boyle & Lating, in press; Flannery,

1998; Everly & Mitchell, 1997; Everly & Boyle, 1997; Mitchell & Everly, in press; Everly, Flannery & Mitchell, in press; Dyregrov, 1997), unfortunately this is fact often overlooked (e.g., see Snellgrove, 1998).

Similarly, there is a misconception that evidence exists to suggest that CISD/CISM has proved harmful to its recipients (e.g., see Snellgrove, 1998), this is a misrepresentation of the extant data. There is no extant evidence that the "Mitchell model" CISD, or the CISM system has proven harmful! The investigations that are frequently cited to suggest such an adverse effect simply did not use the CISD of CISM system as prescribed, a fact that is too often ignored (e.g., see Snellgrove, 1998).

In sum, no one CISM intervention is designed to stand alone, not even the widely used CISD. Efforts to implement and evaluate CISM must be programmatic, not unidimensional (Mitchell & Everly, in press). While the CISM approach to crisis intervention is continuing to evolve, as should any worthwhile endeavor, current investigations have clearly demonstrated its value as a tool to reduce human suffering. Future research should focus upon ways in which the CISM process can be made even more effective to those in crisis.

While the roots of CISM can be found in the emergency services professions dating back to the late 1970's, CISM is now becoming a "standard of care" in many schools, communities, industries, and organizations well outside the field of emergency services (Everly & Mitchell, 1997).

References

Beaton, R. Murphy, S. Johnson, C, Pike, K. & Corneil, W. (1998). Exposure to duty-related incident stressors in urban firefighters and paramedics. *Journal of Traumatic Stress, 11*(4), 821–828.

Caplan, G. (1964). *Principles or Preventive Psychiatry*. NY: Basic Books.

Colen, B. D. (1979). Aircrash rescue-workers also victims psychiatrist says. *Washington Post*, July 9, 1979.

Corneil, D. W. (1993). *Prevalence of Post Traumatic stress disorders in a metropolitan fire department*. Unpublished doctoral dissertation. The Johns Hopkins University, Baltimore.

Dyregrov, A. (1997). The process of psychological debriefing. *Journal of Traumatic Stress, 10,* 589–604.

Everly, G. S., Boyle, S., & Lating, J. (in press). The effectiveness of psychological debriefings in vicarious trauma: A meta-analysis. *Stress Medicine*.

Everly, G. S. & Boyle, S. (1997, April). *A meta-analysis*. Paper presented to the 4th World Congress on Stress Trauma and Coping in the Emergency Services Professions. Baltimore, MD.

Everly, G. S.& Mitchell,J. T.(1997). *Critical Incident Stress Management (CISM): A New Era and Standard of Care in Crisis Intervention*. Ellicott City, MD: Chevron.

Everly, G. S., Flannery, R. & Mitchell, J. T. (in press). CISM: A review of literature. *Aggression and Violent Behavior: A Review Journal.*

Flannery, R. B. (1998). *The Assaulted Staff Action Program: Coping with the psychological aftermath of violence.* Ellicott City, MD: Chevron Publishing.

Helzer, J. Robins, L. & McEvoy, L. (1997). Post-traumatic stress disorder in the general population. *New England Journal of Medicine, 317*, 1630–1634.

Mitchell, J. T. (1983). When disaster strikes ... The critical incident stress debriefing. *Journal of Emergency Medical Services, 13*(11), 49–52.

Mitchell, J. T. (1985). Healing the helper. In Mary Lystad (Ed.) *Role Stressors and Supports for Emergency Workers.* Washington, DC: National Institute of Mental Health, Center for Mental Health Studies of Emergencies (DHHS publication No. ADM 851408).

Mitchell, J. T. & Bray, G. P. (1990). *Emergency Services Stress: Guidelines for preserving the health and careers of emergency services personnel.* Englewood Cliffs, NJ: Brady Publishing – Prentice Hall.

Mitchell, J. T. & Everly, G. S. (in press). CISM and CISD: Evolution, effects and outcomes. In B. Raphael & J. Wilson (Eds.). *Psychological Debriefing.*

Mitchell, J. T. &Everly, G. S. (1996). *Critical Incident Stress Debriefing.- An Operations Manual.* Ellicott City, MD: Chevron Publishing.

NHTSA, National Center for Statistics and Analysis (1996). *An overview of traffic safety facts for 1996.* National Highway Safety Administration Annual Report. Washington, DC: United States Department of Transportation.

NUPE Research department (1991). *Stress and the Ambulance Service*, NUPE Briefings, no. 125, SS / JMK / A8 Stress 2 Research Department Civic House, 20 Grand Depot Road, Woolwich, London SE186SF.

Ravenscroft, T. (1994). *Going Critical: GAIB l Apex and T & G Unions 1994 survey of occupational stress factors in accident and emergency staff in the London Ambulance Service.* London: GMB /Apex and T & G Unions.

Robinson, R. (1994). *Follow-up study of Health and stress in ambulance services Victoria, Australia.*, part 1. Melbourne, Australia: Victoria Ambulance Crisis Counseling Unit.

Snellgrove, T. (1998). Debriefing under fire. *Trauma Lines, 3*(2), 3, 11.

Thompson, I & Suzuki, I. (1991). Stress in ambulance workers. *Disaster Management, 3*(4), 193–197.

Williams, B. (1998). Oklahoma Rescuers are Now Victims. *MSNBC video report aired.* November 25, 1998. http://www.msnbc.com/news/217433.asp

Section 2: Understanding of PTSD

11

The Complex Web of Causation: Motor Vehicle Accidents, Comorbidity and PTSD

SANDRA L. BLOOM, M.D.

Executive Director, The Sanctuary® Horsham Clinic, Ambler, PA & Hampton Hospital, Rancocas, NJ, U.S.A.

Comorbidity, Causality and the Conflict Of Models

An apparently straightforward event occurs when a man swerves to avoid hitting an oncoming car, loses control of his vehicle on an icy road and runs into a tree. The cause is a dangerous patch of highway, the effect is a car accident. But that is about where the simple chain of causality ends. To understand the immediate and long-term impact of the accident on the victim we have to envision a web of causality that embraces multilayered, proximal and distal mechanisms of influence (Krieger, 1994).

The complex and interactive nature of traumatization is reflected in the ways in which clinicians have attempted to define it. Lenore Terr, after studying children who were involved in a mass kidnapping observed that "*'Psychic trauma' occurs when a sudden, unexpected, overwhelmingly intense emotional blow or a series of blows assaults the person from outside. Traumatic events are external, but they quickly become incorporated into the mind*" (Terr, 1990, p.8). Van der Kolk (1989) notes that "*traumatization occurs when both internal and external resources are inadequate to cope with external threat*" (p.393). Both definitions inextricably connect the internal and the external, the personal with the social, the event with the personal interpretation of the event. Clinicians can be quite comfortable with this kind of causal complexity in dealing with a wounded patient because what actually caused the symptoms is less important than treating those symptoms in service of improving the victim's level of function. But the issues of co-existing disorders, pre-existing conditions, and causally related disorders are some of the unhappy points of contact, and often conflict, between men and women of medicine and practitioners of the law.

The requirements of the physician are radically different from those of the lawyer. For him or her, placing blame is largely irrelevant and managing the complex and often tragic experiences of human beings is all that matters. The patient is inevitably connected to his past and everything that has ever happened to him. He is comprised of a vast network of interconnected and reverberating experience, as mind impacts body, body alters mind, past influences present, and all is influenced by biological constitution, psychological interpretations of reality, on-going social interactions and the attribution of meaning acquired through the experience of the individual and the social group. Within the confines of such a reality, how can a physician reasonably answer questions of cause and effect without distorting the perceptions of this reality?

This conflict surfaces with enduring frequency around the issue of motor vehicle accidents, psychological injury, and compensation. In the theatre of the courtroom, the rules of the game inform the players that they must embrace and administer notions of culpability and restitution. If someone can be found to be at fault for causing the disability or distress of another person, than the victim has a right to fair compensation. Expert testimony of physicians is required around the issue of causality and courts usually are looking at "proximate cause" or a "natural and probable cause and effect relationship". But in the law, proximate cause does not necessarily mean proximate in time, and therefore there is much that is open to interpretation (Simon, 1995, p. xxiii). Unlike most other psychiatric labels, a diagnosis of PTSD implies causation and therefore post-traumatic stress disorder has been dubbed the "black hole" of litigation, appearing to present the possibility of easily attributing causality while in practice providing a slippery slope down into a pit of medical and legal confusion.

As our evidence-based understanding accumulates about the complex web of causation that characterizes the aftermath of a traumatic event, physicians and other mental health experts are often unable to give the simplistic cause and effect attributions that the legal system requires. If a person loses an arm in an accident, we can safely say that the severing of the major vessels and tissues connecting the arm to the body caused the amputation and that this severing occurred as a result of the shearing of the car door. But when the question is more subtle and involves not an organ or a body part, but an entire self and that self in a social and relational context, all we can safely discuss is before and after, accompanying and "comorbid" events, vulnerabilities and risk factors, sometimes to the point of absurdity, as far as the legal system is concerned.

In this chapter, I will review what we know thus far about what happens to people after many kinds of traumatic experiences and specifically, after vehicular accidents. We know that exposure to overwhelming stress has multiple effects, that there are risk factors, protective factors, cumulative factors, and possibly constitutional factors that influence how each individual responds to every unique event. But all we can do is speak in generalities. We cannot yet predict how any specific individual will be impacted by any traumatic event. What we can safely say is that exposure to trauma increases the likelihood that victims will suffer from complex and interactive physical, emotional, social, and spiritual/existential problems that ultimately may be diagnosed as medical or psychiatric problems. As we will see throughout this chapter, the subjects of post-traumatic stress, stress-related disorders and comorbid conditions can present a nightmarish situation to the legal system and tax medical experts.

The Complicated Nature of Trauma-Related Disorders

The connection between stress and mental disorder has long been recognized. In the late 70's. Brown & Harris demonstrated that about 60% of persons diagnosed as having a mental disorder had experienced a severely stressful life event in the two weeks preceding the onset of that disorder in comparison to 20% in the comparison group (Brown & Harris, 1978). In the months following a traumatic life event, there is a sixfold greater risk of suicide, a twofold greater risk of depressive disorders, and a slight increase in the risk of developing a schizophrenic disorder, according to Paykel's 1978 review. The connections between depressive disorders, panic disorders, phobic disorders were noted even before there was a diagnosis of "post-traumatic stress disorder" (Horowitz, 1993).

As the field of traumatic stress studies has grown, it has become clear that a variety of factors ultimately effect the outcome of a traumatic event. To obtain a clear picture it is necessary to look at many aspects of the entire system: individual vulnerability and risk factors that exist prior to the traumatic experience; the specific characteristics of the traumatic event; how the individual perceives those characteristics in reference to himself and his own history; the responses of the individual and the social environment during and after the traumatic event including the biological, psychological, social, and philosophical responses (McFarlane & Yehuda, 1996; Shalev, 1996).

Shalev has argued convincingly that PTSD represents a "biopsychosocial trap" in which neurobiological processes specific to traumatic stress combine with the acquisition of fear-conditioned responses to trauma-related stimuli, altered cognitive schemata and social apprehension to produce a vicious cycle of progressive deterioration (Shalev, 1996).

Prevalence of PTSD. In America, where most of the community-wide epidemiological data has been gathered thus far, most individuals will experience a traumatic event sometime in their lifetime. According to population studies of trauma and PTSD, about a quarter of individuals who are exposed to a DSM-IV type stressor go on to develop PTSD, although there is variation depending on the type of stressor. By recent estimates, 5% of men and 10–12 % of women will suffer from PTSD sometime in their lives, and for victims of traumas such as rape, the rate may be as high as 60% to 80%. For at least a third of sufferers, PTSD is a persistent condition lasting many years and over 80% of persons with PTSD suffer from other psychiatric disorders (Solomon & Davidson, 1997). For motor vehicle accidents specifically, Breslau et al.'s (1991) study indicates that about 10% of a sample of young urban adults had suffered a serious road accident and 12% of them went on to develop PTSD. Norris's (1992) study is consistent with this PTSD rate in that of 1000 adults living in the southeast U.S., 25% had experienced a traffic accident and about 12% developed PTSD.

A formal diagnosis of PTSD is not the only diagnosis that can result from a traumatic stressor. Davidson has pointed out that there are at least ten other trauma-related disorders found in DSM-III-R including brief reactive psychosis, dissociative identity disorder, dissociative fugue, dissociative amnesia, conversion disorder, borderline personality disorder, depersonalization disorder, somatization disorder, dream anxiety disorder, and antisocial personality disorder (1993). Additionally, it is clinically well established that survivors of prolonged and repeated trauma develop a syndrome that has been termed "complex post-traumatic stress disorder" (Herman, 1992) or "disorders of extreme stress" not otherwise specified DESNOS – reflecting the multidimensional developmental impact on the entire being of this kind of stress (van der Kolk, 1996).

In 1993, Mayou, Bryant & Duthrie published a study that looked at the psychiatric consequences of road traffic accidents in 188 consecutive road accident victims admitted to an emergency department of the main hospital in Oxford, England. Almost one fifth of the victims suffered from acute stress syndrome with mood disturbance and terrifying memories of the accident. Anxiety and depression usually improved over the twelve months of follow-up, but a tenth of the patients still had mood disorders at one year. But specific post-traumatic symptoms were also common with ten percent of the patients suffering from PTSD and many suffering from phobic travel anxiety that was frequently disabling. According to these researchers, post-traumatic syndromes were not associated with premorbid neurosis but were strongly associated with intrusive memories of the accident that did not occur in patients who had been unconscious or were amnestic for the accident. The victims' mental state at three months was highly predictive of their mental state at one year.

In the same year, Brom, Kleber & Hofman (1993) published another study with similar findings, reporting that 10% of a Dutch cohort of accident victims suffered from PTSD at one month and six months after the accident. In a Swedish study, 84 persons injured in traffic accidents and with moderate to severe injuries were interviewed approximately two years after the accident. Sixty-eight percent of the victims reported that they still suffered from physical sequelae and fifty-seven percent had been or were still suffering from psychological distress after the accident. Sixty-three percent of the accident victims were on the sick list for at least three months as a result of the accident while fifty-eight percent needed some type of handicap aid for some period of time after the accident. For twenty-nine percent of those employed in professions, the traffic accident led to altered working conditions (Andersson, Dahlback & Allebeck, 1994). Green et al. (1993) reported a PTSD rate of 27% in a small series of hospitalized accident victims in Australia. In a report of a severe bus accident in Australia that killed eleven people, 29 survivors were studied (Watts, 1995). Forty-one percent had PTSD and 52% reported severe intrusive or avoidance phenomena, including 31% who had both. These sequelae were associated with being currently distressed by another event and seeing bodies or witnessing the death of someone. Bryant (1997) reported on a series of 1,100 accident survivors in a one-year period in an emergency room in England. A preliminary analysis of the first six months' data indicated that about one in six of those not injured were still have difficulty a year later with work and/or daily tasks and one in five rated the quality of their life as worse than before the accident.

Blanchard and his colleagues at the University of Albany have been researching the effects of motor vehicle accidents and have published a series of articles. A study published in 1994 found that 46% of victims had PTSD. Another 20% had a subsyndromal version of PTSD characterized by the presence of the reexperiencing symptom cluster plus either the avoidance/numbing cluster or the over-arousal cluster of PTSD. In 1995, they reported on 158 victims who sought medical attention after an accident and were assessed for acute psychiatric and psychosocial consequences as well as pre-existing psychopathology at 1–4 months after the accident. They found that 39.2% met criteria for PTSD by DSM-IIIR criteria. Those with PTSD were more subjectively distressed and had more impairment in role function.

DiGallo, Barton & Parry-Jones (1997) looked prospectively at the early psychological consequences of traffic accidents in fifty-seven children and adolescents aged 5–18 years. The children and their parents were interviewed 2–16 days after the accident and then again 12–15 weeks later. Although post-accident stress symptoms had decreased by the second interview, 14% still suffered from moderate or severe PTSD, 17% from serious traffic-related fears and the parents reported increased mood disturbances in their children. Tyano and colleagues (1996) did a seven-year follow-up of child survivors of a bus-train collision and found that high exposure correlated with the highest levels of somatization, depression, phobic anxiety, psychoticism, and more PTSD symptoms. Symptoms of acute stress, and manifestations of fear immediately after the accident were strongly related to long-term maladjustment.

Causative Vulnerabilities and Risk Factors. How vulnerable was the victim to the long-term effects of trauma before the vehicular accident occurred? That is a fundamental question that arises in the courtroom, in the physician's office, and in the workplace. The question of whether or not the accident caused or was caused by a comorbid condition is a pressing one, but is often very difficult to resolve.

In the first place, there are many physical and behavioural factors that make it more likely that accidents will occur. Davidson et al.'s (1985) early work on the relationship between family psychopathology and chronic PTSD may indicate some genetic risk factors. True et al (1993) have demonstrated that genetic vulnerability had a significant impact on symptom liability among a cohort of combat veterans who were twins. It is possible that intrinsic or acquired problems with vital neurohormonal and neurostructural systems may contribute to increased risk for the later development of severe post-traumatic symptomatology after an accident. Recent studies of hippocampal volume have demonstrated a decreased left hippocampal volume in combat veterans and in victims of child abuse (Bremner et al, 1997). Many studies demonstrate that exposure to trauma impacts the HPA-axis, a finding now noted in combat veterans and victims of child abuse (Stein et al, 1997). In addition, medical conditions like certain cardiac disorders, uncontrolled diabetes, cerebrovascular insufficiency, and epilepsy can all increase the likelihood that a motor vehicle accident may occur. Illegal drugs and alcohol are notable in their ability to compromise driving skills, but so too do many prescription drugs. People who suffer from personality disorders that are frequently related to childhood exposure to trauma, often engage in behaviors that put their lives at risk, including deliberate self-harm behaviors and suicide gestures.

Studies support a growing number of other risk factors in the development of PTSD. For instance, in the National Comorbidity Study (Bromet et al, 1998), a risk factor for women was having a history of affective disorder while for men it was history of anxiety disorder and having a parent with a mental disorder. Harsh and abusive childhood environments, as well as other kinds of previous traumatic experiences, increase the risk for PTSD after a later traumatic experience and for many other kinds of comorbid psychological and physical conditions (Bremner et al, 1993; Green et al., 1990a; Kulka et al., 1990; Zaidi & Foy, 1994). Child abuse also increase the risk for many different kinds of personality disorders that then can impact on the way the individual deals with a subsequent traumatic event like an automobile accident. Previous experiences also determine the way an individual interprets their place in the world and how they see themselves in relation to others. The characteristic style and attitudes that people have used in the past to cope with stressful events will influence the way they interpret a recent traumatic event like a vehicular accident (McFarlane & Yehuda, 1996).

A previous history of trauma also may have a cumulative effect that impacts on a recent traumatic event. It is a well-recognized clinical phenomenon that a previous history of trauma appears to exacerbate the effects of a recent trauma, producing the effect of "the straw that broke the camel's back". This topic has been evaluated in several studies related to vehicular accidents. Blanchard et al. (1994) reported that 74% of the PTSD group had a previous trauma and 52% had experienced a previous serious motor vehicle accident. In the subsyndromal group, 90% of them had been in a previous serious accident and 80% had an other previous trauma. Combining these, 87% of the PTSD group and 100% of the sub-syndromal group admitted to a history of previous trauma. In the Blanchard et al. 1995 study, the rate of prior PTSD among the MVA victims who developed either full PTSD or subsyndromal PTSD was 22.4% compared to 3.9% in those who were relatively unaffected. Winje (1996) looked at the relationship between previous trauma and the subsequent reactions to a bus accident. Prior exposure to trauma did not affect the scores on the Impact of Events Scale but was associated with a sustained vulnerability to general psychological distress as measured by the SCL-90. DiGallo & Parry-Jones (1996) also point out the importance of further study relating to pre-accident disposition and vulnerability as it relates to post-accident morbidity.

A powerful vulnerability appears to be the presence of pre-existing psychiatric disorders. In a study by Mayou, Bryant & Duthrie (1993) there was an association between post-traumatic emotional disorders and having pre-accident psychological or social problems. There was also an association between emotional problems and continuing medical complications. In the Blanchard et al 1994 study, of the PTSD group, 48% also met criteria for major depressive disorder and of the PTSD group, 39% had experienced a previous major depression. Of those with PTSD and major depression, 64% had a history of previous depression and in 82% of them, this present depressive episode had begun after the accident. The authors conclude that, "*previous depression seems to predispose the formerly depressed individual to develop PTSD when involved in a serious MVA*" (Blanchard et al, 1994, p.289).

In their 1995 study, Blanchard et al. found that of the PTSD group, 53% also met criteria for major depression, with most of that (81.8%) developing after the accident. Fifty percent of the motor vehicle accident patients with PTSD had a history of previous major depression as compared with 23% of the non-PTSD patients. The MVA-PTSD group had a higher rate of lifetime panic disorder (11.3%) and any anxiety disorder (29%). Personality disorders were also common in this group with 13.3% meeting criteria for at least one disorder compared to 8.6% of controls. Of the victims who were in the midst of a major depression when the accident occurred, 75% developed PTSD, although their symptoms of PTSD were no more severe than those who did not have a history of depression. There was a similar relationship between PTSD and panic disorder. Those victims who developed PTSD were more likely to have a history of a panic disorder (11.3%). The MVA victims were also more likely to have a lifetime history of drug dependence 13.9% vs. 2.1%.

Chubb & Bisson (1996) looked at how patients who already suffered from chronic mental illness fared after a major coach accident. Fifty percent of them had PTSD and the extent of psychological suffering was the most marked in those who suffered from previous depression and anxiety disorders. This effect, however, does not apparently hold for all populations. Resnick and colleagues (1992) studied crime victims and did not find an association between psychiatric diagnoses before the crime and PTSD after the crime except when the person had a prior depression and then was exposed to a high crime stress.

Characteristics of the Event. Although the diagnosis of PTSD requires exposure to an event that involved actual or threatened death or serious injury or a threat to the physical integrity of self or others, some studies have shown that "ordinary" stressors can produce PTSD stressors like marital disruptions, illegal activities of one's children, death of a loved one, money problems, injury (Burstein, 1985; Helzer et al, 1987; Solomon & Caninco, 1990). Green et al.(1990a), reviewed studies up to that point to evaluate the aspects of a traumatic experience that are the most overwhelming, and therefore traumatogenic for the individual. These included: threat to one's life and body integrity; severe physical harm or injury; receipt of intentional injury/harm; exposure to the grotesque; witnessing or learning of violence to loved ones;

learning of exposure to noxious agent; causing death or severe harm to another. Involvement in serious motor vehicle accidents can expose victims to combinations of these stressors, even if the subject escapes the accident physically unharmed. The suddenness of the event, the unexpected nature of the trauma, the intentions of the perpetrator, how long it lasts, how much damage it does to the self and to others, the degree of life threat, the degree of associated humiliation and shame, in addition to actual injury, will all play a role in determining how the traumatic event will impact on the individual.

Later resilience or pathology may also be predicted by how the person deals with the traumatic event itself. Dissociation is commonly associated with traumatic events and can be a protective coping skill, but leads to fragmentation. There is a growing body of evidence to support the clinical impression that dissociation in the face of trauma represents different kinds of physiological reactivity at the time of the traumatic event, may occur more often in those who have experienced prior victimization and is a marker of long-term psychopathology (Bremner & Brett,1997; Cloitre, Scarvalone & Difede,1997; Griffin, Resick & Mechanic,1997). Impaired cognition, panic and freezing at the time of the event can also lead to the perception of impaired ability to cope, shame, guilt and a generalized feeling of ineffectiveness.

Lifton has talked about the "death imprint" that is associated with exposure to death and dying at the time of the traumatic event. He describes this as the radical intrusion of an image or feeling of threat or end to life. The degree of anxiety associated with the death imprint has to do with the inability to assimilate the experiences. The image remains, haunting the victim as he or she struggles to master and integrate the experience (Lifton, 1993). Victims of automobile accidents frequently dissociate at the time of the crash and yet the experience of near-death may leave them feeling fragmented and subject to intrusive experiences of the close call. Clinicians who have worked with accident victims have noticed that victims may persist, consciously or unconsciously, in the feeling that they died during the crash and for treatment to be successful the experience of having died must be integrated with the reality of having survived (Bills, 1998).

The way in which the individual copes with the trauma may also impact on how successful subsequent coping is. Self-efficacy, the term used to describe our belief about what we are capable of doing in any given situation, is influenced by experience and is put to the test when we are caught in dangerous situations like the ones presented at the time of a motor vehicle accident (Bandura, 1982).

Disaster researchers have described the personal devastation that confronts the trauma survivor who loses important aspects of his or her community or social support system. Survivors of motor vehicle accidents in which friends or relatives have been killed lose people in their lives who may provide an important sense of well-being and identity. To the extent that people cannot return to work or to their normal activities, their sense of being a part of a community may also be jeopardized.

Post-Trauma Responses. After the trauma, many normal functions may be radically altered. Memory problems are quite common after a trauma, as is persistent hyperarousal, a tendency to avoid stimuli that reminds the person of the traumatic event, and intrusive phenomena. Physiological hyperarousal and intrusions can dramatically impact on normal cognition and dysregulate affect. The victim's view of him or herself as a competent adult may be drastically altered and attitudes towards self or others may be radically changed. If others have been killed in the trauma, survivors may experience survivor guilt, an apparently paradoxical feeling of self-blame for having survived when others have not. Lifton (1993) has described a phenomenon he calls "failed enactment", the extreme sense of helplessness one experiences at the time of a trauma, and a profound sense of ineffectiveness or inadequate coping resulting from the inability to have prevented the trauma from happening.

Complicating this even further is the issue of social support after a trauma. Social support has repeatedly been found to be a critical component of recovery after trauma or the lack of such recovery. In one study, less psychological support post-trauma was predictive of PTSD whereas more severe injury did not predict PTSD (Perry et al., 1992). Andersson, Bunketorp & Allebeck (1997) have reported on the high rate of psychosocial complications after road traffic injuries and poor social support is one of the risk factors for such complications. When Buckley, Blanchard & Hickling (1996) compared victims of MVA's who developed delayed onset PTSD during a 1-year follow-up interval, MVA victim controls who did not develop PTSD, and a group who met criteria for acute onset PTSD, the delayed onset participants had poorer social support than the controls prior to and after the MVA. Landsman and colleagues (1990) assessed a group of urban trauma victims 3-39 months after their injuries and found that the levels of psychological distress were predicted less by injury severity than by subjective impact of the accident, injury-related financial and employment problems, and family and social environment. Family environment ratings were significantly worse for subjects with elevated levels of psychiatric symptoms.

Rejection, abandonment, blaming on the part of supportive others may lead to a "second injury" (Symonds, 1982), further compounding the effect of the trauma. Accident victims may have post-accident experiences with rescue workers, or hospital personnel that compound the traumatic insult and the hospital itself may be a traumatizing place. The accompanying "sanctuary trauma" is that which occurs when an individual who has suffered a severe stressor next encounters what was expected to be a supportive and protective environment and discovers only more trauma (Silver, 1986).

Finally, traumatic experience, particularly that suffered at the hands of others, shatters the fundamental assumptions upon which we build our sense of reality and safety. We live our day-to-day lives functioning with certain basic beliefs that we simply take for granted – that we are safe, that the world makes sense, that other people can be trusted, that the past is known and the future is predictable (Janoff-Bulman, 1992). Despite newspapers and television reports to the contrary, we don't really believe that tragedy is going to strike us until it happens. But interpersonal trauma can strip us of the certain ground beneath our feet so that for the victim, there is no longer any safety, the world does not make sense, people cannot be trusted, parts of the past or forgotten or erased, and the future is neither predictable nor necessarily benevolent. All of these factors will interact in unpredictable ways with intrinsic vulnerabilities to produce the complicated picture of comorbidity. Solomon, Iancu & Tyano (1997) studied the effects of a bus-train collision on the beliefs and cognitions of 389 young adult survivors, 7 years following the accident. At the time of the accident the survivors had all been adolescents. Exposure to the traumatic accident challenged the survivors' beliefs in a benevolent and a just world. The extent of this change in basic assumptions had a direct relationship to the level of exposure to traumatic stimuli. Changes in these basic cognitive schemata were associated with psychiatric symptoms and problems in functioning.

Psychiatric Comorbidity and PTSD

There is now an abundance of research indicating that there is significant overlap between PTSD and other psychiatric conditions. Some of those premorbid conditions occur immediately after or seemingly along with the PTSD, as in major depression. Others, as in many of the apparently related personality disorders like borderline personality disorder, appear to be a product of the entwined interaction of post-traumatic symptoms, constitutional factors, existing personality, and family environment all interacting with the process of development. Without such a connecting link, many physicians will fail to recognize that many apparently "far-flung" psychological and physical problems may in fact be related to a past history of a traumatic experience, including vehicular accidents. It is this overlap and complexity that makes the discussion of comorbidity and causality so treacherous.

Green and her colleagues (1992) reviewed studies of Vietnam veterans and over three-quarters of the patients with PTSD also met criteria for at least one other diagnosis, most commonly major depression, substance abuse, and antisocial personality disorder. Even in the most conservative study, those with PTSD were two to four times more likely than those without PTSD to have virtually any other psychiatric disorder, particularly somatization (Solomon & Davidson, 1997). According to one study, somatization was found to be 90 times more likely to occur in those with PTSD than in those without PTSD (Davidson et al., 1991). In a study by Breslau and colleagues (1991), those with PTSD were more than six times as likely to have some other psychiatric disorder. The large epidemiological study of Kessler and colleagues (1995) showed that those with PTSD are almost eight times as likely to have three or more disorders – 88% of men and 79% of women with PTSD had a history of at least one other disorder.

Patients with one or more symptoms of PTSD are more likely than those without any mental disorder to experience poor social support, marital difficulties, and occupational problems, as well as more impairment on income and disability measures than even those with major depressive disorder. The people with PTSD symptoms are also more likely to have a number of chronic illnesses, consistent with many other studies of specific trauma groups. Although these patients have a disproportionate utilisation of the health care system, they are reluctant to seek mental health treatment, a finding that has been seen in many other studies as well (Solomon & Davidson, 1997).

In the Kessler study mentioned earlier, men with PTSD were six to ten times more likely and women four to five times more likely to have affective disorders than those without PTSD. Similar figures appear with anxiety disorders with men three to seven times more likely and women two to four times more likely to have another anxiety disorder along with their PTSD. People with PTSD were also two to three times more likely to have a substance abuse disorder. In a number of studies showing the relationship between PTSD and substance abuse, between 25% and 58% of those seeking substance abuse treatment also were comorbid for PTSD (Grady, 1997).

Research reports connecting PTSD with other psychiatric conditions is growing exponentially. There is such a large literature on the connection between trauma and dissociative disorders that the latter are generally considered to be trauma-related disorders. Suggestions have even been made that it is not especially helpful to define the clinical significance of a given person's posttraumatic disturbance in terms of meeting the criteria for a specific DSM-IV stress category because the symptoms are determined by such a wide range of factors, far beyond the description of the stressor itself (Briere, 1997).

Orsillo et al. (1996) found that relative to veterans without PTSD, veterans with PTSD had significantly higher rates of current major depression, bipolar disorder, panic disorder, and social phobia, as well as significantly higher rates of lifetime major depression, panic disorder, social phobia, and obsessive-compulsive disorder. Rogers et al. (1996) studied the prevalence and characteristics of somatoform disorders among 654 subjects with anxiety disorders – 5.5% of the subjects had past or current somatoform disorders. The subjects with somatoform disorders were significantly more likely to have histories of PTSD, lending support to the observation that somatoform disorders are frequently comorbid with PTSD, other anxiety disorders and depressive disorders. Gleason (1993) Orsillo et al. (1996), and Saunders et al. (1992) all have noted the connection between PTSD and obsessive compulsive disorder in several different populations. Bower & Stein looked at civilian trauma and reported on the increased incidence of panic disorder among those exposed to traumatic suffocation. In a study done by Falsetti and Resnick (1997), 69% of a population seeking treatment for trauma-related problems had panic attacks. This association between panic disorder, other anxiety disorders and PTSD has also been noted by Orsillo et al.(1996); Fierman, (1993); Vasile et al. (1997) and others.

Another important aspect of comorbidity between PTSD and other psychiatric disorders is the established connection between trauma and personality disorders. Van der Kolk (1996) points out that the combination of chronic dissociation, physical problems for which no medical cause can be found, and a lack of adequate ability to self-regulate can have profound effect on the ways in which personality develops. Many authors have commented upon the ways early childhood exposure to trauma and loss can skew character formation. The connection between borderline personality disorder and trauma, particularly childhood trauma has been studied by a number of authors (Ellason et al., 1996; Herman, Perry & Van der Kolk, 1989; Perry et al., 1990; Sabo, 1997). What is perhaps even more startling is the recognition that character can be changed even after adulthood. Southwick, Yehuda & Giller (1993) concluded from their study of treatment-seeking Vietnam veterans that war-related PTSD is often accompanied by diffuse, debilitating, and enduring impairments in character that were not present before combat exposure.

Medical Comorbidity and Trauma-related Disorders

Victims of traumatic stress are at risk for many comorbid health problems as well as psychological problems. McFarlane & Yehuda (1996) point out that there are three ways that trauma victims may manifest physical problems: as a direct result of the traumatic experience, as an integral part of the post-traumatic stress disorder, or as a nonspecific response to trauma exposure independent of the PTSD. A great deal more research will need to be conducted before we are able to definitively differentiate among these hypotheses.

Much of our present knowledge regarding the profound connections between environmental events and body physiology derives from the field of "stress studies". As the field of psychoneuroimmunology expands, there is a growing body of information about the relationship between stress, and the immune system that may have serious implications for the study of traumatic stress as well. So far, we know that even mild stress impacts on the immune system (Bachen et al., 1992; Brosschot et al., 1994). In a review article from 1993, Herbert & Cohen assert that there is evidence for a relationship in humans between stress and decreases in functional immune measures. Stress effects the numbers and percentage of circulating white blood cells, immunoglobulin levels, and antibody titers to herpes viruses (Herbert & Cohen, 1993).

Subsequent analyses suggest that objective stressful events are related to larger immune changes than subjective self-reports of stress, that immune response varies with stressor duration, and that interpersonal events are related to different immune outcomes than non-social events. According to an even more recent review by Cohen & Herbert (1996), there is substantial evidence that factors such as stress, negative affect, clinical depression, social support, and repression/denial can influence both cellular and humoral indicators of immune status and function. And, at least in the case of the less serious infectious diseases (colds, influenza, herpes), there is consistent and convincing evidence of links between stress and negative affect and disease onset and progression.

Mood states, compared to a neutral condition, affect the immune system, with some differences between positive and negative moods (Futterman et al, 1994; Kiecolt-Glaser et al., 1993). In two related studies, one of children in day care and another of children entering kindergarten, the development of respiratory illnesses was found to be related to stressful life events (Boyce et al., 1995). Another group looked at conduct disordered, depressed, and normal adolescents and found out that there was a correlation between significant negative life events and lowered natural killer cell activity (Birmaher, 1994). In primates, there is a large body of evidence that disruptions in social relationships have many immunological sequelae, particularly in the young monkey. There is evidence in infant monkeys that normal maternal care is important for the development and maintenance of normal immune function. The immune response of adult monkeys are also affected by aggression within the group (Coe, 1993).

Social support – or the lack of it – has emerged repeatedly in studies of traumatic stress as an important determinant of morbidity. In another group of studies outside of the traumatic stress field, investigators showed that in humans, social support, under experimental conditions of stress, produced less cardiovascular reactivity than a lack of social support (Lepore et al., 1993). A group of Swedish researchers looked at the established connection between social support and mortality. They differentiated between emotional support from very close persons (attachment) and the support provided by an extended network of social connections (social integration). They found that both factors were lower in middle-aged men with coronary heart disease and that this also predicted new cardiovascular incidents (Orth-Gomer, Rosengren & Wilhelmsen, 1993). Buckley, Blanchard & Hickling (1996) have noted that victims of automobile accidents who suffered from delayed onset PTSD had poorer social support before and after the accident. Social support may be a connecting point for many post-trauma physical and psychological adjustment problems.

Outside of the "stress" literature, most of the research connecting trauma-related disorders to health problems has used adult victims of child abuse as subjects. Clinical wisdom reports that the rate of medical comorbidity in this population appears to be quite high. This observation is supported by a number of studies.

Salmon & Calderbank (1996) looked at 275 British undergraduates and surveyed their history of sexual and physical abuse in childhood and their health care utilization, somatization, and hypochondriasis as an adult. Separate groups recalled physical and sexual abuses. Physical abuse predominating in males and sexual abuse in females. Both types of abuse were followed by a greater number of hospital admissions and surgical procedures, somatization, and hypochondriasis in adulthood.

Internists specializing in gastrointestinal disorders have been noticing the connection between chronic disorders and a past history of childhood abuse. One study looked at 239 female patients presenting to a gastroenterology clinic. They found that 66.5% of the women had experienced sexual and/or sexual abuse and that the women with a sexual abuse history had more pain, other somatic symptoms, bed disability days, lifetime surgeries, and functional disabilities than those without sexual abuse. Women with physical abuse also had worse health outcome on most indicators, while rape and life threatening physical abuse seem to have worse health effects than less serious physical violence and milder forms of sexual abuse (Leserman, 1996). Fukudo and colleagues studied irritable bowel syndrome and saw that the IBS patients have an exaggerated responsivity of the gastrointestinal tract to mental stress (Fukudo et al, 1993).

Walker and colleagues (1996) looked at the comorbidity between chronic pelvic pain, irritable bowel syndrome, and a past history of abuse. They found that compared to women with irritable bowel syndrome alone, those with both irritable bowel syndrome and chronic pelvic pain were significantly more likely to have a lifetime history of dysthymic disorder, current and lifetime panic disorder, somatization disorder, childhood sexual abuse and hysterectomy. In a randomized survey of 1599 women, 31.5% of participants reported a diagnosis of gynecologic problems in the past 5 years. Those with problems were more likely to report childhood abuse, violent crime victimization, and spouse abuse (Plichta & Abraham, 1996). Another study looked at the connection between chronic intractable pain and histories of childhood sexual abuse in 112 women sampled from a large university campus health center. Fifty-nine (59) women with chronic back pain were sampled and compared with 53 control subjects obtained simultaneously from the same clinical population. The women with chronic intractable back pain had a significantly higher percentage of childhood sexual abuse experiences than controls (Pecukonis, 1996).

Koss and her associates (1990) looked at the long-term physical health consequences of criminal victimization. Among a population of almost 400 adult women, they found that compared with nonvictims, victimized women reported more distress, less well-being, visited the doctor twice as frequently and had outpatient costs that were 2.5 times greater (Koss et al., 1991). They also studied almost 2300 women in a health maintenance organization. They had a 45% response rate to their survey and 57% of them had been victims of crime. Rape incidence was approximately 15 times higher than the National Crime Survey estimates for women. Medical care had been sought by 92% of crime victims during the first year following the crime and by 100% during the second year.

Amir et al. (1997) investigated fibromyalgia and PTSD. Among the PTSD group, 21% had symptoms of the disorder compared to 0% of the control group. When compared to the PTSD group without fibromyalgia symptoms, these patients reported more pain, lower quality of life, higher functional impairment and suffered more psychological distress. Geisser et al. (1996) examined self-reports of pain, affective disturbance, and disability among pain patients with and without symptoms of PTSD. Patients without PTSD symptoms were further subdivided into persons with no or few symptoms of PTSD whose pain was accident related (Accident/Low PTSD); and patients whose pain was not accident related and did not have PTSD symptoms (No Accident). Both accident-related pain groups were more likely than No Accident patients to be involved in litigation or receiving compensation. Accident/High PTSD patients displayed higher levels of self-reported pain compared to the other two groups. The Accident/High PTSD group also had the highest levels of affective disturbance. Davidson et al. (1991) found an increased incidence of bronchial asthma, hypertension, peptic ulcer associated with PTSD among a large epidemiological sample.

All of these studies indicate that a past history of trauma can impact on post-accident adjustment and health, particularly when the trauma dates back to childhood exposure. It is also well established that a recent trauma can "trigger" the emergence of symptoms related to a long-buried traumatic experience. Herein lies one of the causality dilemmas. If a woman who has been sexually abused as a child is at elevated risk for chronic pain and then is hurt in a car accident, was it the sexual abuse or the accident that "caused" the chronic pain? And what if she had the pain before the accident but continued to work and then after the accident is immobilized? Would the previous trauma ever have been "unearthed" had the automobile accident not occurred? How much do we attribute liability to the past experience and how much to the present? How much of her determination to "make somebody pay" belongs to the present party at fault for the vehicular damage and how much is she taking advantage of an opportunity to make someone accountable for her lifelong pain? Is she malingering? Does the car accident aggravate a pre-existing condition or does the previous history of abuse represent a predisposition, a subject entirely different from an already present disorder? It is clear from the data thus far presented that there is no simple answer for these questions, that this is the dilemma that the web of causation so clearly illustrates.

Course, Comorbidity and MVAs

As is clear, PTSD rarely occurs alone. The rate of psychiatric and medical comorbid conditions is extremely high. In 1997, Mayou, Tyndel & Bryant looked at the psychological outcome of a sample of 111 non-head-injured victims of motor vehicle accident five years after the accident. These victims had been assessed previously in a prospective one-year study. A substantial minority described continuing social, physical and psychological difficulties and a quarter of those studied suffered phobic anxiety about traveling in a car. Little had changed between three months, one year, and five years. The prevalence of PTSD remained approximately ten percent throughout the follow-up period, but most early cases had remitted by five years and a similar number of delayed new onsets had occurred between one year and five years. Physical outcome as well as postaccident intrusive memories and emotional distress predicted the presence of PTSD at five years after the accident. Poor outcome in those who made legal claims, especially those not settled after five years, appeared to be due to their having more serious physical problems. In another article, Mayou (1997) points out that if we look only at formal diagnoses of PTSD, we miss the high rate of travel anxiety and phobia that often occur after vehicular accidents and that have a great impact on everyday life.

In a more recent article (1997), Blanchard et al. looked at 145 individuals who sought medical attention as a result of the accident. They were assessed initially at 1–4 months after the accident and then followed for six months to see how many of the fifty-five who were diagnosed with PTSD and the forty-three with sub-syndromal PTSD would remit. Fifty-five percent of those who showed PTSD initially and sixty-seven percent of those with sub-syndromal PTSD, had remitted at least in part by 6 months. Five percent of the sub-syndromal types had worsened. The variables that largely appeared to predict remission were the severity of the initial symptoms, the degree of initial physical injury, relative physical recovery by four months, and whether a close family member suffered a trauma during the follow-up period. Earlier, Blanchard and colleagues (1996a) reported on 132 victims of automobile accidents and assessed them at 1–4 months after the accident, 6 months later, and 12 months later. Forty-eight met the full criteria for PTSD and of those, half had remitted at least in part at the 6-month assessment and two-thirds by the year assessment. They noted three variables that accounted for the difference between those who improved and those who did not: initial scores on the irritability and foreshortened future symptoms of PTSD and the initial degree of vulnerability the subjects felt in a motor vehicle after the accident.

Buckley, Blanchard & Hickling (1996) did a prospective study of delayed onset PTSD secondary to motor vehicle accidents. The participants had not met criteria for PTSD one to four months after the accident but had developed PTSD during a one-year follow-up interval. Compared with those who did not develop PTSD as well as to those who met criteria for acute onset PTSD, the delayed onset participants were more symptomatic at the time of the initial interview, had poorer social support prior to and after the accident, and for the month prior to the accident had lower Global Assessment of Functioning scores. In another report from the Blanchard group (1996b), using 158 victims of automobile accidents, 70% of the subjects could be classified as PTSD or not with four variables: major depression, fear of dying in the accident, extent of physical injury, and whether litigation had been initiated.

What do we know from recent research on the relationship between car accidents, psychiatric morbidity, and comorbid conditions? Blaszczynski et al. (1998) recently reviewed the literature on the subject and though cautioning that no consistent profile has yet emerged, there are common reported symptoms. These include: depression, anxiety, irritability, driving phobia, anger, sleep disturbances, headache, and post-traumatic stress disorders.

In 1995, Koch & Taylor pointed out that victims of motor vehicle accidents are frequently left with multiple comorbid psychological and physical disorders including PTSD, depression, pain-related conditions, and phobic avoidance of stimuli associated with the accident. Bryant & Harvey (1995) studied 56 Australian patients twelve months subsequent to hospitalization after a vehicular accident. Of this sample, 41% reported significant levels of psychological impairment. Those reporting psychological disturbances had more pain, higher rates of unemployment and substance abuse, avoidance of road transport and compensation claims. Only 44% of these had sought professional help for their conditions

In a study done by Blanchard and colleagues (1996a) four variables combined to predict 64% of the variance in the degree of post-traumatic stress symptoms at twelve months: the presence of alcohol abuse, an Axis-II disorder at the time of the initial assessment, total scores on the hyperarousal and avoidance symptoms of PTSD present at the initial post-accident assessment. In another study by Kuch and colleagues (1994), 55 survivors of traffic accidents with minimal injury and chronic pain were examined. Over thirty-eight percent had simple phobia with onset after the accident. Of these, 23.8% gave a past history of other phobia compared to none of the nonphobics.

Driving phobia is a major problem for many victims after an accident. The inability to drive can impact on the individual's ability to work, to socialize and to actively participate in family life. In the Blanchard et al. 1995 study, all of the driving phobics clustered in the PTSD subgroup, amounting to 15.3% of the PTSD patients who could have been driving at the time of assessment. Over half of the subjects with PTSD who were still driving avoided all driving that was not essential.

The effects of minor head trauma further complicate any analysis of psychiatric comorbidity. In an interesting study reported by Parker & Rosenblum (1996), accident victims who had suffered minor traumatic brain injury were studied twenty months after the accident. There was a loss of 14 points of the Full Scale IQ from estimated pre-injury baseline IQ without evidence of recovery. Personality dysfunctions included cerebral personality disorder and thirty of the thirty-three patients were given a psychiatric diagnosis. The authors caution that the estimation of brain trauma at the time of the accident may be underestimated for many people. In another report by Parker (1996), 31 out of 33 patients suffered an additional psychiatric disorder and manifested a wide spectrum of disorders cerebral personality disorder, persistent altered states of consciousness, PTSD, psychodynamic reactions to impairment, complex reactions expressing neurological, somatic and psychological dysfunctions. He points out that emotional disorders, combined with persistent cognitive loss and other neuropsychological symptoms greatly impair the capacity of the individual to adapt after traumatic injury and then impact on every aspect of the person's life. This relationship between head injury sustained at the time of an accident and consequent psychological problems may turn out to be a complicated one. Fenton and colleagues (1993) have reported on 45 consecutively admitted patients who had sustained a mild head injury with a post-traumatic amnesia duration of less than twenty-four hours. Interestingly, these head injury patients had an average of three adverse life events in the year preceding the injury compared with 1.5 for controls. Thirty-nine percent of the group was diagnosed with a psychiatric disorder at six weeks after the injury. For this group, the mean level of chronic social difficulties was four times that for the non-psychiatric cases. In this study, the emergence of and persistence of post-concussion syndrome was associated with social adversity before the accident.

Headache is another common presenting complaint after a motor vehicle accident. Chibnall & Duckro (1994) looked at the prevalence of PTSD among post-traumatic headache sufferers and noted that nearly 30% of the sample were diagnosed with PTSD. Depression and suppressed anger were significantly higher in subjects with PTSD compared to the rest of the sample and those with PTSD were more likely to have a history of headache prior to the accident.

What Does This High Comorbidity Mean?

Solomon & Bleich (1998) have recently proposed four alternative hypotheses to explain the high comorbidity found in PTSD: They reason that: 1) preexisting disorders could constitute a vulnerability to PTSD; 2) other disorders could be subsequent complications of PTSD; 3) the disorders could co-occur because of shared risk factors; and 4) comorbidity could be the result of a measurement artifact. As we have already seen, there is evidence that supports the first three hypotheses. In many studies of various survivor groups, depression is the most common comorbid condition. In the authors' discussion, they note that for about 65% of the patients they reviewed for lifetime diagnosis, both PTSD and depression emerged simultaneously. For 16%, depression was reported as the first disorder and PTSD as the first for 19%. In considering whether comorbidity could be a measurement artifact, Bleich et al. (1997) looked at patients originally diagnosed with lifetime depression and found that 98% would still be diagnosed as such even after the common symptoms were removed and 70% of those with PTSD would still be so diagnosed. They drew the inference that PTSD and depression are distinctive diagnostic categories. They also note that there is some evidence that biological markers for the two disorders may also be different. To address the question as to whether the threshold for diagnosing comorbid depression should be raised because of symptom overlap, Blanchard et al. (1998) examined data from 107 motor vehicle accident victims. Of the 62 who met PTSD criteria 1–4 months after the accident, 33 also met criteria for major depression and in 27 cases the depression occurred after the accident. Their statistical analysis indicated that PTSD and major depression are correlated but independent responses to trauma. The patients suffering from both syndromes were more subjectively distressed, suffered more role impairment, and remitted less readily over the first six months of follow-up than those with PTSD alone.

There may, of course, be shared risk factors for both disorders including family and genetic vulnerabilities. Davidson et al. (1985) found an increase in affective disorders among untraumatized relatives of PTSD patients. The shared risk may also involve the nature of the stressor. Certainly wartime involvement exposes victims to multiple losses as do motor vehicle accidents.

On the other hand, it may well be that a comorbid condition like substance abuse is related to pre-existing substance abuse and there is some evidence to support that. Abuse of substances certainly increases the risk for traumatic exposure, while it contributes to chronicity after a traumatic event. Many other pre-existing conditions increase the likelihood that PTSD will occur and that the two or several conditions will interact with negative consequences to level of function.

Given the complicated nature of the human response to overwhelming experience it is likely that all four hypotheses will find some confirmation and some disconfirmation. As van der Kolk and colleagues (1996) have pointed out, PTSD and its comorbid conditions should be seen as "*complex, somatic, cognitive, affective and behavioral effects of psychological trauma*" rather than as separate conditions.

Comorbidity, PTSD and Compensation

The issues of litigation, compensation, malingering and secondary gain complicate the entire discussion of comorbidity. Human beings are motivated by both conscious and unconscious needs. Consciously, victims desire compensation for injuries sustained due to the negligence or malice of others and it is this conscious intention that is endorsed and supported by the legal notion of liability and restitution. But there are others who consciously desire to "get something for nothing", who fraudulently claim injury where there is none, or who exaggerate injury in order to increase their claim these are the malingerers. Additionally, there are people who unconsciously exaggerate their disability because it satisfies their unconscious needs such as a desire for vengeance against a previous injurious party who they cannot confront or in order to evoke sympathetic concern from others that is unavailable in any other way.

In 1968, Levine wrote about the "automobile accident syndrome" in discussing the increasing appearance of cases in which minor physical findings were accompanied by major subjective complaints. He attributed the basic motivation to be that of establishing a medical basis in order to receive monetary compensation. This argument is consistent with one that stretches back to at least the last century when railway accidents contributed to the notion of "compensation neurosis" implying that the symptoms would be resolved as soon as the litigation was resolved. This overly simplistic notion has been largely discredited and studies from various survivor groups paint a far more complicated picture. In 1973, Culpan and Taylor published an article on a study in which they attempted to follow-up and classify eighty-two New Zealand accident victims referred by lawyers for psychiatric evaluations. They were able to note the progress of 87% of the original sample. Approximately one-third of the group were disabled by neurotic symptoms which appeared to result from the emotional stress of the accident itself and they classified these patients as suffering from true traumatic neurosis, as it was called at the time. They believed that about half of the group were thought to be unconsciously motivated by the possibility of financial compensation and unlike the first group, they failed to improve or became worse until the time of the settlement of their claim. Six percent of the sample were considered to be outright malingerers with "compensation neurosis" who denied concern about the outcome of their lawsuits.

Smith & Frueh (1996) looked at the relationship between compensation seeking, comorbidity, and the apparent exaggeration of PTSD symptoms among Vietnam combat veterans. They found that there was increased comorbidity, particularly affective disorders, among veterans who exaggerated their symptoms, but there was not a relationship between the symptom exaggerators and those seeking compensation. In another study by Frueh, Smith & Barker (1996), compensation seeking veterans had much higher scores of pathology across a wide range of inventories, but they did not differ in frequency of PTSD diagnoses compared to veterans not seeking compensation.

In 1982, Mendelson reviewed the literature and up to that point 75% of those injured in accidents had failed to return to gainful employment two years after legal settlement. McFarlane investigated the survivors of the Ash Wednesday bush fire disaster in Australia and found similar findings in an eleven year follow-up period (Pitman et al, 1996). In Green et al's (1990b) fourteen-year follow-up of the Buffalo Creek dam collapse of 1972, no significant clinical differences were noted between the litigant and nonlitigant survivor groups. In an Israeli study of combat veterans, veterans who had experienced the most severe traumas and had subsequently developed the most severe symptoms and functional limitations sought compensation. The reported range and severity of symptoms and functional limitations did not diminish with compensation and the social function of both groups before the war was comparable (Solomon et al, 1994). Tarsh & Royston (1985) did a follow-up study of 35 claimants one to seven years after their lawsuits were resolved and compensation was received. All these patients suffered from "accident neurosis" with many somatic symptoms. Few claimants recovered and such recovery as did take place was unrelated to the time of compensation. According to the authors, the legal process and the delays involved caused great distress. Mayou, Bryant & Duthie (1993) studied the differential impact of motor vehicle accidents on victims who were able to sue and those who were not. They found that litigation status did not influence the prevalence of psychiatric disorder, the course of the disorder, or the chronicity of associated disabilities. They found that severe chronic physical and psychological symptoms were also found in the group that was not going to court. In a study by Packard (1992), fifty accident victims who suffered from what had come to be defined as "permanent posttraumatic headaches" were evaluated at least one year after litigation had been settled. Patients with a pre-accident history of headaches, another injury, or head injury were excluded from the study. Only four patients reported any improvement in their headache pattern after settlement of their case.

Binder, Trimble & McNiel (1991) looked at the course of psychological symptoms after a lawsuit and found that a better psychological outcome was associated with a longer time after resolution of the lawsuit, a shorter time between injury and resolution of the suit, and less severe initial psychological symptoms. The finding that a shorter time between injury and resolution of a lawsuit leads to a better prognosis is interesting in that it supports an observation that is frequently observed clinically – that the process of engagement with the legal system can itself be retraumatizing for the victim (Pitman et al, 1996).

Conclusion

Given the existing data, it is impossible to attribute simple cause and effect relationships to the effects of traumatic experience, even in one as seemingly straightforward as a motor vehicle accident. Each person brings individual risk factors and vulnerabilities, including previous life experience, to the accident scene. Each accident then has its unique traumatic aspects that interact with the variable perceptions of every person involved in the accident.

The victims then struggle to cope with the traumatic event and its after effects, while attempting to make some kind of sense out of what has happened to them. For a certain proportion of the population, the attempts to cope will be further complicated by the "biopsychosocial trap" that is post-traumatic stress disorder (Shalev, 1996), as well as a number of other psychological and physical conditions that make a healthy adjustment far more difficult. Given such a complex web of associations, the physician must be willing to be aware and address issues of multicausality that affect the body, mind, family and soul of any victim if he or she is to truly committed to the provision of good care. As for questions of liability and compensation, for now the only useful measure we probably have is before-and-after level of function and the means to address this will continue to evolve and be fought out in the courtrooms of tomorrow.

References

Amir, M., Kaplan, Z., Neumann, L., Sharabani, R., Shani, N. & Buskila, D. (1997). Posttraumatic stress disorder, tenderness and fibromyalgia. *Journal of Psychosomatic Research, 42*(6):607–613.

Andersson, A. L., Bunketorp, O. & Allebeck, P. (1997). High rates of psychosocial complications after road traffic injuries. *Injury*, *28*(8):539–543.

Andersson, A., Dahlback, L. & Allebeck, P. (1994). Psychological consequences of traffic accidents: a two-year follow-up. *Scandinavian Journal of Social Medicine*, *22* (4): 299–302.

Bachen, E. A., Manuck, S. B., Marsland, B. L., Cohen, S., Malkoff, S. B., Muldoon, M. F. & Rabin, B. S. (1992). Lymphocyte subset and cellular immune responses to a brief experimental stressor. *Psychosomatic Medicine*, *54*(6): 673–679.

Bandura, A. (1982). Self-efficacy mechanism in human agency. *American Psychologist*, *37*(2): 122–147.

Bills, L. J. (1998). Personal communication.

Binder, R. L., Trimble, M. R. & McNiel, E. (1991).The course of psychological symptoms after resolution of lawsuits. *American Journal of Psychiatry*, *148*(8): 1073–1075.

Birmaher, B., Rabin, B. S., Garcia, M. R., Jain, U., Whiteside, T. L., Williamson, D. E., al-Shabbout, M., Nelson, B. C. Dahl, R. E. & Ryan, N. R. (1994). Cellular immunity in depressed; conduct disorder; and normal adolescents: role of adverse life events. *Journal American Academy Child Adolescent Psychiatry, 33*(5): 671–678.

Blanchard, E. B., Hickling, E. J., Taylor, A. E., Loos, W. R. & Gerardi, R. J. (1994). Psychological morbidity associated with motor vehicle accidents. *Behaviour Research and Therapy*, *32*(3): 283–290.

Blanchard, E. B., Hickling, E. J., Taylor, E. & Loos, W. R. (1995). Psychiatric morbidity associated with motor vehicle accidents. *Journal of Nervous and Mental Disease*, *183*(8): 495–504.

Blanchard, E. B., Hickling, E. J., Barton, K. A., Taylor, A. E., Loos, W. R., Jones, J. & Alexander. (1996a). One-year prospective follow-up of motor vehicle accident victims. *Behaviour Research and Therapy*, *34*(10): 775–786.

Blanchard, E. B., Hickling, E. J., Taylor, A. E., Loos, W. R., Forneris, C. A. & Jaccard, J. (1996b). Who develops PTSD from motor vehicle accidents? *Behaviour Research and Therapy, 34*(1): 1–10.

Blanchard, E. B., Hickling, E. J., Forneris, C. A., Taylor, A. E., Buckley, T. C., Loos, W. R. & Jaccard, J. (1997). Prediction of remission of acute posttraumatic stress disorder in motor vehicle accident victims. *Journal of Traumatic Stress, 10*(2): 215–234.

Blaszczynski, A., Gordon, K., Silove, D., Sloane, D., Hillman, D. & Panasetis, P. (1998). Psychiatric morbidity following motor vehicle accidents: A review of methodological issues. *Comprehensive Psychiatry, 39*(3): 111–121.

Bleich, A., Koslowski, M., Dolev, A. & Lorer, B. (1997). PTSD and depression: an analysis of comorbidity. *British Journal of Psychiatry, 170*: 479–482.

Bouwer, C. & Stein, J. (1997) Association of panic disorder with a history of traumatic suffocation. *American Journal of Psychiatry, 154*(11): 1566–1570.

Boyce, W. T., Chesney, M., Alkon, A., Tschann, J M., Adams, S., Chesterman, B., Cohen, F., Kaiser, P., Folkman, S. & Wara, D. (1995). Psychobiologic reactivity to stress and childhood respiratory illnesses: results of two prospective studies. *Psychosomatic Medicine*, *57*(5): 411–422.

Bremner, J. D. & Brett, E. A. (1997). Trauma-related dissociative states and long-term psychopathology in posttraumatic stress disorder. *Journal of Traumatic Stress, 10*(1): 37–49.

Bremner, J. D., Southwick, S. M. & Johnson, D. R. et al. (1993). Childhood physical abuse and combat-related posttraumatic stress disorder in Vietnam veterans. *American Journal of Psychiatry, 150*, 235–239.

Bremner, J. D., Randall, P. K., Vermetten, E., Staib, L., Bronen, R. A., Mazure, C. M., Capelli, S., McCarthy, G., Innis, R. B. & Charney, D. S. (1997) Magnetic resonance imaging-based measurement of hippocampal volume in posttraumatic stress disorder related to childhood physical and sexual abuse: a preliminary report. *Biological Psychiatry*, *41*(1): 23–32

Breslau, N., Davis, G. C., Andreski, P. & Peterson, P. E. (1991). Traumatic events and post-traumatic stress disorder in an urban population of young adults. *Archives of General Psychiatry, 48*, 216–222.

Briere, J. (1997). Symptomatology and phenomenology. In *Psychological assessment of adult posttraumatic states ; 1st ed;* J. Briere (Ed.), pp. 25–55; Washington, American Psychological Association

Brom, D., Kleber, R. J. & Hofman, M. C. (1993). Victims of traffic accidents: incidence and prevention of post-traumatic stress disorder. *Journal of Clinical Psychology*, *49*(2): 131–140.

Bromet, E. J., Sonnega, D. & Kessler, R. C. (1998) Risk factors for DSM-III-R posttraumatic stress disorder: findings from the National Comorbidity Survey. *American Journal of Epidemiology, 147*(4): 353–361

Brosschot, J. F., Benschop, R. J., Godaert, G. L., Olff, M., De Smet, M., Heijnen, C. J. & Ballieux, R. E. (1994). Influence of life stress on immunological reactivity to mild psychological stress. *Psychosomatic Medicine, 6*(3): 216–224.

Brown, G. & Harris, T. (1978). *Social Origins of Depression: The Study of Psychiatric Disorder in Women.* Tavistock; London.

Bryant, B. (1997). Road accidents: the impact on everyday life. In *The Aftermath Of Road Accidents: Psychological; Social And Legal Consequences Of An Everyday Trauma,* Mitchell, M (Ed.). (pp. 199–204). Routledge, London

Bryant, R. A. & Harvey, A. G. (1995). Psychological impairment following motor vehicle accidents. *Australian Journal of Public Health, 19*(2): 185–188.

Buckley, T. C., Blanchard, E. B. & Hickling, E. J. (1996). A prospective examination of delayed onset PTSD secondary to motor vehicle accidents. *Journal of Abnormal Psychology, 105*(4): 617–625.

Burstein, A. (1985). Posttraumatic stress disorder (letter). *Journal of Clinical Psychiatry, 46*, 554.

Chibnall, J. T. & Duckro, P. N. (1994). Post-traumatic stress disorder in chronic post-traumatic headache patients. *Headache, 34*(6): 357–361.

Chubb, H. L. & Bisson, J. I. (1996). Early psychological reactions in a group of individuals with pre-existing and enduring mental health difficulties following a major coach accident. *British Journal of Psychiatry, 169*(4): 430–433.

Cloitre, M., Scarvalone, P. & Difede, J. (1997). Posttraumatic stress disorder; self- and interpersonal dysfunction among sexually retraumatized women. *Journal of Traumatic Stress, 10*(3): 437–452.

Coe, C. L. (1993). Psychosocial factors and immunity in nonhuman primates: a review. *Psychosomatic Medicine, 55*(3): 298–308.

Cohen; S. & Herbert, T. B. (1996). Health psychology: psychological factors and physical disease from the perspective of human psychoneuroimmunology. *Annual Review of Psychology, 47*, 113–142.

Culpan, R. & Taylor, C. (1973). Psychiatric disorders following road traffic and industrial injuries. *Australian and New Zealand Journal of Psychiatry, 7*(1): 32–39

Davidson, J. (1993) Issues in the diagnosis of posttraumatic stress disorder. In J. M. Oldham, M. B. Riba & A. Tasman (Eds.), *American Psychiatric Review of Psychiatry* (Vol 12, pp. 141–155). American Psychiatric Press; Washington; D.C.

Davidson, J., Hughes, D., Blazer, D. & George, K. L. (1991). Post-traumatic stress disorder in the community: An epidemiological study. *Psychological Medicine, 21*: 713–721.

Davidson, J., Schwartz, M., Storck, M., Krishnan, R. R. & Hammett, E. (1985). A diagnostic and family study of posttraumatic stress disorder. *American Journal of Psychiatry, 142*: 90–93.

Di Gallo, A., Barton, J. & Parry-Jones, W. L. L. (1997). Road traffic accidents: early psychological consequences in children and adolescents. *British Journal of Psychiatry, 170*: 358–362

Di Gallo; A. & Parry-Jones, W. L. L. (1996). Psychological sequelae of road traffic accidents: an inadequately addressed problem. *British Journal of Psychiatry, 169* (4): 405–407.

Ellason, J. W., Ross, C. A., Sainton, K. & Mayran, L. W. (1996). Axis I and II comorbidity and childhood trauma history in chemical dependency. *Bulletin of the Menninger Clinic, 60*(1): 39–51.

Falsetti, S. A. & Resnick, H. S. (1997). Frequency and severity of panic attack symptoms in a treatment seeking sample of trauma victims. *Journal of Traumatic Stress, 10*(4): 683–689

Fenton, G., McClelland, R., Montgomery, A., MacFlynn, G. & Rutherford, W. (1993). The postconcussional syndrome: social antecedents and psychological sequelae. *British Journal of Psychiatry, 162*, 493–497.

Fierman, E. J., Hunt, M. F., Pratt, L. A., Warshaw, M. G., Yonkers, K. A., Peterson, L. G., Epstein-Kaye, T. M. & Norton, H. S. (1993). Trauma and posttraumatic stress disorder in subjects with anxiety disorders. *American Journal of Psychiatry, 150*(12): 1872–1874.

Frueh, B. C., Smith, D. W. & Barker, S. E. (1996). Compensation seeking status and psychometric assessment of combat veterans seeking treatment for PTSD. *Journal of Traumatic Stress, 9*(3): 427–439

Fukudo, S., Nomura, T., Muranaka, M. & Taguchi, F. (1993). Brain-gut response to stress and cholinergic stimulation in irritable bowel syndrome. A preliminary study. *Journal of Clinical Gastroenterology, 17*(2): 133–141.

Futterman, A. D., Kemeny, M. E., Shapiro, D. & Fahey, J. L. (1994). Immunological and physiological changes associated with induced positive and negative mood. *Psychosomatic Medicine, 56*(6): 499–511.

Geisser, M. E., Roth, R. S., Bachman, J. E. & Eckert, T. A. (1996). The relationship between symptoms of post-traumatic stress disorder and pain; affective disturbance and disability among patients with accident and non-accident related pain. *Pain, 66*(2–3): 207–214.

Gleason, W. J. (1993). Mental disorders in battered women: an empirical study. *Violence and Victims, 8*(1): 53–68.

Grady; K. T. (1997). Posttraumatic stress disorder and comorbidity: Recognizing the many faces of PTSD. *Journal of Clinical Psychiatry, 58* (supplement 9): 12–15.

Green, B. L., Grace, M. C., Lindy, J. D., Gleser, G. C. & Leonard, A. C., et al. (1990a) Risk factors for PTSD and other diagnoses in a general sample of Vietnam veterans. *American Journal of Psychiatry, 147*: 729–733.

Green, B. L., Grace, M. C., Lindy, J. D., Gleser, G. C., Leonard, A. C. & Kramer, T. L. (1990b). Buffalo Creek survivors in the second decade: comparison with unexposed and nonlitigant groups. *Journal of Applied Social Psychology, 20*: 1033–1050.

Green, B. L., Lindy, J. D., Grace, M. C. & Leonard, A. C. (1992). Chronic posttraumatic stress disorder and diagnostic comorbidity in the disaster sample. *Journal of Nervous and Mental Disorders, 180*: 760–766.

Green, M. M., McFarlane, A. C., Hunter, C. E. & Griggs, W. M. (1993) Undiagnosed posttraumatic stress disorder following motor vehicle accidents. *Medical Journal of Australia, 159*: 529–534.

Griffin, M. G., Resick, P. A. & Mechanic, M. B. (1997).Objective assessment of peritraumatic dissociation: psychophysiological indicators. *American Journal of Psychiatry, 154*(8): 1081–1088.

Herman, J. L. (1992) *Trauma and Recovery*. Basic Books; New York

Herman, J. L., Perry, J. C. & Van der Kolk, B. A. (1989). Childhood trauma in borderline personality disorder. *American Journal of Psychiatry*, *146*, 490– 495.

Helzer, J., Robins, L. & McEvoy, L. (1987). PTSD in the general population. *New England Journal of Medicine, 317*, 1630–1634.

Herbert, T. B. & Cohen, S. (1993). Stress and immunity in humans: a meta-analytic review. *Psychosomatic Medicine*, 55(4): 364–379.

Horowitz, M. J. (1993). Stress-response syndromes: A review of posttraumatic stress and adjustment disorders. In J. P. Wilson & B. Raphael (Eds.). *International Handbook of Traumatic Stress Syndromes*. Plenum Press; New York.

Janoff-Bulman, R. 1992. *Shattered Assumptions: Towards a New Psychology of Trauma*. Free Press; New York.

Kessler, R., Sonnega, A., Broment, E., Hughes, M. & Nelson, C. B. (1995). Posttraumatic stress disorder in the National Comorbidity Survey. *Archives of General Psychiatry, 52*, 1048–1060.

Kiecolt-Glaser, J. K., Malarkey, W. B., Chee, M., Newton, T., Cacioppo, J. T., Mao, H. Y. & Glaser, R. (1993). Negative behavior during marital conflict is associated with immunological down-regulation. *Psychosomatic Medicine*, *55*(5): 395–409.

Koch, W. J. & Taylor, S. (1995). Assessment and treatment of motor vehicle accident victims. *Cognitive and Behavioral Practice, 2*(2): 327–342.

Koss, M. P., Koss, P. G. & Woodruff, W. J. (1991). Deleterious effects of criminal victimization on women's health and medical utilization. *Archives of Internal Medicine, 151*(2): 342–347.

Koss, M. P., Woodruff, W. J. & Koss, P. G. (1990). Relation of criminal victimization to health perceptions among women medical patients. *Journal of Consulting and Clinical Psychology, 58*(2): 147–152.

Krieger, N. (1994) Epidemiology and the web of causation: has anyone seen the spider? *Social Science and Medicine, 39*(7): 887–903

Kuch, K., Cox, B. J., Evans, R. & Shulman, I. (1994). Phobias; panic; and pain in 55 survivors of road vehicle accidents. *Journal of Anxiety Disorders, 8*(2): 181–187.

Kulka, R. A., Schlenger, W. E., Fairbank, J. A., Hough, R. L., Jordan, B. K., Marmar, C. R. & Weiss, D. S. (1990). *Trauma and the Vietnam War Generation.* Brunner/Mazel; New York.

Landsman, I. S., Baum, C. G., Arnkoff, D. B., Craig, M. J., Lynch, I., Copes, W. S. & Champion, H. R. (1990). The psychosocial consequences of traumatic injury. *Journal of Behavioral Medicine, 13*(6): 561–581

Lepore, S. J., Allen, K. A. & Evans, G. W. (1993). Social support lowers cardiovascular reactivity to an acute stressor. *Psychosomatic Medicine, 55*(6): 518–524.

Leserman, J., Drossman, D. A., Li, Z., Toomey, T. C., Nachman, G. & Glogau, L. (1996). Sexual and physical abuse history in gastroenterology practice: how types of abuse impact health status. *Psychosomatic Medicine, 58*(1): 4–15.

Levine, H. (1968) The automobile accident syndrome. *Medical Trial Technique Quarterly, 15*(1): 21–27

Lifton, R. J. (1993). From Hiroshima to the Nazi doctors. In J. P. Wilson & B. Raphael (Eds.), *International Handbook of Traumatic Stress Syndromes.* (pp. 11–23). Plenum, New York.

Mayou; R. (1997).The psychiatry of road traffic accidents. In Mitchell, M (Ed.), *The Aftermath Of Road Accidents: Psychological; Social And Legal Consequences Of An Everyday Trauma.* (pp. 235–253). Routledg; London.

Mayou, R., Bryant, B. & Duthrie, R. (1993). Psychiatric consequences of road traffic accidents. *British Medical Journal, 307*(6905): 647–651.

Mayou, R., Tyndel, S. & Bryant, B. (1997). Long-term outcome of motor vehicle accident injury. *Psychosomatic Medicine,* 59(6):578–584.

McFarlane, A. C. & Yehuda, R. (1996). Resilience; vulnerability; and the course of posttraumatic reactions. In B. A. van der Kolk, A. C. McFarlane & L. Weisaeth; L. (Eds.), *Traumatic Stress: The Overwhelming Experience on Mind, Body and Society.* (pp. 155–181). Guilford, New York.

Mendelson, G. (1982) Not cured by a verdict: effect of legal settlement on compensation claimants. *Medical Journal of Australia, 2*(3):132–134.

Norris, F. H. (1992). Epidemiology of trauma: frequency and impact of different potentially traumatic events on different demographic groups. *Journal of Consulting and Clinical Psychology, 60*; 3; 409–418.

Orsillo, S. M., Weathers, F. W., Litz, B. T., Steinberg;, H. R., Huska, J. A. & Keane., T. M. (1996). Current and lifetime psychiatric disorders among veterans with war zone-related posttraumatic stress disorder. *Journal of Nervous and Mental Disease, 184*(5): 307–313.

Orth-Gomer, K., Rosengren, A. & Wilhelmsen, L. (1993). Lack of social support and incidence of coronary heart disease In middle-aged Swedish men. *Psychosomatic Medicine, 55*(1): 37–43.

Packard, R. C. (1992). Posttraumatic headache: permanency and relationship to legal settlement. *Headache, 32*(10): 496–500.

Parker, R. S. (1996). The spectrum of emotional distress and personality changes after minor head injury incurred in a motor vehicle accident. *Brain Injury, 10*(4): 287–302.

Parker, R. S. & Rosenblum, A. (1996). IQ loss and emotional dysfunctions after mild head injury incurred in a motor vehicle accident. *Journal of Clinical Psychology,* 52(1): 32–43.

Paykel, E. (1978). Contribution of life events to causation of psychiatric illness. *Psychological Medicine,* 8, 245–254.

Pecukonis, E. V. (1996). Childhood sex abuse in women with chronic intractable back pain. *Social Work and Health Care, 23*(3): 1–16.

Perry, S., Difede, M. A., Musngi, G. F. & Jacobsberg, L. (1992). Predictors of posttraumatic stress disorder after burn injury. *American Journal of Psychiatry, 149*, 931–935.

Perry, J. C., Herman, J. L., Van der Kolk, B. A. & Hoke, L. A., (1990). Psychotherapy and psychological trauma in borderline personality disorder. *Psychiatric Annals, 20*, 33–43.

Pitman, R. K., Sparr, L. F., Saunders, L. S. & McFarlane, A. C. (1996) Legal issues in posttraumatic stress disorder. In B. A. van der Kolk, A. C. McFarlane, L. Weisaeth (Eds), *Traumatic Stress: The Effects of Overwhelming Experience on Mind; Body and Society.* Guilford, New York. (pp. 378–397).

Plichta, S. B. & Abraham, C. (1996). Violence and gynecologic health in women < 50 years old. *American Journal of Obstetetrics and Gynecology, 174*(3): 903–907.

Resnick, H., Kilpatrick, D. G. & Dansky, B., et al. (1993). Prevalence of civilian trauma and posttraumatic stress disorder in a representative national sample of women. *Journal of Consulting and Clinical Psychology, 61*, 984–991.

Rogers, M. P., Weinshenker, N. J., Warshaw, M. G., Goisman, R. M., Rodriguez-Villa, F. J., Fierman, E. J. & Keller, M. B. (1996). Prevalence of somatoform disorders in a large sample of patients with anxiety disorders. *Psychosomatics, 37*(1): 17–22.

Sabo, A. N. (1997) Etiological significance of associations between childhood trauma and borderline personality disorder: conceptual and clinical implications. *Journal of Personality Disorders,* 11(1): 50–70

Salmon, P. & S. Calderbank. (1996). The relationship of childhood physical and sexual abuse to adult illness behavior. *Journal of Psychosomatic Research, 40*(3): 329–336.

Saunders, B. E., Villeponteaux, L. A., Lipovsky, J. A., Kilpatrick, D. G. & Veronen, L. J. (1992) Child sexual assault as a risk factor for mental disorders among women: a community survey. *Journal of Interpersonal Violence, 7*(2): 189–204.

Shalev, A. Y. (1996) Stress versus traumatic stress: From acute homeostatic reactions to chronic psychopathology. In B. A. van der Kolk, A. C. McFarlane, L. Weisaeth (Eds), *Traumatic Stress: The Effects of Overwhelming Experience on Mind, Body and Society.* (pp. 77–101). Guilford, New York.

Silver, S. M. (1986). An inpatient program for post-traumatic stress disorder: Context as treatment. In C. R. Figley (Ed.], *Trauma And Its Wake, Volume II: Post-Traumatic Stress Disorder: Theory; Research And Treatment,* Brunner/Mazel; New York.

Simon, R. I. (1995). Introduction. In Simon, R. I. (Ed.), *Posttraumatic Stress Disorder in Litigation: Guidelines for Forensic Assessment* (pp. xix–xxvii). American Psychiatric Press, Washington, D.C.

Smith, D. W. & Frueh, B. C. (1996). Compensation seeking; comorbidity; and apparent exaggeration of PTSD symptoms among Vietnam combat veterans. *Psychological Assessment, 8*(1): 3–6.

Solomon, Z. & Bleich, A. (1998). Comorbidity in posttraumatic stress disorder and depression in Israeli veterans. *CNS Spectrums, 3*(7 Suppl 2):16–21.

Solomon, S. & Canino, G. (1990). Appropriateness of the DSM-II-R criteria for post-traumatic stress disorder. *Comprehensive Psychiatry, 31*, 227–237.

Solomon, S. & Davidson, J. R. T. (1997). Trauma: Prevalence; impairment; service use; and cost. *Journal of Clinical Psychiatry, 58*(suppl 9): 5–11.

Solomon, Z., Benbenishty, R., Waysman, M. & Bleich, A. (1994) Compensation and psychic trauma: a study of Israeli combat veterans. *American Journal of Orthopsychiatry, 64*(1): 91–102.

Solomon, Z., Iancu, I. & Tyano, S. (1997). World assumptions following disaster. *Journal of Applied Social Psychology, 27*(20):1785–1798.

Southwick, S. M., Yehuda, R. & Giller, E. L. (1993). Personality disorders in treatment-seeking combat veterans with posttraumatic stress disorder. *American Journal of Psychiatry, 150*, 1020–1023.

Stein, M. B., Yehuda, R., Koverola, C. & Hanna, C. (1997) Enhanced dexamethasone suppression of plasma cortisol in adult women traumatized by childhood sexual abuse. *Biological Psychiatry, 42*(8): 680–686.

Symonds, M. (1982). Victim's response to terror: Understanding and treatment. In Ochberg, F. & Soskis, D. (Eds.), *Victims of Terrorism* (pp. 95–103). Westview; Boulder, CO.

Tarsh, M. J. & Royston, C. (1985) A follow-up study of accident neurosis. *British Journal of Psychiatry, 146*, 18–25.

Terr, L. (1990) *Too Scared To Cry*. Harper and Row; Harper and Row.

True, W. R., Rice, J., Eisen, S. A., Heath, A. C., Goldberg, J., Lyons, M. J. & Nowak, J. (1993). A twin study of genetic and environmental contributions to liability for posttraumatic stress symptoms. *Archives of General Psychiatry, 50*, 267–264.

Tyano, S., Iancu, I., Solomon, Z., Sever, J., Goldstein, I., Toubiana, Y. & Bleich, A. (1996). Seven-year follow-up of child survivors of bus-train collision. *Journal of American Academy of Child and Adolescent Psychiatry, 35*(3): 365–373.

Van der Kolk, B. A. (1989). The compulsion to repeat the trauma: reenactment; revictimization; and masochism. *Psychiatric Clinics Of North America; Vol. 12. Treatment of Victims of Sexual Abuse*; (pp. 389–411). Philadelphia: W. B. Saunders.

Van der Kolk, B. A. (1996). The complexity of adaptation to trauma. In B. A. van der Kolk, A. C. McFarlane, & L. Weisaeth (Eds.), *Traumatic Stress: The Effects of Overwhelming Experience on Mind, Body and Society*. Guilford; New York. (pp.378–397).

Vasile, R. G., Goldenberg, I., Reich, J., Goisman, R. M., Lavori, P. W. & Keller, M. B. (1997). Panic disorder versus panic disorder with major depression; defining and understanding differences in psychiatric morbidity. *Depression and Anxiety, 5 (1): 12–20.*

Walker, E. A., Gelfand, A. N., Gelfand, M. D., Green, C. & Katon, W. J. (1996). Chronic pelvic pain and gynecological symptoms in women with irritable bowel syndrome. *Journal of Psychosomaticatic Obstetrics and Gynaecology, 17*(1): 39–46.

Watts, R. (1995).Posttraumatic stress disorder after a bus accident. *Australian and New Zealand Journal of Psychiatry, 29*(1): 75–83.

Winje, D. (1996). Long-term outcome of trauma in adults: the psychological impact of a fatal bus accident. *Journal of Consulting and Clinical Psychology, 64*(5): 1037–1043.

Zaidi, L. Y. & Foy, D. W. (1994). Childhood abuse experiences and combat-related PTSD. *Journal of Traumatic Stress, 7*(1): 33–42.

12

Who Develops PTSD from Motor Vehicle Accidents, and Who Subsequently Recovers?

EDWARD B. BLANCHARD, Ph.D.

Center for Stress and Anxiety Disorders, State University of New York, Albany, 1535 Western Avenue, Albany, New York, USA

EDWARD J. HICKLING, Psy.D.

Capital Psychological Associates and The Sage Colleges

The two rhetorical questions in this chapter's title frame two of the three topics to be addressed in this chapter. Thus, the topics to be addressed are: (1) Who develops Posttraumatic Stress Disorder (PTSD) from motor vehicle accidents (MVAs) and what are the significant risk factors for developing MVA-related PTSD? (2) what is the natural history of MVA-related PTSD, or who gets better, and what predicts remission? The third topic concerns delayed onset PTSD and addresses what size problem is it and what are the significant risk factors for this manifestation of PTSD?

As in our book, *After the Crash* (Blanchard & Hickling, 1997), we will provide two answers to these questions: the first is what we have learned from our American work in Albany, New York; the second is that provided by a review of the world's English language literature. Lastly, we will give our best guess based upon the two sources.

Who Develops PTSD from MVAs?

The Albany Answer. Since in this book we provide data from two separate MVA survivor cohorts recruited and assessed in the Albany, NY, area, we have titled these Albany Cohort 1 and Albany Cohort 2, respectively. For Albany Cohort 1, the inclusion criteria were: (1) individuals 17 years of age or older; (2) he/she had been in a MVA as driver, passenger, pedestrian or cyclist; (3) 1 to 4 months had elapsed since the MVA; (4) the individual had sought medical attention for the consequences of the MVA within 48 hours of the accident. Only 15% of our sample were actually admitted to a hospital; however, 75% were seen in an emergency room.

We chose the 1 to 4 month window so that the minimum length of time necessary to meet DSM-III-R (American Psychiatric Association, 1987) criteria for PTSD had elapsed and yet the patient was likely to be close enough in time to be able to remember details of the accident and so that years of living with PTSD symptoms were unlikely to distort the subject's recall of what they were like before the accident.

Diagnosis of PTSD was made on the basis of a structured interview developed by the National Center for PTSD, Boston Branch, the Clinician-Administered PTSD Scale (CAPS) (Blake et al, 1990; Weathers & Litz, 1994). The CAPS has good reported reliability and validity. Frequency of the symptom is scored 0 to 4 as is intensity or severity. Individual symptom scores thus range from 0 to 8.

In our own work, we checked for interrater reliability by having a sample of the audiotapes of initial interviews re-scored by an advanced graduate student, blind to all other aspects of the MVA survivor's record. Kappa for diagnostic agreement was 0.810, $p<.0005$. Pearson correlation coefficients for scores on individual symptoms ranged from 0.82 to 0.99, with a mean, using Fisher's r to z transformation, of 0.975, $p<.001$.

We subdivided our sample into three groups: (1) those who met the full criteria for PTSD, (2) those we have termed sub-syndromal PTSD who met the reexperiencing criterion and either avoidance and psychic numbing or hyperarousal criteria, but not both. (3) The last group were termed non-PTSD and met either one symptom cluster or none.

In Table 1 are the characteristics of our sample of 158 MVA survivors. We had 108 females (68.4%) in the sample. The average age was 35.4 years; on average they were 68 days post-MVA. Included were 18 non-Caucasian (11.4%).

We found a high rate of PTSD in our sample, almost 40%. This is one of the higher values for a non-referred sample which has been reported as will be noted in Table 3. Women are over-represented in the PTSD category as you will note. This is consistent with Kessler et al's (1995) National

Table 1. ALBANY COHORT 1. Demographic Characteristics of Sub-Samples of MVA Survivors

Characteristic	Sub-Sample		
	PTSD	Sub-Syndromal PTSD	Non-PTSD
Sub-sample size and (%)	62 (39.2)	45 (28.5)	51 (32.3)
Gender (M/F)	13/49	14/31	23/28
Percent female	79.0%	68.9%	54.9%
Age – Mean	34.8	35.4	36.2
Range	18–73	17–65	17–71
Ethnic Status			
(Caucasian/Minority)	50/12	42/3	48.3
Percent Minority	19.4%	6.7%	5.9%
Days since MVA	69.4	63.4	72.1

Table 2. Summary of Final Logistic Regression to Predict Posttraumatic Stress Disorder in MVA Survivors

Variable	B	sig	Percent Correctly Classification PTSD	Non-PTSD	Total
—	—	—	0	100.0	60.8
Fear of Dying (in MVA)	.014	.0032	40.3	84.4	67.1
Prior Major Depression	.634	.0013	45.2	85.4	69.6
Litigation	.794	.0333	50.0	83.3	70.3
Extent of Injury	.104	.0209	56.5	78.1	69.6
Constant	−2.768				
Total correct Classification =	69.6%				

Adapted from Blanchard et al (1996) *Behaviour Research and Therapy, 34*, 1-10.

Co-Morbidity Study of PTSD and also with the recent large study from Oxford by Ehlers et al (1998). Minorities were also over-represented in the PTSD category. While we believe that the gender difference is true, we are uncertain about the minority issue because of the small sample size.

We examined a large host of pre-MVA and MVA variables to see what predicted who developed PTSD. The values for the individual predictors are in Blanchard and Hickling. We found 4 independent predictors which are shown in Table 2. They are (1) the individual had suffered an episode of major depression prior to the MVA (they were not necessarily depressed at the time of the MVA); (2) The extent of physical injury as measured by the Abbreviated Injury Scale; (American Association for Automotive Medicine, 1985); (3) Extent to which the subject was frightened and feared he/she might die in the MVA on a scale of 0 = not at all frightened to

Table 3. Predictors of who develops PTSD from MVAs

Authors	Population	Assessment and Diagnosis				
		When Assessed Initially	When Diagnosed PTSD	Diagnostic Instrument	Diagnostic Criteria	% PTSD
Feinstein & Dolan, 1991 (UK)	Hospitalized patients w/broken leg (27 MVA)	< 1 week	6 weeks	CIS > 14	DSM-III-R	25% at 6 weeks
Mayou et al, 1993 (UK)	188 consecutive admissions for MVA (n = 63 whiplash)	X = 9.0 days	3 months	PSE	DSM-III-R	8% at 3 mo.
Green et al, 1993 (Australia)	24 hospitalized MVA survivors	In hospital	1 month	DIS and GHQ	DSM-III-R	8%-1 mo. 30%-18 mo.
Epstein, 1993 (USA)	15 hospitalized on trauma unit	Within days of MVA	Within 2 weeks	Structured psychiatric interview	DSM-III-R	40% (4/6 initially, 2/6 at 2-3 Mo. FU)
Bryant & Harvey, 1996 (Australia)	114 successive MVA survivors hospitalized for at least 1 day post-trauma amnesia < 1 day (38 mild head injury)	Within 2 weeks of MVA	Within 2 weeks	IES	IES > 30	31%
Delahanty et al, 1997 (USA)	80 hospitalized MVA survivors	Within 3 weeks of MVA	Within 3 weeks of MVA	SCID	DSM-III-R	24% at 3 weeks
Harvey & Bryant, 1998 (Australia)	92 hospitalized MVA survivors	Average 8 days post-MVA	6 months post-MVA	CIDI	DSM-III-R	25% at 6 mo.
Ehlers et al, 1998 (UK)	967 hospital attendees	Within 8 days post-MVA	3 months post-MVA	PSS Quest.	DSM-IV	23% at 3 mo.
Blanchard et al, 1996 (USA)	158 MVA survivors who sought medical attention	1-4 months post-MVA	1-4 months post-MVA Av. 2 mo.	CAPS	DSM-III-R	39%

Notes: CIS – Clinical Interview Schedule, IES - Impact of Event Scale, PSE – Present State Examination, DIS – Diagnostic Interview Scale, GHQ – General Health Questionnaire, SCID – Structured Clinical Interview for PTSD, CIDI – Composite International Diagnostic Interview, ASD – Acute Stress Disorder, PSS – Posttraumatic Stress Symptom Scale, CAPS – Clinician-Administered PTSD Scale, DSM – Diagnostic and Statistical Manual

100 = extremely frightened and thought he would die or be seriously injured. (4) Whether, by the time of assessment, the patient or the patient's family had contacted a lawyer to explore a legal suit.

Three of these variables are very straightforward and not at all surprising. The litigation variable is more awkward because it is subject to at least two different interpretations: (1) it could be that, having decided on litigation, the MVA survivor portrays him/herself in a very distressed light so as to enhance the possibility of receiving recompense for psychological damages. (2) Alternatively, it could be that the more psychologically distressed the individual is more likely to initiate litigation to seek recompense for their suffering. With correlational data, one can never tell.

The World's Answer. In Table 3 is a summary of the English language literature through the summer of 1998 relevant to this question. To be included the study had to be a prospective follow-up of a non-referred (that is, not selected by medical or legal professionals for evaluation because of MVA-related problems). Included in the table are: the country where the study took place, a description of the sample, when they were initially assessed, when they were initially diagnosed with PTSD (as well as diagnostic criteria used and diagnostic procedures used), *what fraction developed PTSD initially*, and what variables predict initial development of PTSD.

Examining Table 3 several findings emerge. The rate of diagnosing PTSD varies considerably from 8% in Mayou et al (1993) and Green et al (1993) to 39% in Blanchard et al (1996) and 40% in Epstein (1993). The median rate is 25% (Harvey & Bryant, 1998). It should be remembered that this 25% rate of PTSD is for a population who was injured and sought medical attention, usually at the emergency room. Many of the samples were actually hospitalized MVA survivors. However, being admitted to hospital was not especially associated with PTSD since the highest rate (40% in Epstein) and the lowest rate (8% in Green et al) both came from hospitalized samples.

Part of the variability may be due to the diagnostic instrument used. A number of different structured interviews were used as well as the questionable practice of relying upon questionnaires (Bryant & Harvey, 1996; Ehlers et al, 1998). It might be helpful in the future for someone to examine the case finding ability of some of the common instruments.

Another factor possibly affecting the rate of PTSD is when the diagnostic evaluation was made. In 3 of the papers, less than the one-month of symptoms, Criterion E, was used. In others, diagnosis was made 3 months and even 6 months (Harvey & Bryant, 1998) after the trauma. As the next section will show, there is also a natural decay function (or spontaneous remission process) at work in MVA-related PTSD such that cases may have been missed.

Regardless of the precise value, it seems to be a sizable percentage of those injured in MVAs, and thus constitutes a notable, but until recently largely ignored, public health problem.

Who Recovers from MVA-Related PTSD?

The Albany Answer. We attempted to re-interview our entire sample at points 6 months and 12 months after the initial assessment. We also sought to re-interview only those initially diagnosed with PTSD at the 18-month follow-up point. In addition to using the CAPS to re-assess for the symptoms of PTSD, we adapted Keller et al's (1987) Longitudinal Interval Follow-up Evaluation (LIFE) procedures to track individual symptoms of PTSD and Axis I co-morbidity on a week-by-week basis, and psychosocial variables on a month-by-month basis. The LIFE utilizes personally meaningful calendar anchors (birthdays, anniversaries) as well as widely known anchors (holidays such as Labor Day, Independence Day, Christmas, etc.) to help patients date the time of changes in symptoms.

In Table 4 are the demographic characteristics of the samples who were re-assessed at 6 months (91.8% of total) and at 12 months (83.6%), as well as those of the drop-outs.

Although we held a very good percentage of our sample in the study for the 6-month (91.8%) and 12 month (83.6%), there was a disproportionate loss of participants among those with PTSD (11.3% at 6 months versus 6.3% of others; 22.6% at 12 months versus 12.5% of others). Neither of these is statistically significant although the 12-month data show a trend ($p = .09$). Overall drop-outs tended to be younger, more likely to be single and to be minority.

The important answer to the question of who recovers are given in Table 5 for both those initially diagnosed with full PTSD and those diagnosed with sub-syndromal PTSD.

As one can see in Table 5, slightly over half (54.5%) of those with an initial diagnosis of PTSD had remitted in part (23.6%) or fully (30.9%) by the 6-month follow-up point and two-thirds (66.7%) had remitted at least in part by the 12-month follow-up. There was little additional apparent remission at 18 months but this conclusion must be drawn cautiously since only 56.5% of the sample were re-assessed at that point.

In Tables 6 and 7 are the results of the logistic regression analyses to predict remission of PTSD (either fully or in part) for the 6-month and 12-month follow-up assessments, respectively.

The 6-month predictors are fairly straightforward: those with more severe PTSD symptoms (higher initial CAPS scores) and more severe initial physical injury (initial AIS score) were less likely to remit. Also, the occurrence of

Table 4. Demographic and Diagnostic Information on Completers and Dropouts at Each Assessment

Variable	Sample				
	Initial	6-Mo. Completers	6-MO Dropout	12-Mo Completers	12-Mo Dropout
Initial Diagnosis					
PTSD	62 (39.2%)[1]	55 (37.9%)	7 (11.3%)[2]	48 (36.4%)[1]	14 (22.6%)[2]
Sub-Syndromal	45 (28.5%)	43 (29.7%)	2 (4.4%)	42 (31.8%)	3 (6.6%)
Non-PTSD	51 (32.3%)	47 ((32.4%)	4 (7.8%)	42 (31.8%)	9 (17.6%)
TOTAL	158	145	13 (8.2%)	132	26 (16.4%)
Gender (M/F)	50/108	48/97	2/11	44/88	6/20
(% Female)	(68.4%)	(66.9%)	(84.6%)	(66.7%)	(76.9%)
Age (SD)	35.4 (12.5)	36.0 (12.7)	29.3 (7.7)	36.2 (12.6)	31.7 (11.8)
Ethnicity					
Caucasian/Minority	140/18	131/14	9/4	123/9	17/9
(% Minority)	(11.4%)	(9.7%)	(30.8%)	(6.8%)	(34.6%)

Note [1] Percentages of the total sample at that assessment. For follow-ups, the frequencies are of those available based on initial diagnosis.
Note [2] Percentages for dropouts are percent of initial diagnostic subsample who dropped out.

Table 5. Remission Data for Initial Full PTSD and Sub-Syndromal PTSD at 6, 12 and 18 Months

Initial Diagnosis	Follow-up Status	Follow-up Point 6 Month	12-Month	18-Month
PTSD	PTSD			
n=62	n (%)	25 (45.4)*	16 (33.3)	12 (34.3)
	Sub-PTSD			
	n (%)	13 (23.6)	7 (14.6)	5 (14.3)
	Non-PTSD			
	n (%)	17 (30.9)	25 (52.1)	18 (51.4)
	Percent Re-assess.	88.7%	77.4%	56.5%
Sub-Syndromal				
PTSD	PTSD			
n=45	n (%)	2 (4.7)	3 (7.1)	—
	Sub-PTSD			
	n (%)	12 (27.9)	9 (21.4)	—
	Non-PTSD			
	n (%)	29 (67.4)	30 (71.4)	—
	Percent Re-assess.	95.6%	93.3%	

*Percentages in columns represent percent of sub-sample assessed at that follow-up point.

Table 6. Summary of Logistic Regression to Predict Remission of PTSD Among MVA Survivors Over 6-Months Follow-up

Variable	B	Sig	Cummulative % Correct Classification		
			PTSD	Sub-PTSD or Non-PTSD	Total
—	—	—	0	100.0	54.6
Initial CAPS Score	.0520	.0083	60.0	80.0	70.9
New Trauma to Family	2.4868	.0096	64.0	83.3	74.6
Abbreviated Injury Scale Score	.1252	.1084	72.0	86.7	80.0
Physical Injury Quotient (Mo. 4)	2.7914	.0427	80.0	86.7	83.6
CONSTANT	–6.2987	.0005			
Total Correct Classification = 83.6%					

From E. B. Blanchard et al (1997), *Journal of Traumatic Stress, 10*, 215-231.

a new traumatic event within the participant's immediate family predicted lower likelihood of remission. Finally, the relative degree of recovery from all of the physical injuries by month 4 predicted recovery, that is, the less physical healing, the less psychological healing. These data and others lead us to see the intimate interconnection or reciprocal relations of healing of the "psyche" and the "soma".

Table 7. Prediction of Remission of MVA-PTSDs at 12-Month Follow-up

Predictor	B	Sig.	Percent Correctly Identified		
			PTSD	Less than PTSD	Overall
Base Rate	—	—	0	100	66.7
Initial CAPS-13 Irritability	.5251	.0069	50.0	78.1	68.8
Initial CAPS-11 Foreshortened Future	.4723	.0124	56.3	90.6	79.2
Vulnerability in Auto. at Initial Assessment	.0379	.0419	62.5	87.5	79.2
CONSTANT	−6.6571	.0010			
Total Correct Classification = 79.2%					

From: Blanchard et al (1996) *Behaviour Research and Therapy, 34*, 775-786.

12-Month Follow-up. The prediction of remission by the 12-month follow-up was much less straightforward. Three variables emerged in the logistic regression as significant predictors: (1) the degree of irritability at the initial assessment as rated on the CAPS, (2) the degree to which the participant reported a sense of foreshortened future on the CAPS, and (3) the degree of vulnerability the participant experienced when riding in a vehicle (0 = no vulnerability to 100 = extreme vulnerability) at the time of the initial assessment. Altogether 62.5% of those who remained PTSD and 87.5% of those who had remitted fully or in part were correctly identified for an overall correct classification rate of 79.2%.

The World's Answer. In Table 8 is summarized the English language literature from prospective follow-up studies of MVA survivors.

Of the six studies (it is not possible to discern remission in Harvey and Bryant's (1988) 6-month prospective follow-up of MVA survivors), five show substantial remission 6 to 12 months after the MVA with a range from 38.5% to 67% with a mean of 50%. There was no remission in the Australian sample of Green et al (1993).

Prediction of remission of PTSD has lagged behind prediction of the risk factors for developing it. However, the large scale Oxford study by Ehlers et al (1998) identified 10 different, independent predictors which held up in cross validation analyses. None is outstandingly strong; the degree of vari-

Table 8. Remission of MVA-related PTSD and its prediction

Authors	Population	% Initial PTSD	Follow-up Interval	% PTSDs Remitted	Predictors
Feinstein & Dolan, 1991 (UK)	Hospitalized for broken leg	25%	6-Mo.	5/12 41.7%	N/R
Mayou et al, 1993 (UK)	188 consecutive admissions for MVA	8% at 3-mo.	12-Mo.	5/13 38.5%	N/R
Green et al, 1993 (Australia)	24 hospitalized MVA survivors	8% at 1-mo.	18-Mo.	No remission	N/R
Delahanty et al, 1997 (USA)	80 hospitalized MVA survivors	24% at 3-wks.	12-Mo.	10/19 52.6%	Self-responsible, remit more readily than other responsible.
Ehlers et al, 1998 (UK)	781 hospital attendee MVA survivors	23% at 3-mo.	12-Mo.	49.7%	1. Negative interp. of intrusions. 2. Persistent health problems. 3. Rumination. 4. Pre-MVA emotional problems. 5. Persistent financial problems. 6. Thought suppression. 7. Anger. 8. Dissociation. 9. Litigation. 10. Gender.
Blanchard et al, 1996 (US)	48 MVA survivors who sought medical attention and had PTSD 1-4 mo. post-MVA.	39% at 1-4 mo.	12-Mo.	67%	1. Initial irritability. 2. Initial foreshortened future. 3. Initial sense of vulnerability. - - - - - - - - - - - - - - Self-responsible remit more readily.

ance accounted for is in the range of 1 to 4%. More work is needed to replicate their findings. (But it will be difficult to mount such a large scale study as theirs.)

One prediction which has been replicated is the finding by Delahanty et al (1997) that those MVA survivors with PTSD who saw themselves as responsible for the MVA remitted more quickly than those who saw someone else as responsible. A recent re-analysis of the Albany Cohort-1 data (Hickling et al, 1999), replicated this finding.

Delayed Onset PTSD

The official nomenclature (DSM-IV, American Psychiatric Association, 1994) recognizes that not all cases of PTSD are present immediately after the exposure to the trauma by describing Delayed Onset PTSD as the appearance of the full syndrome 6 months or more after the trauma.

The Albany Answer. Since we were using the LIFE methodology to track the individual symptoms of PTSD over the follow-up intervals, it was possible to know with some accuracy at what point a MVA survivor, who initially did not meet the criteria for PTSD, did, in fact, meet it.

We found 7 cases of delayed onset PTSD in our Albany Cohort 1. All of these cases had sub-syndromal PTSD at the initial assessment. This means that over 15% of those with sub-syndromal developed delayed onset PTSD, and that delayed onset was present in 4.4% of our total sample.

In our sample, variables which predicted delayed onset PTSD were having sub-syndromal PTSD at the initial assessment, at pre-MVA a lower level of social support and lower level of overall functioning, the overall severity of symptoms as measured by the CAPS and particularly the presence of avoidance. This work is summarized in Buckley et al (1996).

We should also note that we could find a proximal stressor in only 3 of the 7 cases; in the other 4, we could identify nothing which logically would lead a patient to worsen.

The World's Answer. This crossing over of sub-syndromal, or sub-clinical, PTSD into full-blown PTSD was also noted in Green's series from Australia. Other individuals who have looked at delayed onset are Professor Mayou who found 3.4% of his total sample, Green who found 21%, and Professor Ehlers who found 6.2% (see Table 9).

Table 9. Delayed onset of MVA-related PTSD

Authors	Population	% Delayed Onset PTSD	Predictors
Mayou et al, 1993 (UK)	188 consecutive admissions for MVA	3.4% 6/174	N/R
Green et al, 1993 (Australia)	24 hospitalized MVA survivors	20.8% 5/24	Initial sub-syndromal PTSD
Ehlers et al, 1998 (UK)	967 hospital attendees	6.2% 34/549	Persistent health problems. Negative interpretation of intrusions. Emotional problem pre-MVA. Rumination.
Buckley et al, 1996 (USA)	158 MVA survivors	4.4% 7/158	Initial sub-syndromal PTSD. Initial level of PTSD symptoms (CAPS score). Pre-MVA lower level of social support. Pre-MVA lower overall functioning (GAS rating).

For the most part, the overall percentage of the samples studied who develop delayed onset PTSD is small (3 to 6%). However, compared to the total percentage of MVA survivors who develop PTSD initially, the delayed onset group represent an additional 10 to 20% of cases.

Initial sub-syndromal PTSD is a clear risk for later escalating to full PTSD as shown both by Green et al (1993) and Buckley et al (1996).

Conclusions

It seems clear that personal injury MVAs, especially those with more serious injury warranting attendance at the ER or hospital, have large psychological and psychosocial consequences. As Table 3 shows, about 25% of individuals injured in MVAs are likely to develop PTSD in the short term and another 5% are likely to develop it later.

Fortunately, about half of those with initial PTSD have remitted fully, or in part, by a year later, usually with no formal treatment. Those who do not remit spontaneously over the first year seem destined to have a very slow recovery and clearly are in need of psychological and medical care.

References

American Association for Automotive Medicine. (1985, Revision). *The Abbreviated Injury Scale*. Des Plaines, IL: American Association for Automotive Medicine.

American Psychiatric Association. (1994). *Diagnostic and Statistical Manual of Mental Disorders*, 4th Edition. American Psychiatric Association: Washington, DC.

American Psychiatric Association. (1987). *Diagnostic and Statistical Manual of Mental Disorders* (3rd Edition, Revised). American Psychiatric Association: Washington, DC. American Psychiatric Press.

Blake, D., Weathers, F., Nagy, L., Kaloupek, D., Klauminzer, G., Charney, D. & Keane, T. (1990). *Clinician Administered PTSD Scale* (CAPS). National Center for Post-Traumatic Stress Disorder, Behavioral Science Division-Boston, Boston VA, Boston, MA.

Blanchard, E. B. & Hickling, E. J. (1997). *After the Crash: Psychological Assessment and Treatment of Survivors of Motor Vehicle Accidents*. American Psychological Association, Washington, DC.

Blanchard, E. B., Hickling, E. J., Barton, K. A., Taylor, A. E., Loos, W. R. & Jones-Alexander, J. (1996). One-year prospective follow-up of motor vehicle accident victims. *Behaviour Research and Therapy, 34*, 775–786.

Blanchard, E. B., Hickling, E. J., Forneris, C. A., Taylor, A. E., Buckley, T. C., Loos, W. R. & Jaccard, J. (1997). Prediction of remission of acute post-traumatic stress disorder in motor vehicle accident victims. *Journal of Traumatic Stress, 10*, 215–234.

Blanchard, E. B., Hickling, E. J., Taylor, A. E., Loos, W. R. & Forneris, C. A. (1996). Who develops PTSD from motor vehicle accidents? *Behaviour Research and Therapy, 34*, 1–10.

Bryant, R. A. & Harvey, A. G. (1996). Initial posttraumatic stress responses following motor vehicle accidents. *Journal of Traumatic Stress, 9*, 223–234.

Buckley, T. C., Blanchard, E. B. & Hickling, E. J. (1996). A prospective examination of delayed onset PTSD secondary to motor vehicle accidents. *Journal of Abnormal Psychology, 105*, 617–625.

Delahanty, D. L., Herberman, H. B., Craig, K. J., Hayward, M. C., Fullerton, C. S. & Ursano, R. J. (1997). Acute and chronic distress and posttraumatic stress disorder as a function of responsibility for serious motor vehicle accidents. *Journal of Consulting and Clinical Psychology, 65*, 560–567.

Ehlers, AQ., Mayou, R. A. & Bryant, B. (1998). Psychological predictors of chronic posttraumatic stress disorder after motor vehicle accidents. *Journal of Abnormal Psychology, 107*, 508–519.

Epstein, R. S. (1993). Avoidant symptoms cloaking the diagnosis of PTSD in patients with severe accidental injury. *Journal of Traumatic Stress, 6*, 451–458.

Green, M. M., McFarlane, A. C., Hunter, C. E. & Griggs, W. M. (1993). Undiagnosed post-traumatic stress disorder following motor vehicle accidents. *The Medical Journal of Australia, 159*, 529–534.

Harvey, A. G. & Bryant, R. A. (1998). The relationship between acute stress disorder and posttraumatic stress disorder: A prospective evaluation of motor vehicle accident survivors. *Journal of Consulting and Clinical Psychology, 66*, 507–512.

Hickling, E. J., Blanchard, E. B., Buckley, T. C. & Taylor, A. E. (1999). Effects of attribution of responsibility for motor vehicle accidents on severity of PTSD symptoms, ways of coping and recovery over six months. *Journal of Traumatic Stress, 12*, 345–353.

Keller, M. B., Lavori, P. W., Friedman, B., Nielsen, E., Endicott, J., McDonald-Scott, P. & Andreasen, N. C. (1987). A longitudinal interval follow-up evaluation: A comprehensive method for assessing outcome and prospective longitudinal studies. *Archives of General Psychiatry, 44*, 540–548.

Kessler, R. C., Sonnega, A., Bromet, E., Hughes, M. & Nelson, C. B. (1995). Post-traumatic stress disorder in the National Comorbidity Survey. *Archives of General Psychiatry, 52*, 1048–1060.

Mayou, R., Bryant, B. & Duthie, R. (1993). Psychiatric consequences of road traffic accidents. *British Medical Journal, 307*, 647–651.

Weathers, F. W. & Litz, B. T. (1994). Psychometric properties of the Clinician-Administered PTSD Scale, CAPS-I. *PTSD Research Quarterly, 5*, 2–6.

13

Psychophysiological Dimensions of Motor Vehicle Accident Survivors

EDWARD B. BLANCHARD, EDWARD J. HICKLING, TODD C. BUCKLEY, and CONNIE H. VEAZEY

Center for Stress and Anxiety Disorders, University at Albany, Albany, NY, USA

One of the relatively unique aspects of our work with motor vehicle accident (MVA) survivors at Albany has been our focus on psychophysiological assessment. This research topic which relies on measurement of peripheral physiological responses, usually those mediated by the autonomic nervous system, to trauma-related cues, has been the subject of research attention among PTSD researchers for over 15 years.

Most of the early work was conducted with Vietnam veterans with combat-related PTSD, including studies from our laboratory using an audiotape of combat sounds played at progressively greater sound levels (Blanchard, Kolb, Pallmeyer & Gerardi, 1982; Blanchard et al, 1986). Other approaches used a videotape depicting ever more threatening combat scenes with an accompanying sound track (Malloy et al, 1983) and idiosyncratic audiotapes depicting the trauma (Pitman et al, 1987). (For a recent review of this psychophysiological assessment literature, see Blanchard & Buckley, 1998).

The Albany Psychophysiology Studies

We have published a pair of studies (Blanchard et al, 1994); Blanchard et al, 1996) on the psychophysiological assessment of MVA survivors with our so-called Albany Cohort-1 participants. Fortunately, we have been able to replicate the essential findings of that work with our new set of MVA survivors, whom we have termed, Albany Cohort-2. The basic methodology was the same with both cohorts.

Response Measures

In the first studies we measured heart rate (HR) in beats per minute (bpm) and both systolic and diastolic blood pressure (SBP and DBP, respectively) with a Dinamapp Critikon 1990 which was programmed to take readings once per minute. The values are provided as a digital display on the device and are printed on a paper tape. We also measured electrodermal activity using a Grass Instruments Company Model 7 polygraph and a 7P1 bridge circuit. The exact level of skin resistance level was read from the potentiometer after centering the pen. Silver-silver chloride electrodes, filled with conductive gel, were attached to the ventral surfaces of the index and middle finger.

Finally, we measured forehead muscle activity (electromyogram [EMG]) with a Grass 7P3 AC preamplifier interfaced with a 7P10 integrator. Electrodes were attached approximately 2.5 cm above the eyebrow, centered over each eye, with a ground electrode midway in between. The forehead was cleaned thoroughly; Grass EC-2 electrode paste was the conductive medium.

For the Cohort-2 study, we dropped the forehead EMG measurement since it did not yield much in the Cohort-1 studies.

Assessment Conditions

We have used relatively standard conditions in all of the studies. They are described in Table 1 for the Cohort-1 studies.

For Cohort-1, we used both idiosyncratic audiotapes, modeled after the procedure of Pitman et al (1987), and a generic videotape depicting a series of auto crashes, most filmed from inside of the vehicle.

Thus, our stressor conditions were (1) mental arithmetic, as a standard cognitive stressor which tends to elicit a mild pressor response from most individuals, (2-3) two idiosyncratic audiotapes, both describing the participant's MVA in the second person (e.g., "you see the red car coming

Table 1. Psychophysiological Test Conditions

Adaptation: 2–7 min
Polygraph and Dynamapp calibrated
Baseline (BL): 5 min
"Please sit quietly with your eyes closed."
Mental math: 3 min
"Please count backwards by 7s starting at 250."
Return to BL-1: 5 min
"Please sit quietly with your eyes closed."
Audiotape 1: 3 min
"Please listen to this audiotape."
Return to BL-2: 5 min (same instructions as return to BL-1)
Audiotape 2: 3 min (same instructions as Audiotape 1)
Return to BL-3:5 min (see instructions as return to BL-1)
Eyes open: 2 min
"Please sit quietly with your eyes open."
Videotape: 3 min
"Please watch this video."
Return to BL-4: 5 min (same instructions as return to BL-1)
Relax: 2 min

right at you") with a slight variation between the two tapes, and (4) the standard videotape. Rest periods designed to allow the participant to return to a baseline level of physiological responding were interspersed.

As will be clear from the section below, the generic videotape of MVA crashes was not especially provocative. It was dropped for the Cohort-2 study in the interest of saving time.

An example of an audiotape script is contained in Table 2.

Albany Cohort-1

The participants in our initial psychophysiological studies of MVA-related PTSD included the MVA survivors we described earlier, subdivided into those with full PTSD, those with sub-syndromal PTSD, and those without PTSD, as well as 93 non-accident controls, selected to match the MVA sample on age and gender. They had had no MVAs of any kind over the past 12 months. Demographic characteristics are contained in Table 3.

Details of the various statistical analyses are available in Blanchard et al (1994) and Blanchard et al (1996). Neither forehead EMG nor electrodermal activity yielded much in the way of significant differential responding among

Table 2. Example of Audiotape Script

Now I want you to imagine this scene in your mind's eye. I want you to try to recreate it and make it just as real as you can in your imagination. It's early Friday morning on January 16, 1996. You are going to work when you realize you need gas. You stop on the corner of Rosendale Road and Route 7 to get gas. Since the traffic is so heavy on Route 7 you decide to take the back way on Rosendale to Buhrmaster. You are going down Rosendale Road about 10 m.p.h. when you see the front end of a truck coming right at you. There is no where for you to go to get away from the truck. The next thing you remember is seeing the other driver get out of his truck and walk away from you and your van. You see smoke coming out of the engine of your van. Your driver's door is jammed shut, and your tools are on the other side of you. You grab your cellular phone and dial 911. It takes you a few minutes to describe to the operator where you are. It seems forever before the paramedics arrive. You are in and out of consciousness. Your head is pounding and you are in pain. You keep shaking your right arm. The paramedics arrive and tell you not to move. One paramedic is throwing your tools out onto the road to get you out. You then remember driving by your house and wanting to call your wife.

.........*Now take that scene away.*

Now, I want you to imagine again, just recreate this scene right in your mind's eye, make it as real and as vivid as you can. You are on your way to work when you stop to get gas. It is early on a Friday morning in January. You are in your van. You decide to take a back way to avoid traffic. The road is small and curves sharply to the left. You see the front end of a truck headed right for you. You try to get off of the road, but there is no where to go. The truck hits you, and you see your hammer crash through your windshield. The next thing you remember is seeing the driver of the truck get out of his truck and walk to the other side of the road. You then notice smoke coming from your van, and you realize you cannot get out. You are afraid you might burn. One of your tool racks is on your right side and the driver's door is jammed shut. You reach for your cellular phone and dial 911. It takes you a few minutes to describe to the operator where you are. It seems like forever until the paramedics arrive. During this time, you are in and out of consciousness. Someone comes and asks how you are doing. Your head is pounding and you keep shaking your right arm. The paramedics arrive and tell you not to move. One paramedic is taking your tools and throwing them on the road to get you out. You are put on a board and in a neck brace. You then remember driving by your house, and you want to call your wife. One of the paramedics calls her for you......Now take that scene away.

groups or within groups across the stressors. There was some differential responding for the BP measures; however, by far the strongest results came with HR.

In Figure 1 are the mean HR responses (that is, the HR value for the stressor minus the HR value from the immediately preceding baseline condition [see Table 1]) for the 4 groups of participants at the 4 stressor conditions.

Comparisons across the 4 participant groups for Mental Arithmetic, Audiotape-2, and the videotape were non-significant; however, the comparison for Audiotape-1 was highly significant ($F[3,155] = 6.61$, $p = .0003$).

Table 3. ALBANY COHORT 1 Demographic Characteristics of Sub-Samples of MVA Survivors and Non-MVA Controls

Characteristic	Sub-Sample			
	PTSD	Sub-Syndromal PTSD	Non-PTSD	Non-MVA
Sub-sample size	62	45	51	93
Gender (M/F)	13/49	14/31	23/28	28/65
Percent female	79.0%	68.9%	54.9%	69.9%
Age – Mean	34.8	35.4	36.2	37.7
Range	18–73	17–65	17–71	20–78
Ethnic Status				
(Caucasian/Minority)	50/12	42/3	48/3	84/9
Percent Minority	19.4%	6.7%	5.9%	9.7

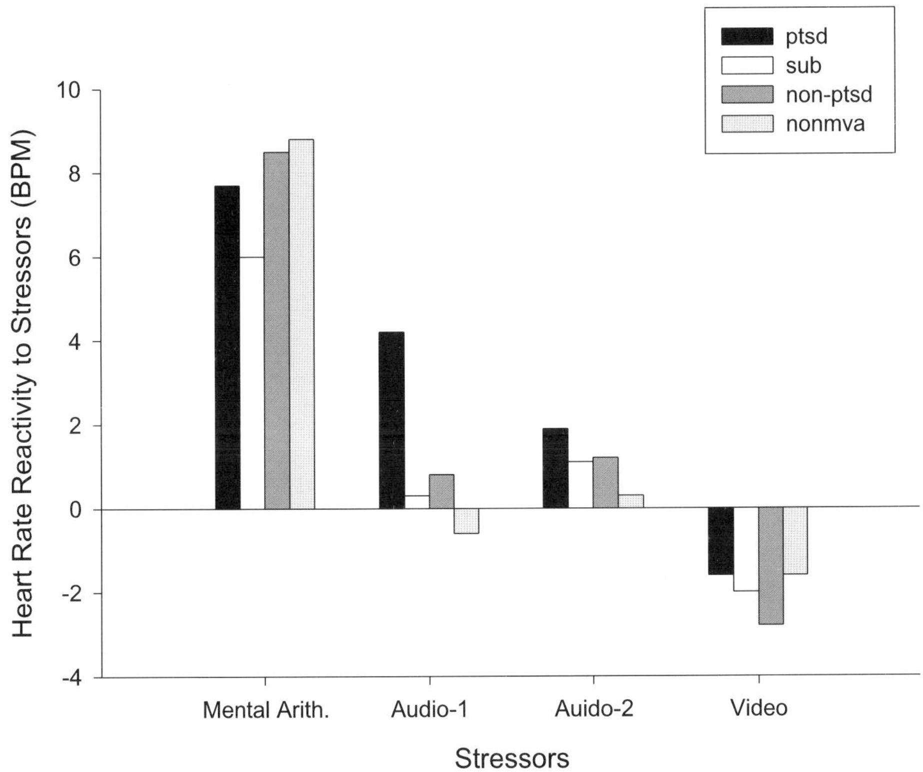

Figure 1.

We sought to learn if these results might have value at the level of the individual patient, rather than just finding group mean differences. Relying only upon the HR data for Audiotape-1, and using as a cut-off score +2.0 bpm (that is, the HR value to Audiotape-1 minus the HR value to "Return to Baseline-1"), we find a sensitivity of 65.6, a specificity of 68.6, and a diagnostic efficiency of 67.9 when comparing those with full PTSD to the other three groups combined. This translates to 40 of 61 MVA-PTSD participants being correctly identified.

Discussion. Correctly identifying 65.6% of those MVA survivors with PTSD with a single cut off value for a single measure, HR response to Audiotape-1, can be viewed two ways: it could be seen as a very strong result when a simple non-self-report measure is correct almost two-thirds of the time. Alternatively, one would not want to throw out the structured interview since the psychophysiological measure misses one-third of those with PTSD, and also has a fair degree of false positives.

One could probably achieve better separation of PTSDs from the others if multiple physiological responses to multiple stressors were combined in a discriminant function. In our clinical experience, we find that practicing clinicians would never use these elegant multivariate equations. So, if one wants a simple answer to the non-verbal diagnostic question, it is not very accurate but of some value.

Prediction of 12-month clinical status. One other interesting aspect of these data is this: we examined those initially diagnosed with PTSD (and all the others) at 12 months. We then sought to see how the initial psychophysiological data, that is, measurements about 2 months after the accident predicted clinical status 12 months later. In Blanchard et al (1996) we showed clearly that the early psychophysiological data could predict later clinical status. Those initial PTSDs who remained PTSD 12 months later were more reactive initially than those who had remitted fully or in part. We could correctly classify 76% of the total sample.

Albany Cohort-2

The Albany Cohort-2 is primarily a work in progress. By that we mean that we are in the midst of recruiting another cohort of MVA survivors; in this paper we present data on 63 individuals who were assessed in our Center between January 1, 1997, and July 29, 1998. This sample differs from Cohort-1 in several important ways. First, we are recruiting MVA survivors with PTSD into a treatment trial. Second, they were selected if they were more than 6

Table 4. ALBANY COHORT 2 Demographic Characteristics of Sub-Samples of MVA Survivors

Characteristic	Sub-Sample		
	PTSD	Sub-Syndromal PTSD	Non-PTSD
Sub-sample size and %	43 (68%)	11 (18%)	9 (14%)
Gender (M/F)	8/35	3/8	1/8
Percent Female	(81%)	(73%)	(89%)
Age – Mean	37.7	37.5	38.5
Range	(20–53)	(20–55)	(21–62)
Ethnic Status			
(Caucasian/Minority)	41/2	8/3	7/2
Percent Minority	(4.6%)	(27.2%)	(22.2%)
Months since MVA			
Mean	14.4	12.9	12.3

months but less than 30 months post-accident. Third, we have pre-screened potential subjects by telephone using the PTSD Checklist (PCL) (Weathers et al, 1993), in an effort to maximize the fraction of the sample who met criteria for full PTSD or fairly severe sub-syndromal PTSD. Fourth, there is no non-MVA sample.

The demographic characteristics of this sample are presented in Table 4.

Several things are notable about this sample: (1) females are over represented in the non-PTSD sub-samples as are minorities; (2) the average time since the MVA is about 14 months rather than two months with Cohort-1; (3) the average age is about the same.

Procedures. The psychophysiological assessment for Cohort-2 is very similar to that described earlier. We have made two major changes: the MVA videotape condition was deleted and measurement of forehead EMG was deleted. Thus, we continued to measure HR, SBP, DBP and skin resistance level, using the same equipment.

Results. Again, the most interesting results emerge with HR. In Figure 2 are the mean HR responses (e.g., HR for Audiotape-1 minus the preceding baseline) for the three groups of subjects for the three stressors.

A two-way ANOVA with repeated measures was significant ($F[4,118] = 2.42$, $p = .050$). Follow-up one-way ANOVAs across the 3 sub--groups for each stressor were significant for Audiotape-1 ($F[2,54] = 6.79$, $p = .002$) and Audiotape-2 ($F[2,53] = 3.06$, $p = .055$) but not for mental arithmetic. Individual comparisons on Audiotape-1 were significant between

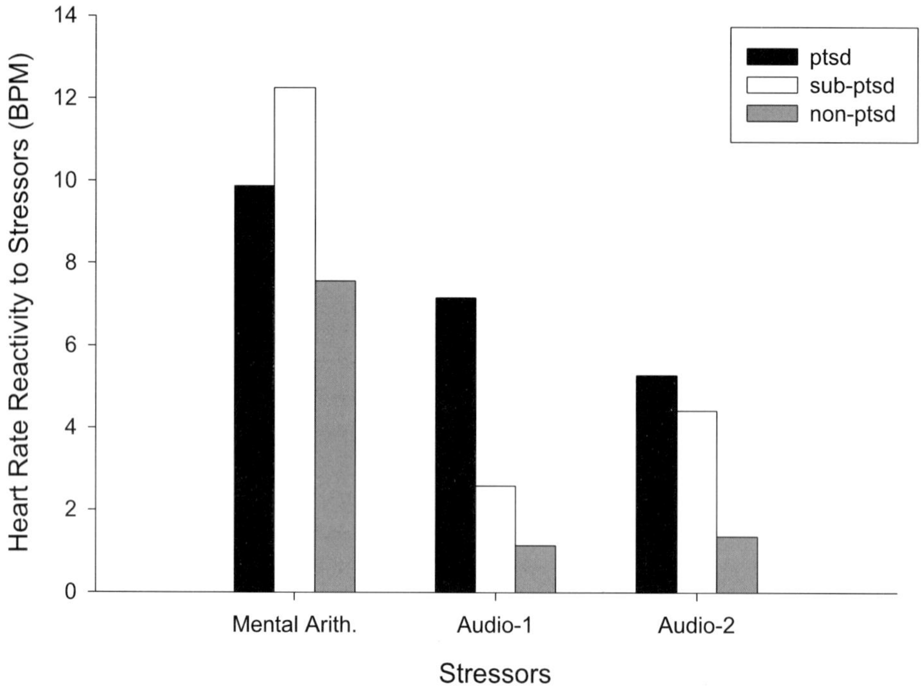

Figure 2.

PTSD and sub-syndromal PTSD ($p = .017$) and between PTSD and non-PTSD ($p = .003$). For Audiotape-2, only the difference between PTSD and non-PTSD was significant ($p = .025$).

Again, examining the individual subject data, we find fairly good separation with the +2.0 bpm to Audiotape-1. Even better separation was found by combining the response scores to Audiotape-1 and Audiotape-2 and using a +5.0 bpm cut off. These data are presented in Figure 3.

Thirty-two out of 40 (80%) PTSDs are correctly identified. As is usual there are a number of false positives among the group with current sub-syndromal PTSD and the non-PTSD set of MVA survivors.

Discussion. It seems clear that MVA survivors who meet the full criteria for PTSD continue to be noticeably reactive (especially with changes in HR) to idiosyncratic audiotaped descriptions of their accidents almost 14 months after the MVA. This replication of the finding from those with acute (about 2 months post-MVA) PTSD, with more chronic cases of PTSD, is gratifying, as is the fact that again good identification of the individual case is available.

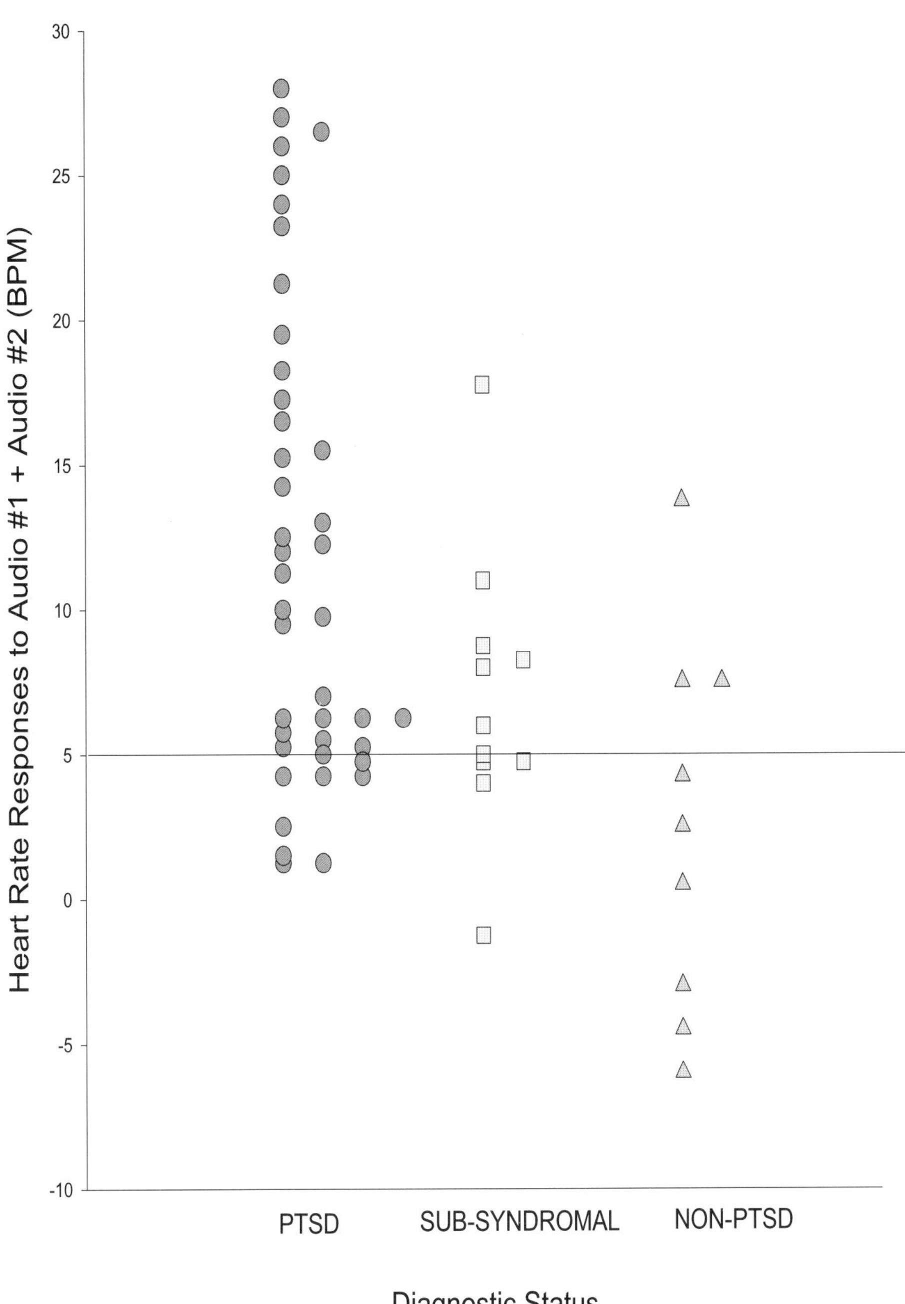
Heart Rate Responses to Audio #1 + Audio #2 (BPM)
30
25
20
15
10
5
0
-5
-10
PTSD
SUB-SYNDROMAL
NON-PTSD
Diagnostic Status

Figure 3.

The results seem consistent with both Keane et al's (1985) conditioned emotional response model of PTSD and Foa & Kozak's (1986) cognitive fear structure models of PTSD. If the emotional response or fear structure has not been treated, the physiological arousal and other symptoms of PTSD seem to persist.

References

Blanchard, E. B., Hickling, E. J., Buckley, T. C., Taylor, A. E., Vollmer, A. & Loos, W. R. (1996). The psychophysiology of motor vehicle accident related post-traumatic stress disorder: Replication and extension. *Journal of Consulting and Clinical Psychology, 64*, 742–751.

Blanchard, E. B., Hickling, E. J., Taylor, A. E., Loos, W. R. & Gerardi, R. J. (1994). The psychophysiology of motor vehicle accident related post-traumatic stress disorder. *Behavior Therapy, 25*, 453–467.

Blanchard, E. B., Kolb, L. C., Gerardi, R. J., Ryan, P. & Pallmeyer, T. P. (1986). Cardiac response to relevant stimuli as an adjunctive tool for diagnosing post-traumatic stress disorder in Vietnam veterans. *Behavior Therapy, 17*, 592–606.

Blanchard, E. B., Kolb, L. C., Pallmeyer, T. P. & Gerardi, R. J. (1982). A psychophysiological post-traumatic stress disorder in Vietnam veterans. *Psychiatric Quarterly, 54*, 220–229.

Foa, E. B. & Kozak, N. J. (1986). Emotional processing of fear: Exposure to corrected information. *Psychological Bulletin, 99*, 20–35.

Keane, T. M., Zimering, R. T. & Caddell, J. N. (1985). A behavioral formulation of post-traumatic stress disorder in Vietnam veterans. *the Behavior Therapist, 8*, 9–12.

Malloy, P. F., Fairbank, J. A. & Keane, T. M. (1983). Validation of a multimethod assessment of post-traumatic stress disorders in Vietnam veterans. *Journal of Consulting and Clinical Psychology, 51*, 488–494.

Pitman, R. K., Orr, S. P., forgue, D. F., deJong, J. B. & Claiborn, J. M. (1987). Psychophysiologic assessment of post-traumatic stress disorder imagery in Vietnam combat veterans. *Archives of General Psychiatry, 44*, 970–975.

Weathers, F. W., Litz, B. T., Herman, D. S., Huska, J. A. & Keane, T. M. (1993, October). *The PTSD Checklist: Reliability, Validity, & Diagnostic Utility.* Paper presented at the annual meeting of the International Society for Traumatic Stress Studies, San Antonio, TX.

14

Psychosocial Effects of Motor Vehicle Accidents

EDWARD J. HICKLING
Capital Psychological Associates and The Sage Colleges

EDWARD B. BLANCHARD, ELIZABETH MUNDY and CONNIE H. VEAZEY
Center for Stress and Anxiety Disorders, University at Albany, Albany, NY, USA

While a great deal of attention has been paid to the psychological impact of trauma, very little has been written on the psychosocial effects of motor vehicle accidents (MVAs). This chapter will describe the findings for two distinct samples of subjects from the Albany Motor Vehicle Accident Project. The particular focus of the chapter will be on the psychosocial effects of MVAs and how the MVA can have a pervasive effect on many aspects of an individual's life. It will then outline a method to assess and follow those changes.

The major evaluation tool within our study for the psychosocial effects of MVAs has been the longitudinal interval follow-up evaluation (LIFE Base) of Keller, Lavori, Friedman, Nielson, Endicott, McDonald-Scott & Andreason (1987). As part of our initial assessment study of MVA survivors, we modified Keller et al's scale to assess subjects for the month before their accident, for the current symptom status, and for follow-up studies across

Table 1. ALBANY COHORT 1 Demographic Characteristics of Sub-Samples of MVA Survivors and Non-MVA Controls

Characteristic	Sub-Sample			
	PTSD	Sub-Syndromal PTSD	Non-PTSD	Non-MVA
Sub-sample size	62	45	51	93
Gender (M/F)	13/49	14/31	23/28	28/65
Percent female	79.0%	68.9%	54.9%	69.9%
Age – Mean	34.8	35.4	36.2	37.7
Range	18–73	17–65	17–71	20–78
Ethnic Status				
(Caucasian/Minority)	50/12	42/3	48/3	84/9
Percent Minority	19.4%	6.7%	5.9%	9.7

time. The LIFE Base provides a measure of performance within the work, school, home, family, friends, and recreational aspects of an individual's life. When the assessment addressed the quality of social relations, we were primarily looking for first degree relatives, that is, either parent, siblings, children, and spouse/partner. The LIFE Base evaluation utilizes a 5-point scale, ranging from 1 = very good, high level of performance to 5 = very poor performance. For purposes of our study we averaged the ratings across all first degree relatives to derive the measure of perceived social support. The quality of relationships with friends and the quality of recreational activities were, again, assessed using this same 5-point scale. This evaluation was performed to assess major role functioning. Work was considered full-time if they were employed 30 hours or more per week or if applicable how they were performing within the school or within the home setting.

Cohort 1

The Albany MVA Research Project initially performed a comprehensive assessment study of MVA survivors. Cohort 1 consisted of 158 MVA survivors who had sought medical attention because of their MVA and were initially seen 1–4 month post-MVA, followed up at 6, 12, and in some cases, 18 months later. Cohort 1 is described in Table 1 along with a non-MVA control group.

Table 2. ALBANY COHORT 2 Demographic Characteristics of Sub-Samples of MVA Survivors and Non-MVA Controls

Characteristic	Sub-Sample		
	PTSD	Sub-Syndromal PTSD	Non-PTSD
Sub-sample size and %	43 (68%)	11 (18%)	9 (14%)
Gender (M/F)	8/35	3/8	1/8
Percent Female	(81%)	(73%)	(89%)
Age – Mean	37.7	37.5	38.5
Range	(20–53)	(20–55)	(21–62)
Ethnic Status			
(Caucasian/Minority)	41/2	8/3	7/2
Percent Minority	(4.6%)	(27.2%)	(22.2%)
Months since MVA			
Mean	14.4	12.9	12.3

Cohort 2

Cohort 2 is an ongoing treatment study in which we are recruiting MVA survivors who are 6–30 months post-MVA into a randomized controlled clinical treatment trial. Those who are admitted into the treatment trial suffer from PTSD or a reasonably severe sub-syndromal presentation of PTSD. The data that will be presented here is for the first 18 months of that treatment trial through July 15, 1998. Cohort 2 is described in Table 2.

Subjects are entered into the study after a telephone screen using the PCL (Weathers et al., 1993). Those not thought likely to meet inclusion criteria are not admitted into the study. The preponderance of Cohort 2 subsequently are individuals who have PTSD. We consider sub-syndromal PTSD as individuals who are showing significant dysfunction as a result of their motor vehicle trauma but do not exhibit sufficient symptoms to render a full diagnosis of PTSD. In particular, if individuals reach criteria for two (Criterion B, C or D) but not all three of the criteria for PTSD, they are considered to have sub-syndromal PTSD (see Blanchard & Hickling, 1997).

The data in Table 3 describes the LIFE Base scores for employment or major role function for individuals who have either PTSD, sub-syndromal PTSD, non-PTSD, or were non-MVA subjects in our initial study.

As you will note, there is a full scale unit difference between PTSD and the sub-syndromal PTSD suggesting a very dramatic difference. Additionally, there is a very significant difference between all three groups and PTSD in terms of their impairment in employment.

Table 3

EMPLOYMENT OR SELF-EMPLOYMENT

1 = No impairment – high level (e.g., has worked as much as someone in his social situation would be expected to work, and worked at a high level).

2 = No impairment – satisfactory level (e.g., has worked as much as someone in his social situation would be expected to work, and worked at a satisfactory level).

3 = Mild impairment (worked somewhat less than someone in his social situation would be expected to work and/or had mild difficulties in carrying out work activities).

4 = Moderate impairment (has missed a lot of work and/or has had considerable difficulties in carrying out work activities).

5 = Severe impairment (has missed a great deal of work when someone in his social situation would have been expected to work and/or has been virtually unable to carry out his work activities when he did work).

Cohort 1

PTSD	Sub-PTSD	Non-PTSD	Non-MVA
3.1_a	2.1_b	1.9_b	1.4_c

Note: Means which share a subscript letter do not differ at the .05 level by Duncan's test.

Table 4

RELATIONSHIPS WITH FAMILY

1 = Very good, e.g., experiences very close emotional relationships with this family member. Feels only very minor or occasional need to improve quality of relationship, which is usually close and satisfying.

2 = Good, e.g., feels close emotionally to this family member. May occasionally prefer not to be with them because of dissatisfaction with them or be actively working with them to improve relationship.

3 = Fair, e.g., thinks that relationship needs to be closer emotionally even when no conflict is present. May withdraw from this person due to dissatisfaction. For those relatives not living with the subject, contacts with them by choice are less frequent than feasible or rarely enjoyed very much when made.

4 = Poor, e.g., feels great deficit in emotional closeness. Regularly prefers to avoid contact with them. For those family members out of the household, subject avoids seeing as much as possible and derives little pleasure from contact when made.

5 = Very poor, e.g., feels no emotional closeness with this (these) family member. Completely avoids those family members living out of household or almost always hostile when in contact.

Cohort 1

PTSD	Sub-PTSD	Non-PTSD	Non-MVA
2.3_a	2.1_b	$1.9_{b,c}$	1.8_c

Table 5

RELATIONS WITH FRIENDS

1 = Very good, e.g., had several special friends that he saw regularly and frequently and was fairly close to.
2 = Good, e.g., had at least two special friends that he saw from time-to-time and was fairly close to.
3 = Fair, e.g., had only one special friend that he saw from time-to-time and was fairly close to, or contacts limited to several friends that he was not very close to emotionally.
4 = Poor, e.g., had no special friends he saw from time-to-time and was fairly close to, or contacts limited to one or two friends that he was close to.
5 = Very poor, e.g., had no special friends and practically no social contacts.

Cohort 1

PTSD	Sub-PTSD	Non-PTSD	Non-MVA
2.4_a	1.8_b	1.9_b	1.6_c

Table 6

RECREATIONAL ACTIVITY

1 = Very good, e.g., has at least 2 activities which he/she enjoys fully and frequently.
2 = Good, e.g., participates in several activities and does not always enjoy them fully; or participates in fewer activities or less frequently than optimal but enjoys participation.
3 = Fair, e.g., occasional participation in recreational activities or hobbies, or limited enjoyment when participation occurs.
4 = Poor, e.g., some participation in recreational activities or hobbies, and derives very little enjoyment from such activities.
5 = Very poor, e.g., no involvement in recreational activities or hobbies.

Cohort 1

PTSD	Sub-PTSD	Non-PTSD	Non-MVA
3.3_a	2.4_b	2.2_b	1.8_c

Relationships with family show a consistent pattern where individuals with PTSD or sub-syndromal PTSD, again, have higher scores (that is, less close relationships) with the PTSD group having a statistically significance difference between the other groups and sub-syndromal PTSD having significant differences from the non-MVA controls in terms of relationships with relatives and mates.

When one looks at the effect of a diagnosis of PTSD on the relationship with friends, again, you see the same pattern with individuals with PTSD having poorer relations than those without PTSD for friendships. The same pattern is found for their ability to participate in and enjoy recreational activities. Again, there is almost a full unit difference between those with PTSD and the others in the recreational activities.

The only other study that we are aware of that has investigated the psychosocial effects of MVA survivors, was that of Mayou et al (1993), when they examined individuals with PTSD during a year-long follow-up study. He found that those individuals with PTSD, when compared to other MVA survivors, had greater levels of impairment on measures of leisure and the effect on work. Taking Mayou et al's (1993) study and our results, together, one finds support for the notion that meeting the criteria for PTSD subsequent to a MVA, generally implies that there will be a major impact on the individual's life.

Cohort Study 2

As mentioned earlier, Cohort 2 involves 63 subjects who have been assessed for our controlled treatment study. Individuals, again, are compared on the same LIFE Base measures but in this case they are compared at three points in time: prior to their MVA, in the two months right after the MVA, and at the time of the assessment.

Prior to the MVA the treatment, there was no significance difference found between individuals who subsequently developed PTSD, sub-syndromal PTSD, or non-PTSD on LIFE based measures. Once the accident occurred, there was a dramatic difference for all groups from their pre-accident level of functioning. By the time the same individuals were assessed for treatment, those who had PTSD, were found to have significantly greater impairment in employment and major role performance than those with sub-syndromal PTSD or with non-PTSD.

When one examines the relationships with family members, a similar pattern is found. There is no significant difference among groups prior to the MVA. Those who have developed PTSD following their accident were significantly different than those with sub-syndromal PTSD or non-PTSD. Finally, by the time they were entered into our study, there is a significant difference, again, for those with PTSD and the other two groups.

The relationship with friends reveals a similar trend having fairly good relationships with friends prior to the MVA, with a significant change following the MVA. Those with PTSD, again, report much more difficulty in friendships. The impact on recreation is, again, very similar with individuals who are doing at least two things they fully enjoy frequently being present before the accident, being dramatically changed for all groups at the time

Table 7

EMPLOYMENT OR SELF-EMPLOYMENT

1 = No impairment – high level (e.g., has worked as much as someone in his social situation would be expected to work, and worked at a high level).

2 = No impairment – satisfactory level (e.g., has worked as much as someone in his social situation would be expected to work, and worked at a satisfactory level).

3 = Mild impairment (worked somewhat less than someone in his social situation would be expected to work and/or had mild difficulties in carrying out work activities).

4 = Moderate impairment (has missed a lot of work and/or has had considerable difficulties in carrying out work activities).

5 = Severe impairment (has missed a great deal of work when someone in his social situation would have been expected to work and/or has been virtually unable to carry out his work activities when he did work).

Cohort 2

	Pre-MVA	Post-MVA	Current
PTSD	$1.37_{a,1}$	$3.90_{b,1}$	$3.09_{c,1}$
Sub-syndromal	$1.14_{a,1}$	$3.77_{b,1}$	$2.15_{c,2}$
Non-PTSD	$1.10_{a,1}$	$3.5_{b,1}$	$1.78_{c,2}$

Values in a row which share a letter subscript do not differ.
Values in a column which share a number subscript do not differ.

of the accident. The PTSD group, however, continues to evidence difficulty while the sub-syndromal and non-PTSD group show less impact by greater than one full unit score than the other two groups.

Taken together, individuals following a MVA who develop PTSD do significantly worse on all the scales of the LIFE Base measures. The quality of their life is significantly impacted and the ability to draw support from significant aspects of their life including family, friends, work, and pleasurable outlets, all are significantly diminished.

Driving Behavior

One last area we considered in our psychosocial data, is the effect of the MVA on subsequent driving behavior. As you will see in Table 11, subjects from our first cohort study have shown significant impact on their driving behavior following their MVA. The PTSD group has a significantly greater impact that occurs much more frequently than those who do not develop PTSD. In many Western countries many of us are bound by motor vehicle

Table 8

RELATIONSHIPS WITH FAMILY

1 = Very good, e.g., experiences very close emotional relationships with this family member. Feels only very minor or occasional need to improve quality of relationship, which is usually close and satisfying.

2 = Good, e.g., feels close emotionally to this family member. May occasionally prefer not to be with them because of dissatisfaction with them or be actively working with them to improve relationship.

3 = Fair, e.g., thinks that relationship needs to be closer emotionally even when no conflict is present. May withdraw from this person due to dissatisfaction. For those relatives not living with the subject, contacts with them by choice are less frequent than feasible or rarely enjoyed very much when made.

4 = Poor, e.g., feels great deficit in emotional closeness. Regularly prefers to avoid contact with them. For those family members out of the household, subject avoids seeing as much as possible and derives little pleasure from contact when made.

5 = Very poor, e.g., feels no emotional closeness with this (these) family member. Completely avoids those family members living out of household or almost always hostile when in contact.

Cohort 2

	Pre-MVA	Post-MVA	Current
PTSD	$2.17_{a,1}$	$2.50_{b,1}$	$2.49_{b,1}$
Sub-syndromal	$1.75_{a,1}$	$1.76_{a,1}$	$1.76_{a,2}$
Non-PTSD	$1.94_{a,1}$	$2.31_{a,1}$	$2.23_{a,1}$

Values in a row which share a letter subscript do not differ.
Values in a column which share a number subscript do not differ.

Table 9

RELATIONS WITH FRIENDS

1 = Very good, e.g., had several special friends that he saw regularly and frequently and was fairly close to.

2 = Good, e.g., had at least two special friends that he saw from time-to-time and was fairly close to.

3 = Fair, e.g., had only one special friend that he saw from time-to-time and was fairly close to, or contacts limited to several friends that he was not very close to emotionally.

4 = Poor, e.g., had no special friends he saw from time-to-time and was fairly close to, or contacts limited to one or two friends that he was close to.

5 = Very poor, e.g., had no special friends and practically no social contacts.

Cohort 2

	Pre-MVA	Post-MVA	Current
PTSD	$1.63_{a,1}$	$3.02_{b,1}$	$3.04_{b,1}$
Sub-syndromal	$1.40_{a,1}$	$1.86_{b,2}$	$1.33_{a,2}$
Non-PTSD	$1.60_{a,1}$	$2.44_{b,1}$	$2.10_{a,3}$

Values in a row which share a letter subscript do not differ.
Values in a column which share a number subscript do not differ.

Table 10

RECREATIONAL ACTIVITY
1 = Very good, e.g., has at least 2 activities which he/she enjoys fully and frequently.
2 = Good, e.g., participates in several activities and does not always enjoy them fully; or participates in fewer activities or less frequently than optimal but enjoys participation.
3 = Fair, e.g., occasional participation in recreational activities or hobbies, or limited enjoyment when participation occurs.
4 = Poor, e.g., some participation in recreational activities or hobbies, and derives very little enjoyment from such activities.
5 = Very poor, e.g., no involvement in recreational activities or hobbies.

Cohort 2

	Pre-MVA	Post-MVA	Current
PTSD	$1.38_{a,1}$	$4.33_{b,1}$	$3.54_{c,1}$
Sub-syndromal	$1.33_{a,1}$	$3.36_{b,2}$	$2.53_{c,2}$
Non-PTSD	$1.40_{a,1}$	$2.88_{b,2}$	$2.40_{b,2}$

Values in a row which share a letter subscript do not differ.
Values in a column which share a number subscript do not differ.

use as a required way to live and survive. The number of MVA survivors who actually drive will in all likelihood continue to be fairly high with very few individuals following MVAs stopping driving altogether. However, as you will note from Table 11, there is a dramatic amount of distress reported for an individual with PTSD who drives. While the DSM-IV diagnosis does not allow one to diagnose a specific phobia if the PTSD trauma subsumes the driving behavior, we have found it important to designate a driving phobia for individuals where and when it occurs. Since individuals may be continuing driving but with significant distress, we have termed a phrase "driving reluctance" to describe individuals who continue to drive but only with a great deal of difficulty. We have kept a narrow definition of driving phobia as someone who has given up all driving other than that which is critical and necessary or that they endure, but with considerable anxiety and apprehension. These definitions may change for us across time. The number of individuals with PTSD are significantly greater for those who avoid the site of the MVA, avoid highway driving, avoid pleasure driving, and report noticeable reluctance in driving. The impact, therefore, on driving is uniformly worse for individuals with PTSD than either those with sub-syndromal PTSD or those with non-PTSD.

Table 11. Effects of Accident on Driving Behavior of Motor Vehicle Accident Groups

Measure	MVA Sub-Groups			Comparisons	
	PTSD	Sub-Syndromal PTSD	Non-PTSD	PTSD vs. Sub and Non	
				o^2	p
Does not drive (no license, injuries)	3 (4.8)	1 (2.2)	6 (11.8)		ns
Driving Phobia	9 (15.3)	0 (0)	0 (0)	14.46	.00014
Driving Reluctant					
Avoids MVA Site	20 (33.9)	9 (20.4)	4 (8.9)	8.11	.0044
Avoids highways, etc.	14 (23.7)	6 (13.6)	2 (4.4)	6.47	.011
Avoids driving/riding for pleasure	26 (44.1)	6 (13.6)	1 (2.3)	17.02	.00004
Any noticeable driving reluctance	55 (93.2)	35 (79.5)	8 (17.8)	12.23	.00047

Note: Values in parentheses represent the percentage of the subsample of possible drivers [eliminating those in first row] which the tabulated frequencies represent.

Adapted from Table 8, Blanchard et al, "Psychiatric Morbidity Associated with Motor Vehicle Accidents", *The Journal of Nervous and Mental Disease*, 1995, Vol. 183, No. 8, 495-504. Copyright by Williams & Wilkins. Adapted by permission of the publisher and the author.

The effect of PTSD on psychosocial functioning is considerable. The change in driving behavior can be extremely devastating in areas where there are limited public transportation in widely-spread communities. For many of us in the United States, daily travel by car is a necessity if we are to have any chance of a normal lifestyle. We have found many individuals who will endure the driving to go to work because of the need or, again, who are willing to endure the drive to visit their physician. Overall, the LIFE Base interview has proven to be a very efficient method for describing changes in psychosocial behavior. We also believe that inquiring about driving behavior would be a very useful and important in quantifying and demonstrating changes in the psychosocial aspects of an individual's lifestyle. It is hoped that the Cohort 2 treatment study will be able to demonstrate improvement within the psychosocial aspects of behavior at a future time, when the data is available for analysis.

References

Blanchard, E. B. & Hickling, E. J. (1997). *After the Crash: Assessment and treatment of motor vehicle accident survivors.* American Psychological Association, Washington, D.C.

Keller, M. B., Lavori, P. W., Friedman, B., Nielsen, E., Endicott, J., McDonald-Scott, P. & Andreasen, N. C. (1987). A longitudinal interval follow-up evaluation: A comprehensive method for assessing outcome and prospective longitudinal studies. *Archives of General Psychiatry, 44*, 540–548.

Mayou, R., Bryant, B. & Duthie, R. (1993). Psychiatric consequences of road traffic accidents. *British Medical Journal, 307*, 647–651.

Weathers, F., Litz, B. T., Herman, D. S., Huska, J. A. & Keane, T. M. (1993, October). *The PTSD Checklist: Reliability, validity and diagnostic utility*. Paper presented at the annual meeting of the International Society for Traumatic Stress Studies, San Antonio, Tx.

15

The Bendigo Road Accident Research Project: Predicting Who Suffers Psychological Trauma in the First Year After a Road Accident

SUE JEAVONS BA (Hons) M Phil Ph D

La Trobe University, Bendigo

Background

I became interested in this area whilst working as a clinical psychologist at a rehabilitation centre in Bendigo, a city of approximately 80,000 people in central Victoria, Australia. The particular focus of my work there was a pain management clinic and many of the participants had sustained injuries in road accidents. I noticed that a number of them had emotional issues and posttrauma symptoms that had not been recognised or treated, although in some cases a considerable time had passed since the accident.

Some people were very embarrassed about their symptoms as family and friends tended to say things like "You should be over this now", so that if they suffered nightmares, phobic anxieties about travel or other symptoms, they feared they were going crazy. This further reduced the likelihood of these symptoms being discussed with health practitioners. Education about the "normality" of these symptoms after a traumatic experience was sometimes a great relief for sufferers.

I therefore decided to do some research into psychological trauma in road accident victims as, at this time (early 1990s), there was relatively little literature in the area. Most of the published research was from large metropolitan centres yet many accidents occur in country areas. This project was one of the first to be carried out in a rural area.

The First Study – A Retrospective Postal Survey

As a basis to finding out the extent of posttrauma symptoms in the road accident population, a postal survey was planned to a sample from the Bendigo hospital. In general the study aimed to determine the extent of post-traumatic stress symptoms following road accidents and identify the characteristics of road accident victims with respect to demographic variables such as age, gender and marital status; accident variables such as length of time since the accident, severity of the accident and of injury, as well as injury of others in the accident.

A sample of 350 16–70 year olds who had attended the hospital, either to the Accident and Emergency or been admitted, from 3 months to 2 years previously were selected to receive the following questionnaires:

1. The Late Effect of Accidental Injury Questionnaire (LEAIQ: Malt, Blikra & Høivik, 1989). This questionnaire was specifically designed to assess the biological, psychological and social effects of traumatic injuries. It was modified slightly to improve suitability for Australian conditions and to be specific to road accident respondents.
2. The General Health Questionnaire, 28 item version (GHQ-28) (Goldberg & Hillier, 1979). This is a self administered questionnaire screening for diagnosable psychiatric disorder.
3. The Impact of Event Scale (IES) (Horowitz, Wilner & Alvarez, 1979). This scale is widely used in trauma research and measures subjective distress with subscales of intrusion and avoidance.
4. The Post-traumatic Stress Disorder Interview (PTSD-I) (Watson, Juba, Manifold, Kucala, & Anderson, 1991). This is a diagnostic measure based on DSM IIIR which was in use when the study was commenced.

Replies were received from 80 people, giving a response rate of 23%. There were 33 men and 47 women with a mean age of 39 years. Some of these people had been in relatively minor accidents, 41% were not admitted to hospital. Half of the sample were drivers, 31% were passengers, the remainder were motorcyclists, cyclists and pedestrians.

Sixty three percent of the sample reported permanent physical changes as a result of the accident and a similar number that they had reduced physical function. Half stated that their bodily health was worse.

Occupationally, 55% reported a change in occupation following the accident, of these 67% attributed the change to the accident. Approximately 30% of the sample were not able to work.

Socially, half the sample reported reduced pleasure from leisure, 35% reported reduced contact with others and 29% worse relationships with family or partner. Psychological health was claimed to be worse in 67% of cases but few had received counselling.

According to the screening scoring of the General Health Questionnaire, with a cut off of 5/6, 44% of the sample could be regarded as "cases". The mean score for the Impact of Event Scale was 23.71 (SD = 19.14) which was not significantly different from that of a sample of workers exposed to a gunman randomly shooting in an office building (Creamer, Burgess, Buckingham & Pattison, 1989). Using the Post-traumatic Stress Disorder Interview as a diagnostic measure indicated that 14% of people had a current diagnosis of post-traumatic stress disorder (PTSD).

What this brief section of the obtained results showed was that there were definite effects on people's physical and psychological health following accidents and this extended to their personal and family relationships, their occupations and leisure time.

There were limitations to this study as it was retrospective and there was a low response rate. However it had shown that this was an area worthy of further study and so a larger scale prospective study was planned. More details of the postal survey can be found in Jeavons, Greenwood and Horne (1996, 1998).

The Second Study: A Prospective Repeated Measures Study

The second study was planned as a prospective study which aimed to take a cohort of accident survivors as soon as practicable after their accidents and follow them up for 12 months, with contact at 3 and 6 months also. As my clinical experience had shown that even people with relatively minor accidents could suffer symptoms of psychological disorder, a broad spectrum of levels of injury was sought. Some studies reported in the literature in this area have relied on samples admitted to major trauma units (Gordon, Blaszczynski, Silove, Sloane & Hilman, 1996; Green, McFarlane, Hunter & Griggs, 1993) or referred for medico-legal assessment after the accident (Kuch, Swinson & Kirby, 1985). I aimed to get as representative a sample as possible by contacting everyone who attended the Bendigo Hospital over the study period of 4 months and inviting them to take part in the study.

The first study showed that a minority of those with psychological disorder had received any counselling. Also few hospital emergency departments appear to offer any follow up, especially for psychological issues, to patients on being discharged. Other Australian studies (Horne 1995; Watts, Horne, Sandells & Petrie, 1996) have identified the need for counselling following accidents. Thus a major aim of the second study was to attempt to identify factors, from information gained at the time of the accident, which could enable prediction of which people were at risk of developing psychological disorder so they could be targeted for preventive counselling. A particular focus of this prediction was to examine the role of physical injury as there have been inconsistent reports in the literature about the relationship between injury and subsequent trauma symptoms.

Green (1994) and Epstein (1993) both reported that survivors with and without PTSD showed no significant differences on severity of injury and Pilowsky (1992) cited case studies illustrating psychological disability despite minimal injury. Blanchard, Hickling Barton et al. (1996) reported injury to be a predictor of PTSD at 12 months and Blanchard, Hickling, Mitnick Taylor, Loos and Buckley (1995) found a correlation of .31 between physical injury and PTSD.

Burstein (1989), Goldberg and Gara (1990) and Smith (1989) confirmed the existence of psychological disorder such as PTSD following accidents but have not found it to be related to factors such as previous psychiatric history or severity of injury.

A series of studies by the Albany researchers (Blanchard, Hickling Mitnick, et al., 1995; Blanchard, Hickling, Taylor, & Loos, 1995; Blanchard, Hickling, Taylor, Loos, & Gerardi, 1994; Blanchard, Hickling, Vollmer, Loos, Buckley, & Jaccard, 1995; Blanchard, Hickling, Taylor, Loos, Forneris, & Jaccard, 1996) found PTSD incidence of 39%–46% in people referred for medical attention following accidents. After 4 months there was a reduction of a quarter in those meeting PTSD criteria. A group of "sub-syndromal" PTSD sufferers was also identified. Those who had PTSD were more likely to have experienced previous trauma, to have concurrent or previous depression and to be more subjectively distressed than those who did not. Four factors found to predict PTSD were prior major depression, fear of dying, severity of injury and initiation of litigation (Blanchard, Hickling, Taylor et al., 1996).

In an Oxford prospective study, Mayou, Bryant and Duthie (1993) identified almost a quarter of 188 accident victims as having psychiatric problems one year later. PTSD was diagnosed in 11% and was not associated with neuroticism, previous psychological problems or baseline depression. The rating of horrific intrusive memories at the post accident interview was the principal predictor of PTSD.

The theoretical context selected for this study was one of cognitive appraisal which focuses on the basic assumptions and beliefs held by an individual which are not usually seriously challenged at a deep level but may be shattered by a traumatic event and the coping strategies used to manage such an event. Coping may be problem or task focussed, which includes purposeful efforts at solving a problem or attempting to alter a situation, or emotion-focussed in which the person uses self-oriented emotional reactions or changes the way of appraising or interpreting the threat. Endler and Parker (1990) also add avoidance-focussed coping, which they describe as activities of a cognitive or practical nature (i.e. distraction and social diversion) aimed at avoiding the stressful situation. Endler and Parker (1992) claimed that individuals have personal preferred patterns of coping reactions to stressful situations. The subjective experiences of the participants were also investigated in relation to subsequent trauma reactions.

The sample was obtained by following up everyone aged 18–70 who attended the Bendigo Hospital following road accidents over a 4 month period. Seventy-two people of the 96 contacted, returned useable questionnaires. There were 38 men and 34 women aged 18 to 62 ($M = 32$). Sixty-two people completed both the 3 and 6 month follow ups and 58 the 12 month.

Those who were still in hospital were visited on the wards, completing questionnaires at the time if possible. Those discharged were telephoned to arrange an interview which was conducted by phone if the person lived away from the area. Interviews were generally conducted within 2 weeks of the accident. Follow-up was conducted at 3, 6 and 12 months by post.

The questionnaires included three measures to assess psychological trauma as used in Study One, the GHQ-28, the IES and the PTSD-I. A broad based view of psychological trauma was intended, rather than just a diagnosis of PTSD. Additionally two questionnaires were used for the cognitive appraisal aspects of the study.

4. The Coping Inventory for Stressful Situations (CISS) has subscales of task, emotion and avoidance coping (Endler & Parker, 1990).

5. The World Assumptions Scale (WAS) has subscales of meaningfulness and benevolence of the world and self worth (Janoff-Bulman, 1989).

All questionnaires were administered initially after the accident and at 3, 6 and 12 months.

Other information was obtained from a structured interview covering demographic, accident and subjective variables. This asked for details of the respondent, his/her accident and personal reactions to it. Information was also provided by a hospital doctor from the patients' records and consisted of ratings of severity of injury, likelihood of a loss of consciousness having occurred, triage rating (priority on a 1–5 scale where 1 is the most urgent) and Glasgow coma score (a measure of response to neurological stimuli between 1 and 15 where 15 is highest level of response) on arrival at the hospital.

In looking at the scores on the psychological trauma measures, there was a significant change over the 12 month period in the PTSD-I and IES ($p < .001$) as well as the GHQ ($p < .03$). If the GHQ-28 is used as a screening measure, according to the "case" method of scoring with a cut off of 5/6, initially after the accident 51% of people could be diagnosed with non psychotic psychiatric disorder. At 3 months 34% were "cases", at 6 months 18% and 12 months 19% of the sample. According to the PTSD-I, 6 people (8.3%) could be diagnosed with PTSD at 3 months; 5 people (8%) at 6 months and 5 people (8.6%) at 12 months. The Impact of Event Scale has been used as a diagnostic measure (Bryant & Harvey, 1995) although there are no norms for use of the scale in this way. The means for this sample initially ($M = 27.7$, SD = 18.1) did indicate levels of distress, still present to a lesser degree at 12 months ($M = 13.4$, SD = 18.7).

At 12 months some difficulty driving was reported by 41.5% of the sample and some difficulty as a passenger by 53.5%. Participants were asked to rate their emotional recovery from 0 (not at all) to 4 (complete). Ratings were 1–3.5%, 2–8.8%, 3–40% and 4–47%. Only 8.8% reported receiving any counselling.

One of the major aims for the study was to find factors that, taken immediately after the accident, could be used to identify those vulnerable to subsequent psychological trauma. Stepwise multiple regression analyses were used for the prediction of trauma related symptoms at 3, 6 and 12 months. There were 3 dependent variables (GHQ-28, IES and PTSD-I) for each occasion. Due to the ratio of participants to variables, a series of analyses was used. Five groups of conceptually-related variables were entered and significant variables re-entered into the final model for each time period. The following groups of predictor variables were identified for inclusion in the analysis:

1. Demographic: age, sex, marital status, presence of relationship, family history of psychological/psychiatric treatment, personal history of treatment, previous traumatic incident, recovery from this;

2. Accident: accident severity, whether admitted, length of admission, whether driver/passenger/motorcyclist/cyclist/pedestrian, injury severity self- and doctor-rated, number of others involved in the accident, injury of others known and not known, Glasgow coma score, loss of consciousness, triage rating;

3 & 4. Subjective experience (two groups): Group 1– distress immediately after the accident, distress at being in hospital, perceived life threat, concurrent stress at the time of the accident, self blame for the accident, responsibility for the accident, practical and emotional support; Group 2–were all options for a question regarding experience at the moment of accident/injury and included: do not remember anything, did not think would be seriously injured, thought would be seriously injured, thought would die, concern for others, fear, distress, and shock; and,

5. Coping (CISS) and World Assumptions (WAS): Task coping, emotion coping, avoidance coping, social diversion, distraction, meaningfulness, benevolence, and self worth.

Results showed that for 3 month trauma measures, the variables found to have predictive value were : Emotion focused coping, perceived threat to life or the expectation of injury, at the time of the accident. These were able to predict 12% of variance in GHQ-28, 34% in IES and 38% in PTSD-I.

For 6 month trauma measures, the variables of emotion focussed coping, previous psychological treatment, self rated injury, thinking one might die, avoidance in the form of social diversion, assumption of benevolence (WAS) and accident distress were able to account for 27% of variance in GHQ-28 scores, 49% in IES and 77% in PTSD-I.

For 12 month trauma measures, the variables of emotion focussed coping, number of days spent in hospital, accident distress, fear at the time of the accident and whether driver, passenger etc accounted for 33–47% of variance in GHQ scores, 26–45% of IES and 44–58% of PTSD-I depending on the manipulation of the number of days admitted to hospital variable which was very skewed. These results are summarised in Table 1.

The relationship between injury and trauma scores varied across measures and time. There were four possible ways in which severity of injury was measured: self ratings and doctor's ratings from patients' records, both of which were on a mild, moderate or severe scale; triage scores on arrival at hospital and the number of days that the patient was admitted to hospital. Correlations generally between these measures and the trauma scores were low. The only significant correlation for triage rating was with 3 month PTSD-I ($r = .26$, $p = < .05$). There were no significant correlations with doctor's ratings of injury. Self ratings were significant for GHQ at 12 months ($r = .30$, $p < .01$); IES at 6 months ($r = .30$, $p < .01$) and 12 months ($r = .27$, $p < .05$); and PTSD-I at 12 months ($r = .34$, $p < .01$). Number of days admitted was significantly correlated with all 12 month measures (GHQ-$r = .46$, IES $r = .47$ and PTSD-I $r = .53$–all $p < .01$).

Overall, there were three main findings from this study:

Table 1. Summary of Multiple Regression Results: Variables With Significant Relationships to GHQ-28, IES and PTSD-I at 3, 6 and 12 Months and Adjusted R^2 From Final Multiple Regression Analyses

Scale	3 Month	6 Month	12 month
GHQ-28	Emotion Coping	Emotion Coping Psych. Treat. Injury (self rated)	Emotion coping Days admitted
	R^2 adj .12	R^2 adj .27	R^2 adj .33–.47
IES	Emotion Coping Lifethreat	Emotion Coping Injury (self r/d) Psych.Treatment Social Diversion	Days admitted Fear at accident Emotion Coping
	R^2 adj .34	R^2 adj .49	R^2 adj .26–.45
PTSD-I	Emotion Coping Lifethreat Expect Injury	Emotion Coping Psych. Treat. Thought Die Social Diversion Injury (self r/d) WAS Benevolence Acc. Distress	Emotion Coping Days admitted Accident distress Driver/passenger etc
	R^2 adj .38	R^2 adj .77	R^2 adj .44–.58

i. even when a high proportion of the sample were not seriously injured or admitted to hospital, these road accident survivors still suffered psychological trauma symptoms. Whilst the overall trauma scores decreased over the 12 months, the percentage with PTSD remained relatively constant at about 8%.

ii. information gained soon after the accident, allowed prediction, with 12–77% accuracy depending on the scale used, of who is likely to suffer psychological disorder from 3 to 12 months post accident.

iii using emotion focussed coping, being distressed, fearing losing one's life and subjective experiences were important, rather than demographic or accident variables such as severity of the accident or number of people involved. Injury did prove to have some predictive ability for trauma related symptoms later on, especially self rated injury and number of days spent in hospital.

The factors found to be important in the prediction of trauma symptoms at 3, 6 and 12 months post-accident changed with the passage of time. There was also variation in the predictability for each measure. This study aimed to use a range of trauma measures and not only PTSD diagnosis. The PTSD-I had the strongest overall predictability and was highest at 6 months. The GHQ-28 was least predictable at 3 and 6 months but was equal to the IES at 12 months. It is not clear why measures had stronger predictability later in the year. Those with higher scores at 3 months were those whose expectations of death or injury were greatest and who relied on emotion focussed coping. By 6 months those with higher scores were still those who coped emotionally but also had a history of psychological or psychiatric treatment and rated their own injury high. At 12 months emotion coping continued to be a strong predictor as well as the length of time admitted to hospital and fear and distress at the accident scene.

It could have been expected that accident variables such as severity of the accident, whether driver or passenger, and number of others in the accident may have been important in determining severity of trauma, but the results did not support this. Feeling responsibility for the accident and degree of social support following the accident also were not important predictors of trauma. In this sample injury levels and number of fatalities were generally low, so this may be an artifact of the sample. Gender also was not a predictor, in contrast to Blanchard (1998) and Ehlers, Mayou and Bryant (1998) who found women to be over represented in those with PTSD following accidents.

Previous psychiatric/psychological treatment contributed some predictive strength in this study in line with previous literature (Blanchard et al., 1994; Blanchard, Hickling, Taylor et al., 1996; Blanchard, Hickling, Taylor, et al., 1995; McFarlane 1988, 1989; and Smith, North, McCool, & Shea, 1992). It was not explored in depth in this study and so is not directly comparable with other studies.

Emotion-focussed coping is described by Endler and Parker (1990) as self oriented emotional reactions to reduce stress. These may include emotional responses such as blaming, getting angry, self preoccupation or fantasizing which may actually increase the stress. This appears to be a logical link for these people as overall, relying on emotion focussed coping soon after the accident was the strongest predictor for post accident trauma.

One particular focus for this study was the relationship between injury and psychological trauma. Previous reports in the literature have been inconsistent and different means of measuring injury have been used (Blanchard et al., 1994; Epstein 1993; Goldberg & Gara , 1990; Green, 1994; Pilowsky, 1992). Malt, Høivik & Blikra's (1993) three year follow-up with injured road accident victims reported nervousness to be statistically associated with severity of injury. Blanchard, Hickling, Mitnick, et al. (1995) reported a correlation of .31 between physical injury and PTSD whilst Blanchard, Hickling, Barton et al. (1996) reported that sheer extent of physical injury was a predictor for degree of post-traumatic stress 12 months post-accident, results supported by the present study. Thus it appears that injury became more important in the longer term. It is also important to note that subjects' own ratings of injury rather than doctors' ratings were important. Later on time spent in hospital was a predictor, although only 24% of victims had been admitted to hospital.

Why then do we see this difference over time in the way that injury measurements predict trauma? The focus on subjective experience variables underlying this study, was supported by the finding that victims' own perceptions of their degree of injury are important in the shorter term. However by 12 months post accident, for those with serious injury who spent a longer time in hospital, ongoing pain and disability may be constant reminders of the trauma, as suggested by Blanchard and Hickling (1997). This may hinder emotional recovery from the accident.

One of the advantages of this study is that the participants were consecutive hospital attendees rather than only seriously injured patients or those referred for medico-legal assessment. This broad cross section of respondents should allow generalisability of results, although few of the sample were seriously injured. It would be useful to repeat the study with a bigger sample and to refine measures of psychological trauma to include the range of symptoms experienced by this population and further examine the role of physical injury in subsequent trauma.

These results make a start towards enabling identification of which road accident victims are likely to suffer psychological sequelae 3,6 and 12 months after their accidents. This means hospitals could follow up those people for preventive counselling in an attempt to reduce longer term distress.

References

Blanchard, E. B. (1998). *Who gets better? Can we tell?* Paper presented at Road Accidents and the Mind Conference, Bristol UK, 1–3 September.

Blanchard, E. B. & Hickling, E. J. (1997). *After the crash. Assessment and treatment of motor vehicle accident survivors.* Washington DC: American Psychological Association.

Blanchard, E. B., Hickling, E. J., Barton, K. A., Taylor, A. E., Loos, W. R. & Jones-Alexander, J. (1996). One year prospective follow-up of motor vehicle accident victims. *Behaviour Research and Therapy, 34,* 775–786.

Blanchard, E. B., Hickling, E. J., Mitnick, N., Taylor, A. E., Loos, W. R. & Buckley, T. C. (1995). The impact of severity of physical injury and perception of lifethreat in the development of post-traumatic stress disorder in motor vehicle accident victims. *Behaviour Research and Therapy, 33,* 529–534.

Blanchard, E. B., Hickling, E. J., Taylor, A. E. & Loos, W. (1995). Psychiatric morbidity associated with motor vehicle accidents. *The Journal of Nervous and Mental Disease, 183,* 495–504.

Blanchard, E. B., Hickling, E. J., Taylor, A. E., Loos, W. R., Forneris, C. A. & Jaccard, J. (1996). Who develops PTSD from motor vehicle accidents? *Behaviour Research and Therapy, 34,* 1–10.

Blanchard, E. B., Hickling, E. J., Taylor, A. E., Loos, W. R. & Gerardi, R. J. (1994). Psychological morbidity associated with motor vehicle accidents. *Behaviour Research and Therapy, 32,* 283–290.

Blanchard, E. B., Hickling, E. J., Vollmer, A. J., Loos, W. R., Buckley, T. C. & Jaccard, J. (1995). Short term follow-up of post-traumatic stress symptoms in motor vehicle accident victims. *Behaviour Research and Therapy, 33,* 369–377.

Bryant, R. A. & Harvey, A. G. (1995). Avoidant coping style and post-traumatic stress following motor vehicle accidents. *Behaviour Research and Therapy, 33*, 631–635.

Burstein, A. (1989). Post-traumatic stress disorder in victims of motor vehicle accidents. *Hospital and Community Psychiatry, 40,* 295–297.

Creamer, M., Burgess, P., Buckingham, W. & Pattison, P. (1989). *The psychological aftermath of the Queen Street shootings.* Melbourne, Australia: Department of Psychology, University of Melbourne.

Ehlers, A., Mayou, R.A. & Bryant, B. (1998). Psychological predictors of chronic posttraumatic stress disorder after motor vehicle accidents. *Journal of Abnormal Psychology, 107,* 508–519.

Epstein, R. S. (1993). Avoidant symptoms cloaking the diagnosis of PTSD in patients with severe accidental injury. *Journal of Traumatic Stress, 6,* 451–458.

Endler, N. S. & Parker, J. D. A. (1990). *Coping Inventory for Stressful Situations (CISS): manual.* Toronto, Canada: Multi-Health Systems, Inc.

Endler, N. S. & Parker, J. D. A (1992). The multidimensional assessment of coping: concepts, issues and measurement. In G. L. van Heck, P. Bonaivto, I. Deary, & W. Nowack (Eds.), *Personality Psychology in Europe* (Vol 4, pp. 377–390). Amsterdam: Swets & Zeitlinger.

Goldberg, L. & Gara, M. A. (1990). A typology of psychiatric reactions to motor vehicle accidents. *Psychopathology, 23,* 15–20.

Goldberg, D. P. & Hillier, V. F. (1979). A scale version of the General Health Questionnaire. *Psychological Medicine, 9,* 139–145.

Gordon, K., Blaszczynski, A., Silove, D., Sloane, D. & Hillman, K. (1996, October). *Psychological reactions to motor vehicle accidents: A preliminary report.* Paper presented at the International Congress on Stress and Health, Sydney, Australia.

Green, B. L. (1994). Psychosocial research in traumatic stress: An update. *Journal of Traumatic Stress, 7,* 341–362.

Green, M. M., McFarlane, A. C., Hunter, C. E. & Griggs, W. M. (1993). Undiagnosed post-traumatic stress disorder following motor vehicle accidents. *The Medical Journal of Australia, 159,* 529–534.

Horne, D. (1995). Detection and assessment of PTSD by health and legal professions. *Psychiatry, Psychology and Law, 2,* 65–73.

Horowitz, M., Wilner, N. & Alvarez, W. (1979). Impact of Event Scale: A measure of subjective stress. *Psychosomatic Medicine, 41,* 209–22.

Janoff-Bulman, R. (1989). Assumptive worlds and the stress of traumatic events: Applications of the schema construct. *Social Cognition, 7*, 113–136.

Jeavons, S., Greenwood, K. & Horne, D. (1996). Reported consequences following road accidents. *Australian Journal of Primary Health-Interchange, 2*(2), 21–28.

Jeavons, S., Greenwood, K. & Horne, D. (1998). Psychological symptoms in rural road trauma victims. *The Australian Journal of Rural Health, 6,* 52–57.

Kuch, K., Swinson, R. P. & Kirby, M. (1985). Post-traumatic stress disorder after car accidents. *Canadian Journal of Psychiatry, 30,* 426–427.

Malt, U. F., Blikra, G. & Høivik, B. (1989). The Late Effect of Accidental Injury Questionnaire (LEAIQ). *Acta Psychiatrica Scandinavica, 353*(80), 113–130.

Malt, U. F., Høivik, B. & Blikra, G. (1993). Psychosocial consequences of road accidents. *European Psychiatry, 8,* 227–228.

Mayou, R., Bryant, B. & Duthie, R. (1993). Psychiatric consequences of road traffic accidents. *British Medical Journal, 307*, 647–651.

McFarlane, A. C. (1988). The aetiology of PTSDs following a natural disaster. *British Journal of Psychiatry, 152,* 116–121.

McFarlane, A. C. (1989). The aetiology of post-traumatic morbidity: Predisposing, precipitating and perpetuating factors. *British Journal of Psychiatry, 154,* 221–228.

Pilowsky, I. (1992). Minor accidents and major psychological trauma: A clinical perspective. *Stress Medicine, 8,* 77–78.

Smith, R. S. (1989). Psychological trauma following automobile accidents: A review of literature. *American Journal of Forensic Psychology, 7*(4), 5–20.

Smith, E. M., North, C. S., McCool, R. E. & Shea, J. M. (1990). Acute postdisaster psychiatric disorders: Identification of persons at risk. *American Journal of Psychiatry, 147,* 202–206.

Watson, C. G., Juba, M., Manifold, V., Kucala, T. & Anderson, P. E. D. (1991). The post-traumatic stress disorder interview: Rationale, description, reliability and concurrent validity of a DSM-III technique. *Journal of Clinical Psychology, 47,* 179–188.

Watts, R., Horne, D., Sandells, J. & Petrie, M. (1996). The need for acute hospitals to provide counselling following motor vehicle accidents. *Australian Health Review, 19* (3), 93–103

Section 3: Legal Issues

16

Compensation for Psychological Injuries in England

BERNIE ROWE

Lyons Davidson Solicitors, Bristol, UK

MARK RIVERS

Lyons Davidson Solicitors, Bristol, UK

NORMAN COTTINGTON

Highway Motor Policies, London, UK

CAROL PARSONS

Lyons Davidson Solicitors, Bristol, UK

Introduction

Seldom is there much argument over the fundamental legal principle that the blameless victim of a road accident should be fairly compensated for losses sustained. Put as a statement of principle this seems only fair.

Although some other jurisdictions have introduced (and in other cases abandoned) "no fault" schemes the idea of a universal 'no fault' compensation system for road or other accident victims has never gained widespread support in the UK.

The social welfare system provides sickness, unemployment and other social benefits as a safety net to protect against the worst effects of poverty. Free medical treatment from the National Health Service ensures that medical treatment is available to all who need it.

Occasionally, suggestions for a system of compensation based upon the fact of injury, rather than the cause of it, emerge but then fade quickly away.

Thus, compensation payments in English Civil Law remain dependent upon finding a defendant who can be shown to have owed the victim a duty of care, to have breached that duty thus causing injury resulting in loss to the victim.

As in so many things in life the principle is easy, the devil is in the detail. In psychological injury the problems are nearly always encountered in establishing the extent and consequence of the psychological components of an injury and the cause of it.

This paper will not attempt the impossible task of describing in a few pages the legal process used in England to determine a disputed claim for psychological injuries. Indeed to do so would not only attempt the impossible but would be misleading, as most claims settle long before the issue of court proceedings. The intellectual cut and thrust of the court room, the battle between experts, the forensic scrutiny of the nightmares experienced by the victim can attract "rubber neckers" just as much as the original crash at the intersection. But this is not the way claims are resolved. Only 5,000 of the 100,000 or more personal injury actions started every year go to trial in England. A disproportionate number involve disputes that focus on psychological or psychiatric injuries.

The reason is simple to find. It is because judges, lawyers and the law itself has been uncomfortable with claims where the largest value component concerns not a provable physical injury but something less certain, less measurable and less understood; an injury to the mind.

In this chapter we will look at a number of challenges, new and old, that face the claimant and defendant and their representatives in the handling of claims for psychological injuries.

The topic that uses up most of the time, energies and money of all those involved in the claims process is that of ascertaining and verifying the extent and cause of an injury. Once this has been achieved the task of quantifying the losses will generally become much easier. This is then the theme for contributions from a number of different perspectives. Norman Cottington, Claims Manager of the largest Lloyds Motor Syndicate explains his dilemma in facing claims. One of my partners, Mark Rivers, considers the points that should occupy the mind of the alert Personal Injury Solicitor in setting out to prove a claim for psychological injuries. As is apparent, both lawyer and insurer crave solid evidence to identify the injury and the cause. With this in mind Carol Parsons takes a look at expert witnesses and how their role will be changed by the new Civil Procedure Rules that came into force on 26 April 1999.

But first a few words about new challenges and old systems. In April 1999 the most radical, some say revolutionary, changes to the conduct of civil litigation took place for more than a 100 years.

The new Civil Procedure Rules implement most, if not all, of Lord Woolfs report on Access to Justice. The report found that civil litigation was too expensive and took too long. The answer, a new set of rules aimed at making the cost of civil litigation proportionate to the issues at stake. High on the hit list of past practice has been the way in which the use of experts was seen to have increased cost and delay in civil litigation.

This was not so much an attack upon experts as an attack upon the way in which experts had become increasingly "tainted" by those who instruct them. The subtle, and not so subtle, pressure exerted by those who instructed and paid experts was seen as having eroded the independence and thus, credibility of the expert witness. In many cases the expert witness was openly spoken of as part of a litigants team. The expert witness too often was suspected as being partisan, whether the suspicion was soundly based or not. Mutual suspicion breeds more litigation not less. Lord Woolf's report and the new rules seeks to break the bond between expert and party. The primary duty of an expert witness in giving evidence, is to the court.

Psychological injuries cannot exist without medical reports. Without the clinicians report there is no provable injury and thus no compensation. The lawyer and the courts want medical opinion to fit the legal framework and determine simple questions of cause and effect. The clinician knows that the human mind and our understanding of it is not so simple!

In the past 5 years the appellate courts in England have struggled with changing attitudes on when to compensate for psychological injury, especially when it was the only injury sustained in an accident.

Whilst the courts had overcome the 19th century view expressed in *Victorian Railway Commissions v Coultas* 1888[1] that compensation was not recoverable for psychological injury because of evidential difficulties in establishing the *cause* of psychiatric symptoms, they remained uneasy about compensating for psychiatric injury unless it was allied to a physical injury.

It was not until 1996[2] when the House of Lords decided (on a majority of 3–2) that English law should finally demolish the distinction between physical and psychological injury. Lord Lloyd avoided any future ambiguity by stating boldly:–

"There is no justification for regarding physical and psychiatric injury as different 'kinds of damage'".

The acceptance that psychiatric injury is as real as physical injury has not disposed of the long held fear that to fully recognise psychological injury will *'open the floodgates'* of claims for compensation. In turn this revives concerns about the evidential difficulties of identifying the cause of psychiatric symptoms, even if we are now better placed to identify and clarify the symptoms.

So, where are we now in English Law as applied to claims for psychological damage? Lord Steyn as recently as December 1998 in *White -v- Chief Constable of South Yorkshire*[3] said;

"My Lords, the law on the recovery of compensation for pure psychiatric harm is a patchwork quilt of distinctions which are difficult to justify".

Lord Hoffman in the same case was less charitable in his approach when he observed:

"Your Lordships are now engaged not in the bold development of principle, but in a practical attempt under adverse conditions, to preserve the general perception of the law as a 'system of rules which is fair between one citizen and another'".

For my own part, I invite you to decide whether Lord Wilberforce was expressing hope or despair when he said of injuries of the mind;

"... the area of ignorance seems to expand with that of knowledge."[4]

The Insurers Dilemma

The dilemma I face regularly is how to deal with compensation claims for injuries for which there is no or only questionable evidence.

I would first like to stress one further dilemma, and that is that I am very much misunderstood! My wife understands me, my problem is that I and all of my insurance colleagues are misunderstood by the general public, the legal fraternity and it would appear most, if not all doctors and Consultants.

It is not our sole task in life to settle all claims as cheaply as possible, nor to dispose of claims at figures below that to which the claimant is legitimately entitled.

Our role as defendants is to properly identify those persons who have suffered injury and are entitled to compensation and to ensure that they receive proper and adequate compensation as quickly as possible. It is with those objectives in mind that I have publicly advanced the cause of rehabilitation and co-operation with claimant's solicitors, with a view to breaking down the adversarial barriers so as to provide support and assistance to those injured claimants at the earliest opportunity. It was with this purpose that I originated the concept of immediate needs assessment in the United Kingdom and went on to encourage the introduction of the Disability Assessment Unit. The Unit provides independent reports outside of the litigation arena, with the sole objective of arranging early visits to injured claimants, so as to identify their immediate needs and assist with their motivation, independence and mobility. I continue to chair the working party that was responsible for the working practices of the unit and which is made up of both claimant and defendant lawyers, together with insurers.

I firmly believe that it is to an insurers advantage to attend to these matters in a sympathetic and co-operative manner. If we can assist with rehabilitation, whether that be towards independent living or vocational rehabilitation, it can at the end of the day have advantages for everyone. I call that common sense! The individual claimants benefit from this proactive approach, whilst having the added advantage of having their claims settled much earlier and go on to enjoy a much better quality of life than would previously have been expected. Increasingly there are signs that Claimant lawyers and defendant insurers can work constructively to improve the recovery and outcome for those who have suffered injury.

But that is not the problem. The insurers dilemma is when dealing with claims arising from muscular, whiplash or PTSD type injuries, being those that are not easy to objectively verify on examination.

In describing myself and my colleagues as being sympathetic toward injured parties, it must be accepted that our task must also be to ensure that we are not dealing with fraudulent or exaggerated claims. Historically, such claims are more likely to be presented as whiplash or PTSD or psychiatric in nature. The dilemma we have is in recognising the genuine from the exaggerated, the malingerer from the downright fraudulent.

It is no problem to us to equate adequate and proper compensation to someone who has suffered a visible injury, such as a fracture to any part of their anatomy, a laceration, nerve injuries, loss of any senses or simply bruising. The problem that we have is in dealing with whiplash type injuries or PTSD/psychiatric injuries such as I have described above. The problem is that there is nothing there to be seen, and therefore nothing that we can easily identify or relate to.

If I receive a medical report that tells me that someone has suffered a fractured femur, was detained in hospital for a short period whilst an intermedllary nail was inserted and thereafter provides me with a history of partial/full weight bearing to an eventual recovery and return to work after a period of say three months, I have no difficulty in relating to it. I can quantify that injury and I can offer fair and proper compensation.

The problem arises when a report is received from an Orthopaedic Consultant who examines a claimant nine months after the accident, which tells me according to the history given by the claimant, that they attended their GP four days after the event and were given analgesics, that there was nothing to find on examination apart from some discomfort on palpation and then goes on to provide a prognosis to the effect that the party sustained a minor whiplash injury, that caused discomfort for six months following the accident and is still exhibiting minor symptoms which should die down within the course of the next twelve months. An identical prognosis would likely have been provided if the report took place within three months, nine months or two years of the accident occurring. I can guarantee that minor symptoms would still have been exhibited!

The alternative is the report I receive from a Consultant following an interview with a claimant nine months after the event, and which provides a diagnosis of PTSD and/or anxiety disorder. More often than not the PTSD diagnosis is provided by a Consultant from totally the wrong discipline. It is not uncommon to have a PTSD diagnosis added on to an Orthopaedic Consultant's report or even included within the General Practitioner's notes. Often the diagnosis has no regard to the diagnostic and statistical manual of mental disorders nor any reference made to the subject's individual history. More often than not, reports are prepared without reference to any pre-accident medical records and it is therefore impossible for the individual Consultant to know whether any symptoms that are exhibited were pre-accident in their nature.

At best these reports are based totally and exclusively on the individual's own verbal account given at the time of the examination and there is nothing to see on examination that can either support or question that verbal history. The best that can be said for the Consultant concerned is that their report has been prepared on the basis that the history given was honest.

The insurer's dilemma is what to do with these reports. We cannot afford to compensate people simply because they say they are entitled to it and upon the assumption that every claim that is presented to us is unquestionably honest.

It is necessary for us to investigate but that in itself is expensive. A disclosure of all pre and post accident medical records is essential if any merit is to be given to a Consultant's diagnosis and therefore to enable us to properly quantify an award of damages. Solicitors acting for the individual will frequently refuse insurers access to those records, and that being the case, it is necessary for us to instruct Consultants of our own choosing to medically examine the claimant in the sure knowledge that there is nothing to find on examination.

It is true to say that more often than not we will find that the claimant at no time attended the hospital following the accident in which they were involved, nor did they attend their own General Practitioner. This despite the severity of the symptoms they describe to the Consultant on examination. Indeed, despite the severity of the symptoms they describe, there will be no evidence that they sought any medical attention at all! In many cases where the records are disclosed, there will be some relevant pre-accident history. It may be a pre-accident history of depression, mental disorders or disruption to family life following divorce, or perhaps even the loss of a close family relative.

There are in many cases a history of previous accidents for which compensation is still being claimed for what was then described as a permanent disability. All matters that are often excluded from the original Consultant's report.

The disclosure of a pre-accident history as described above does not exclude the fact that an injury may still have been sustained in the accident under review. Our task is to try and identify whether an injury was suffered in the accident and if so, the extent to which that injury may have been exacerbated by the pre-existing condition ... not an easy task!

On occasions, we have to resort to more practical forms of investigation which sometimes includes surveillance. A video film will often show far more than any medical report. Often it will show a claimant doing all of those things that they are described in the medical report as no longer being capable of doing.

I have recently attended to a claim for a police officer who alleged he had suffered PTSD in the accident, to the extent that it was necessary for him to take early retirement from the police force.

This police officer was travelling in a patrol car, which was travelling at no more than twenty five miles per hour, when our policyholder negligently reversed out of a driveway and collided with the side of the police car in which the officer was a near side passenger. This was not a major accident. The damage to the police car was repaired for less than £100 and yet we were led to believe that the impact was such that an experienced and capable police officer, with an exemplary record, was traumatized to the extent that he was no longer able to continue with his duties.

Were this claim to be accepted at face value, that is, were we to have accepted the medical evidence that was presented, we would be facing a claim for the personal injuries suffered and the loss of earnings and future loss that was to be experienced that would run into hundreds of thousands of pounds. At a conservative estimate it was necessary for us to reserve £350,000.

With such a large sum involved and based upon the flimsy evidence produced, we found it necessary to investigate.

It transpires that the medical and employment record showed that this officer had a history of problems. He had been involved in violent affrays on two previous occasions which traumatized him to the extent that he took lengthy periods off work on both occasions. He had been turned down for promotion on two previous occasions because of his poor sickness record and eventually his solicitors were forced to concede that the road traffic accident was certainly not the cause of his early retirement. Whether our road traffic accident had any effect on him at all we will never know. It was impossible to argue that it might possibly have been traumatic for him and might possibly have precipitated the inevitable.

Personally, I do not believe he suffered at all, but that our road traffic accident proved to be fortuitous and an ideal opportunity to accelerate the inevitable. We nonetheless ended up having to pay him £10,000 plus his solicitor's costs and all of the not inconsiderable expenses we had incurred in investigating his claim. In comparison to the potential of this claim, our expenditure of £20,000 may not seem very much, but to put it into context I would suggest that you equate it with what you pay for your own comprehensive motor insurance premium.

It must of course be said, that a great many people do genuinely suffer minor personal injuries in road traffic accidents. I would not suggest for one moment that minor whiplash injuries or psychological trauma do not occur but the percentage of exaggerated and even possibly fraudulent claims in this area has been shown to be a very large percentage of those presented to us and this inevitably creates scepticism. Indeed, it can be shown that certain solicitors have presented claims to us where none exist purely with a view to justifying profit costs.

We can show examples where claims have been presented for injury to a vehicle owner who was not even in the vehicle when it was struck whilst parked and unattended. That particular claim for injury was withdrawn. Similarly, we have an example where a personal injury payment was made to a claimant through his solicitors, only to have the cheque returned on the basis that the claimant says that no injury was suffered. He was apparently a born again Christian and could not find it in his conscience to accept money that had been obtained under false pretences. Sadly, such honesty is rare.

Without doubt, it would aid our ability to attend to claims properly if all medical reports were deemed unacceptable and inadmissible should they be presented without due regard for the pre and post-accident medical history. Perhaps the new rules and the Protocols that came into existence in April, 1999 will be of some value here and assist us in attending to these claims fairly.

In conclusion, the Insurer's Dilemma is that it is in everybody's interests to be considerate and co-operative when attending to personal injury claims. At the same time however, it must be recognized that insurers have a duty to defend themselves and their policyholders against fraudulent and exaggerated claims for of course inevitably, the more that we accept those claims the more there will be and ultimately the more we all pay.

Legal Considerations: Who Gets Paid?

When a lawyer first takes instructions from an accident victim the psychological affects of the accident upon the victim need to be at the forefront of the lawyer's mind.

If there is likely to be a psychological component or the only component of a claim it is essential to focus at an early stage on the question of causation. The Plaintiff will need to satisfy the court that there is a causal link between the negligent act of the defendant and the psychiatric harm sustained.

Before deciding this, one should always have in mind the possibility of the following as alternative or additional factors in diagnosing their condition and the cause of it:–

1. Previous psychiatric history.
2. Familial history.
3. Multiple causal factors e.g. divorce, work stress etc.
4. Successive injuries.
5. Intervention by a third party.
6. Natural events.

If one is satisfied that there is a causal link then any psychiatric or psychological disorder can give rise to a claim, *provided that* it is accepted that the disorder had a traumatic event as its foundation or, in the case of a pre-existing disorder, its exacerbation was caused by a traumatic event.

Of course when one is seeing a client or a patient for the first time it is not easy to compartmentalize them into a neat diagnostic category. People who have suffered a similar type of event will experience sometimes widely different levels of symptoms ranging from the mildest reaction to the most extreme.

The temptation to put a certain type of behaviour down to a 'difficult personality' when something more sinister may provide the explanation, must be resisted.

Many will present with a whole gamut of symptoms which may include some or all of the following;[5]

1. Perception of physical symptoms.
2. Effects on mental state
   a) organic (cognitive impairment)

b) emotional
3. Quality of life:work, leisure, marital, family etc.
4. Use of medical services
5. compliance with medical care.
6. Effects on close relatives

It is the job of the lawyer, assisted by medical practitioners, to make legal sense of the patient's history. For the purpose of establishing a legal claim it assists considerably if we can fit them within one of the diagnoses set out within the International Classification of Diseases (10th revision) or the American Psychiatric Association's Diagnostic & Statistical manual (DSM IV).

From a legal standpoint in the United Kingdom this is all the more important since the case of *Nicholls v Rushton*[6] decided that compensation is not available for 'shock and shaking up' *unless* a physical injury was also suffered. This principle has now been refined so that there needs to be a recognised psychological diagnosis if a claim for compensation is to succeed.

So, how do we determine who gets paid? Remember that what follows is not an exhaustive list and we all need to keep an open mind!

Cognitive Impairment

Lawyers tend to like something they can measure! This goes some way to explaining why the recovery of damages for cognitive impairment has been established for some considerable time in one's daily case load compared to the rather more esoteric psychiatric disorders. The experienced injury lawyer will be used to obtaining appropriate reports to assess the effects of traumatic brain injuries. A claimant's performance can be measured according to recognized benchmarks, although we rarely have the benefit of pre morbid test results of a similar nature against which to compare the results and so we have to fall back on the "imperfections" of historical evidence from family and friends. Anecdotal evidence is recognised by the judiciary in this area and accepted readily by them when assessing damages.

Nervous Shock Cases

This legal principle has been most recently dissected and redefined by the case of *Alcock v Chief Constable of South Yorkshire Police*[7] which arose out of the Hillsborough disaster. For the most part damages are recoverable if caused by shock involving the "*sudden appreciation by sight or sound of a horrifying event which violently agitates the mind.*" (Lord Ackner)

The Claimant in such cases will be a primary victim if he is within the range of foreseeable injury or is a participant directly involved in the event or has a reasonable fear of immediate personal injury to himself. For example he could be the driver of a car involved in a life threatening accident who walks away physically unscathed but suffers post traumatic stress disorder.

Alternatively the Claimant will be a secondary victim if he is a spectator or bystander such as a parent watching through a window as a child is run down in the street outside.

In primary victim cases the "eggshell skull" principle applies. That is, it is not necessary to ask whether the Plaintiff is a person of ordinary fortitude or phlegm. If he has a personality which renders him peculiarly vulnerable to a psychological reaction to an event which would leave most people unscathed, he still gets compensated.

In secondary victim cases however, one must clear the additional hurdles of 'control mechanisms' erected by the courts in a series of recent cases to limit those who can claim. Secondary victims will have to show that although not directly at risk of injury they nevertheless sustained psychiatric injury as a result of:–

1) being present at the accident or its immediate aftermath;
2) having close ties of love and affection with a victim of the accident (such ties will be assumed between spouses and as between parent and child);
3) the psychiatric injury having been caused by direct perception of the accident or its immediate aftermath and not upon hearing of it from someone else.

Rescuers form a distinct category. The law recognizes that they may be professional rescuers or ordinary members of the public who attempt to rescue.

Provided that the rescuer has played an active part in the rescue operation, they can recover for Nervous Shock caused by their attempts to rescue.[8]

The House of Lords however has recently seriously curtailed the circumstances in which a rescuer can recover damages for a purely psychological injury. In *Frost v Chief Constable of South Yorkshire Policy*[9] 4 police officers who had been involved in rescuing spectators at the Hillsborough Football Stadium disaster in 1989 sought damages for psychiatric injury sustained as a result. In his leading judgment Lord Steyn said;

> "*In order to contain the concept of rescuer within reasonable bounds for the purposes of the recovery of compensation for pure psychiatric harm the Plaintiff must at least satisfy the threshold requirement that he objectively exposed himself to danger or reasonably believed that he was so doing*".

The four police officers admitted that in their rescue acts none were exposed to danger and none thought they were so exposed therefore their claims failed. There will be many such cases where the emergency services come across the aftermath of an horrific event which has had equally devastating results but where the danger element has subsided. They will now go without compensation.

Post Traumatic Stress Disorder (PTSD)

The term and definition first appeared in 1980 in DSM III although this was really the bringing together of a range of disorders which were recognized as capable of having adverse stress from a traumatic event at their root.

One should be aware that PTSD can arise and be compensated for in a number of non stereotypic events. For example in *Ackers v Wigan Health Authority*[10] the Plaintiff suffered awareness during a Cesarean section procedure under general anaesthetic as a result of which she suffered a number of psychiatric reactions such as depression and phobia of hospitals. She recovered £12,000 for pain and suffering and £1,700 for the cost of therapy.

We are all familiar with the criteria for the diagnosis of PTSD but there are some interesting legal implications to some of them which need to be considered when looking at who is entitled to compensation.

Firstly, the previous diagnosis according to DSM III required an event which was '*outside the range of usual human experience*'. This requirement probably had at its root the original perception of the need to define a reaction demonstrated by American servicemen who had returned from the conflict in Vietnam. Its omission from DSM IV is significant as it now brings in a whole raft of events which were arguably not appropriate to a compensation claim before. The most common example of course is the low speed car crash.

The language used in the second requirement of paragraph A that '*the persons response involved intense fear, helplessness or horror*', is very similar to that used in Nervous Shock cases and we should look again at Lord Ackner's definition of nervous shock for comparison.

Experience suggests that this requirement is all too easily assumed in medico legal reporting without any detailed consideration of whether or not it has in fact been satisfied.

We often hear of clients re-living the traumatic event as if they were there, thereby complying with the criteria of Paragraph B. The descriptions are often vivid and colourful. They can often be very distressing. It is important to be able to distinguish this from other symptoms of different disorders or 'ordinary shock' which is non compensatable.

In paragraph F we have an addition which was not present in DSM III;

"The disturbance causes clinically significant distress or impairment in social, occupational or other important areas of functioning".

Psychologists might debate whether or not the question of disability should form part of the diagnosis but it is a critical feature for lawyers to consider, as the extent of the disability broadly determines how much the Plaintiff is going to receive in compensation.

Acute Stress Disorder

If you come to the conclusion that PTSD is not a valid diagnosis, it is important to consider whether the Plaintiff is suffering from any other disorder. Acute Stress Disorder was first introduced by DSM IV and is a valid diagnosis for symptoms lasting for a short period of time but it is rarely diagnosed or pleaded as part of a claim for compensation. There is no reason to suppose that the disability, however short lived, cannot be quite debilitating. Nor is it being too flippant to say that almost any injury commands an award of £1000 nowadays and even moderate to severe symptoms lasting for a month or two should not be dismissed as insignificant from a medico-legal point of view.

It is worth noting that some professionals find it difficult to justify a distinction between Acute Stress Disorder and "normal" reactions to an adverse event which are non compensatable[11] but if the Plaintiff fits within the diagnostic criteria which exist for Acute Stress Disorder, the likelihood is that he will be compensated for it.

Pathological Grief Disorder

The ordinary grief which one experiences at the loss of a loved one is not compensatable except in accordance with the Bereavement provisions in S1A of the Fatal Accidents Act 1976.

Trying to asses whether and to what extent someone's reaction is excessive compared to "normal", presupposes one can define normal in this context. This is difficult in itself but there is often the added complication that a number of other illnesses may be present.

In addition it will be necessary to establish that the Pathological Grief Disorder has set in as a result of the death and not as a result of intervening events which occur after death but which transform the normal grieving process into something pathological.

For example Stephen O'Brien in his article "The validity of the diagnosis of PTSD"[12] examines the case where a patient suffers a pathological grief disorder after witnessing the death of her common law husband in a road traffic accident. Prior to the event there had been a dispute with the husband's family which, after his death, resulted in them ignoring her existence or her importance to her husband. She did not suffer from PTSD despite the severity of the event. On the balance of probabilities this patient was suffering from a genuine disability but brought on as a result of the family's treatment of her after the event and not the event itself.

Phobic Travel Anxiety

It is extremely common for clients to describe nervousness, anxiety or fear when travelling as a passenger after an accident. In addition, they will describe the use of imaginary brakes or holding onto the dashboard, a fear of returning to driving or of driving over long distances.

Symptoms such as these may justify a diagnosis under the DSM or ICD criteria.

In severe cases the effect may be most debilitating affecting social relationships, leisure activities and the ability to function capably at work. This may have a significant effect on the level of compensation to which the Plaintiff is entitled. If the effect is likely to be long lasting the benefits of counselling or a course of driving lessons should be considered.

Workplace Stress

We should just remind ourselves once again of Lord Ackner's definition of Nervous Shock;

> "*the sudden appreciation by sight or sound of a horrifying event which violently agitates the mind*"

Damages are not usually recoverable for psychiatric illness caused by the accumulation over a period of time of more gradual assaults on the nervous system. (but see Criminal Injuries Compensation Authority post).

An extension to these principles was established in *Walker v Northumberland County Council*[13]. In this case the Plaintiff recovered damages for a nervous breakdown he suffered as a result of unreasonable pressure put on him during his employment in relation to his workload. It seems as though reports are now being published on a regular basis citing the high proportion of employees who operate under conditions of stress in their working environment. Time away from work is now more routinely described as being due to stress related illnesses and litigation in this area is bound to increase substantially over the next decade.

Retraumatisation

R. K Pitman, L.F Sparr, L.S.Saunders and A.C. Mcfarlane[14] describe the ability of the litigation process to retraumatise the psychologically damaged Claimant by forcing them to relive the experience again and again through interviews with lawyers, consultants etc. This can lead to two distinct problems;

a) " thwarting of characteristic efforts at avoidance thus resulting in the resurgence of intrusive ideation and increased arousal"
b) " acceptance of inadequate settlements through the wish to avoid such retelling"

Certainly we now recognise as lawyers that clients who "go quiet" i.e. not contacting you for months, failing to give instructions or reply to correspondence and so on, may be displaying avoidance behaviour to retraumatisation without knowing that they have a psychological injury. The last thing they need in such circumstances is a letter telling them that if you do not hear from them in 14 days you will close their file! By the same token, medico legal professionals must be sympathetic to the possibility of retraumatisation in their dealings with their clients or patients. Where the line is to be drawn on legal causation of symptoms resulting from retraumatisation is unclear. If symptoms flow from treatment then this should be part of the claim. Where symptoms result from repeat medico-legal examinations as part of the litigation process there exists an argument that the cause of the symptoms is not the accident but the way in which the litigation has been handled. In reality, a judge is likely to take the view that once litigation is finished the symptoms will disappear once the cause of them has been removed. Whether the judge is justified in taking this view is not for me to say!

Masking

All professionals dealing with this area of injury should not lose sight of the need to recognise symptoms which might;

a) present subtly, and/or
b) might be masked by some other condition/medication

For example a diagnosis of concussional syndrome in hospital may be forgotten about in a severe and long lasting PTSD case and we should all be vigilant for signs of loss of concentration, memory or ability to multi task which might represent an underlying organic brain dysfunction.

Similarly a client with a pre existing history of depression may be on medication for that depression which may be masking either the fact of PTSD as a consequence of the accident or, more likely, the disability associated with it.

This simply serves to emphasise the need for precise diagnosis and attribution of symptoms and disabilities in a theatre of injury which may involve multiple disorders.

Delayed Onset

The delayed onset of symptoms for a significant period is always likely to result in a problem case. One needs to take extra care therefore to consider the likely areas of dispute namely the genuineness of the Claimant's symptoms, the possibility of any intervening causative events and whether the defendant could be expected to have foreseen the possible psychological consequences of the negligent act although the latter may be more a matter of legal argument.

It is particularly important when preparing a case where delayed onset is involved to consider the client's past medical records in some detail. The case will look weak and ill prepared if their relevance is not considered fully in the first report on causation.

Children

Studies suggest that the rate of psychiatric disorder associated with head injury in children is higher than for the population at large. Where Post Traumatic Amnesia lasts for over 1 week the rate has been found to be 2–3 times the population base rate (Brown et al, 1981).

Very different responses to those experienced with adult patients are recorded, often dominated by psychosocial factors and family relationships in particular. Serious mental illnesses are rarer although the incidence probably increases with age.

The personality disorders displayed will often have common themes for example;

- apathy
- loss of initiative
- lack of inhibition of sexual or aggressive behaviour
- carelessness about dress or hygiene

It is essential that a report is prepared by someone specialising in child or adolescent psychiatry. It will be particularly important for them to consider the likely effect of their symptoms on their schooling and the development of their interpersonal relationships with family and friends. Careful consideration should be given to treatment and full and frank discussion with parents is essential. Recognition of the two extremes of parental reaction is required, that is those who think their child is coping well when they are not and those who are over-protective which may hinder the child's ability to come to terms with what has happened.

Crimes of Violence

From 1st April 1996 the Criminal Injuries Compensation Act (1995) introduced a scheme for the compensation of victims of crime. Applications can be made on behalf of children under 18 by an adult with parental responsibility.

Compensation is now awarded under a tariff system and there are a number of categories which are relevant to this paper:

	£
• *Brain Damage* –	
– Moderate impairment of social/intellectual functions	15,000
– Serious impairment etc.	40,000
– Permanent: Extremely serious (no effective control of functions)	250,000
• *Disabling but temporary mental anxiety* (medically verified)	1,000
• *Disabling mental disorder lasting up to 28 wks*	2,500
• *Disabling mental disorder 28 wks. to 1 year*	4,000
• *Disabling mental disorder >1 year but not permanent*	7,500
• *Permanently disabling mental disorder confirmed by psychiatric diagnosis*	20,000

The notes state that;

"Shock or Nervous shock may be taken to include conditions attributed to PTSD, depression or similar generic terms covering:–

a) such psychological symptoms as anxiety, tension, insomnia, irritability, loss of confidence, agoraphobia and pre-occupation with thoughts of guilt or self harm.

b) related physical symptoms such as alopecia, eczema, enuresis or psoriasis. Disability in this context will include impaired work (or school) performance, significant adverse effects on social relationships and sexual dysfunction."

New Ways of Thinking

Until relatively recently those involved in the compensation process have been required to look at the victim of an accident in almost entirely physical terms. Function in ones arms, legs or whatever part of the body that has been subjected to a traumatic insult can be measured objectively and the level of disability in occupational or domestic environments assessed.

The greater acceptance of the validity of psychological injury is encouraging all of us to look at the client/patient in more holistic terms. We can associate with patterns of behaviour affecting the way in which other people interact with them and the levels of sympathy or stigmatisation they might attract.

The fact that someone can physically drive a car shortly after an accident does not mean they can continue to cope on a psychological level with a job that requires them to drive long distances and continually re-experience anxiety at the possibility of a repeat.

The fact that someone is physically capable of doing the shopping or cleaning the house does not mean that they do not require assistance with some domestic tasks on a permanent or semi-permanent basis during periods when they are suffering from a chronic depressive reaction to what has happened to them.

We need to weigh in the balance the benefits and disadvantages of counselling, the likely effect of protracted legal action on the client's recovery as well as the knock on effect on their spouse and other family and their employment. These are just some of the challenges facing those of us who practice in an area of the law which is still subject to considerable change.

Medical Experts in the English Courts

Under the principles of English Law, the general rule is that a witness may only testify as to matters actually observed by him and may not give his opinion about those matters. The one exception to this rule arises in the case of "expert" witnesses. In civil cases s. 3(1) of the Civil Evidence Act 1972 provides that an expert may give his opinion *"on any relevant matter on which he is qualified to give expert evidence*". The expert need not have personal knowledge of every relevant matter within the field of his expertise, his testimony may be based on academic books or articles, professional publications, research data from his peers and other verifiable records.

When asked to prepare a report for the purposes of litigation, the expert must be conscious of the fact that the requirements of a Medico-Legal report are clearly different to providing an assessment of a patient for medical purposes. There will undoubtedly be issues relevant to the court which must be dealt with by the expert, areas which he would not normally consider in a clinical environment. The person being examined is not his patient and is therefore not able to rely on the usual Doctor–Patient privilege of confidentiality. Indeed, once the report has been disclosed to the other side all privilege in relation to its contents are waived. It is worth remembering however, that a report prepared for the purposes of litigation remains privileged until such time as it is disclosed to the other side.

The duty of the Instructing Solicitor is clearly to his client. Whilst every solicitor is under a similar duty not to mislead the court, he will be failing in his duty to his client if he does not present the case in the most favourable light possible. This in turn may lead to a conflict of interest between the solicitor and the expert. The Court will not tolerate an expert witness who although sceptical about a case nevertheless submits a favourable report, because he knows that is what his Instructing Solicitor is expecting.

The duty of an expert witness is to provide the court with an independent and unbiased expert opinion on matters which are likely to be outside the experience or knowledge of the Judge; the expert should be unaffected by the litigation process, deal only with matters within his expertise, state the reasons for his opinion having dealt with all the material facts whether or not they assist the client's case, state clearly if the report is provisional only, communicate any change of opinion without delay to the other side and the Court and ensure that any documents referred to in the report are provided to the other side and the court[15]. An expert must never mislead the court either intentionally or by failing to deal with a matter relevant to the facts in issue. Post Woolf, this duty has been embedded within the new Civil Procedure Rules.

Heralded as the most radical change in English civil procedure in over 100 years, Lord Woolf's new Civil Procedure Rules make far reaching changes. All experts whose evidence is to be used in court now have an overriding duty to the Court to assist on matters within their expertise, beyond any obligation that expert may have to the person who instructed him or is to pay him[16]. At the end of his report an expert must certify that he understands this duty to the court and that he has complied with it[17]. In the event that an expert requires assistance in the carrying out of his duty, he may apply to the court for directions[18]. In doing so he need not notify either party to the litigation. Experts need to be aware of the Practice Direction which supplements the Civil Procedure Rules relating to experts and assessors. Importantly, the Direction stipulates the manner in which the report should be presented to the Court. Highlighting the duty of an expert to assist those who must decide the facts, the report should be addressed to the Court and not the person who commissioned the report.

> "*1.1 An expert's report should be addressed to the court and not to the party from whom the expert has received his instructions.*"[19]

Furthermore, the Direction supplements the new Rules on what should be included in the expert's report.

> "*1.2 An expert's report must;*
> (1) *give details of the expert's qualifications*
> (2) *give details of any literature or other material which the expert has relied on in making the report*
> (3) *say who carried out any test or experiment which the expert has used for the report and whether or not the test or experiment has been carried out under the expert's supervision*
> (4) *give the qualifications of the person who carried out any such test or experiment, and*
> (5) *where there is a range of opinion on the matters dealt with in the report*
> (i) *summarise the range of opinion, and*
> (ii) *give reasons for his own opinion*
> (6) *contain a summary of the conclusions noted*
> (7) *contain a statement that the expert understands his duty to the court and has complied with that duty (rule 35.10(2)), and*
> (8) *contain a statement setting out the substance of all material instructions (whether written or oral). The statement should summarise the facts and instructions given to the expert which are material to the opinions expressed in the report or upon which those opinions are based (rule 35.10(3))*[20]

Expanding on the requirement that an expert must now specifically certify the accuracy of his report, Paragraph 1.3 of the Practice Direction states that the report must contain a statement verifying the truth of the report, in addition to complying with Paragraph 1.2 (7) and (8) above. The form to be adopted for the statement of truth is as follows;

> "*1.4 I believe that the facts I have stated in this report are true and that the opinions I have expressed are correct*"[21]

To knowingly mislead the court by making a false statement, perverts the course of justice. If an expert verifies a report by signing the statement of truth, without an honest belief that it's contents are true, he will be guilty of contempt of court and can be punished accordingly.[22]

A major change that will transform lower value claims is that there is now a general requirement for expert evidence to be given in written format only unless the court specifically directs otherwise.[23] In Fast Track cases i.e. injury claims with an estimated value of between £1,000–£15,000, it will be the norm for expert evidence to be in the form of written reports. If detailed cross examination is likely then the increased cost of this exercise will have to be justified and the case would be moved into the higher value multi track.

At the heart of the new rules is the requirement that the court and parties should seek to further the 'Overriding Objective' of the rules to deal with cases justly.[24]

What is new is that the concept of 'justly' is defined by a number of criteria which must be considered by the court in managing the proceedings.

Part of the overriding objective is to ensure that the parties are able to deal with one another on an equal footing and this principle clearly extends to those instructed on their behalf as experts. Rule 35.9 and Paragraph 2 of the "Practice Direction – Experts and Assessors" provide that, where a party has access to information not reasonably accessible to the other side, the court may direct that they provide a statement recording the details of such information. Furthermore, the statement must be comprehensive enough to enable assessment and understanding of the significance of the information held.

Woolf introduces the novel concept to English litigation, of joint experts. In an attempt to shorten court proceedings the Court is now in a position to insist that evidence is to be given by a single joint expert.[25] In cases where an expert cannot be agreed by the parties the court may intervene and select an expert of its own choice. Each party may give its own instructions to the expert, as may the Court. Experts will need to be clear as to what is expected of them and instructing parties will need to ensure that their instructions are coherent and unambiguous. If an expert is unclear as to what is expected of him he will be unable to fulfill his duty to the court and in turn, the court will ultimately be unable to evaluate the claim. Instructions are not privileged and will be brought before the court in the body of the report. This should be borne in mind by the Instructing Solicitor when composing his instructions.

Discussions between experts instructed by each party is to be encouraged under the new Rules.[26] Again, in order to reduce the amount of oral testimony given at a hearing, the Court will hope that by getting experts to "talk" agreement may be reached on various issues. The more issues agreed, the fewer will need to be dealt with during court time. It should be noted, that any issues discussed by the experts may not be referred to at trial unless both sides agree. Where experts agree certain points, the agreement will not become binding until such time as the parties consent to be expressly bound by the matters agreed.

It remains open for a party to instruct their own expert, unless otherwise directed by the court. In such cases, the other party may wish to make enquiries of the expert instructed. This is covered in the new rules. Rule 35.6(1) provides as follows;

> *"35.6 (1) A party may put to –*
> *a) an expert instructed by another party; or*
> *b) a single joint expert appointed under rule 35.7,*
> *written questions about his report."*

In all cases such questions must be submitted within 28 days of service of the report and must only be for the purpose of clarification of the report unless the court or the other party agree otherwise. Thus questions are not intended to be a means by which instructions may be supplemented or amended in the light of what has already been written by the expert. A party has only one opportunity of asking written questions and care should be taken to ensure that the questions are worded so as to allow clear answers. This is of particular importance as the answers may be treated as part of the expert's report. Once again, clarity of communication is of paramount importance not only in the preparation of instructions to an expert but also in any subsequent communication.

If an expert fails to reply to a request for written answers, the court may determine that the expert's report cannot be relied upon or alternatively may impose costs sanctions. Another new feature of the new rules is that they seek to regulate pre litigation procedure. This is achieved through Pre-action Protocols. In his final Access to Justice Report in 1996 Lord Woolf commented that the development of pre-action protocols was to be recommended "*... to build on and increase the benefits of early but well informed settlement which genuinely satisfy both parties to the dispute*".

The Pre-Action Protocol for Personal Injury claims requires the court to treat the standards set out in the protocol as the normal reasonable approach to pre-action conduct. The language used makes it clear that, to ignore the protocol invites criticism by the court and probably result in the imposition of adverse sanctions. Indeed, the court's ability to impose immediate and unilateral costs sanctions on a party, regardless of whether or not they ultimately succeed in the litigation, may well prove to be the incentive, if one is needed, to work within the 'best practice' models set out in the Protocols.

What does this mean for experts?

Paragraph 2.11 of the Protocol encourages the joint selection of, and access to, experts, although the ability for each party to seek and obtain their own expert's report remains. What has changed is the courts ability to decide what expert evidence should be admissible. The courts are being encouraged to reduce the amount of expert evidence that is allowed, the cost of experts being seen as one of the main causes of extra cost and delay in the conduct of civil litigation.

Under the Personal Injury Protocol a party intending to instruct an expert must first provide the other party with a list of experts he considers to be suitable. The claimant (as a plaintiff is now called) must also ensure that the other party is granted full access to the claimant's medical records. The defendant can object to any of the experts on the list supplied. One should then be selected from those that remain who is then instructed by the claimant. If the other party objects to any expert listed, they must do so within 14 days. Where none of the experts listed are acceptable then both parties may instruct experts of their own choice.

Gone are the days of pro-plaintiff/pro-defendant experts, or so it is hoped. In a new era where co-operation amongst litigants is encouraged it is the responsibility of the parties to comply with the spirit of the Protocol by taking reasonable steps to ensure that there is at least one expert on the list who they agree should provide a report. If the parties are unable to achieve this then the Court is likely to intervene and choose an expert for them. A litigant who is seen to be "playing the rules" will be given short shrift by the Court; a costs order will generally be the appropriate sanction to discipline litigants but where needed courts will have the ability to strike out the claim or part of it.

Where the other party has not objected to the nomination of a particular expert, he cannot later use other expert evidence unless the other party agrees or the court so directs. Written questions may be put to the expert instructed via those who instructed him, although the expert should send the answers to both parties simultaneously.

In the event that a medical report has been provided to the other side in compliance with the protocol, proceedings should be delayed for 21 days to allow an opportunity for settlement of the claim.

The emphasis is on co-operation between the parties. The previous adversarial nature of English civil proceedings had, in its worst guise, created a system in which an injured person seeking compensation, could wait many years for settlement or trial. Old rules allowed each side to obtain its own expert evidence, often leading to numerous examinations by experts. This in itself could further traumatize the accident victim. Although it will take some time for practitioners and experts alike to come to terms with the new rules, they are claimant friendly. The instruction of a single joint expert straight away eliminates the additional trauma a claimant experiences in being examined by the defendant's nominated expert. The new rules seek to promote greater communication between the parties and so create an environment in which more can be agreed. Where agreement is possible, so it will identify those areas in dispute which can be more easily resolved by the courts if need be.

References

1 [1881] 13 A C 222
2 *Page v Smith* [1996] A.C. 155
3 [1998] 1 AER 1
4 *McLoughlin v O'Brian* [1983] A.C. 410, 422–423
5 R Mayou and M C Sharpe '*Psychiatric Illnesses associated with physical disease*' 1995 Vol 1 No. 2 Bailiere's Clinical Psychiatry
6 (1992) *The Times* 19 June CA
7 [1992] 1 A.C. 310
8 *Chadwick v British Railways Board* [1967] 2 AER 945
9 *The Times* 4th Dec 1998
10 [1986] *Current Law Yearly* 1048
11 For example see Dr O'Brien – *Journal of Personal Injury Litigation* [1994] *Journal of Personal Injury Litigation* 257 @273
12 *The Journal of Personal Injury Litigation* [1994] 257 @ 271
13 [1995] 1 ALL ER 737
14 "Legal issues in PTSD" in "*Traumatic Stress*" – B.A.van der Kolk et al.
15 *Ikarian Reefer' National Justice Compania Naviera SA v Prudential Assurance Co. Ltd.* [1993] Vol 2 Lloyds Rep pg. 18 QB per Mr Justice Cresswell
16 *Civil Procedure Rules*, Part 35 Experts and Assessors, Rule 35.3
17 *Civil Procedure Rules*, Part 35 Experts and Assessors, Rule 35.10(2)
18 *Civil Procedure Rules*, Part 35 Experts and Assessors, Rule 35.14(1)
19 Part 35 Practice Directions Experts and Assessors
20 Part 35 Practice Directions Experts and Assessors
21 Part 35 Practice Directions Experts and Assessors
22 Part 22 of the *Civil Procedure Rules* provide further guidance on statements of truth and is also supplemented by a Practice Direction.
23 *Civil Procedure Rules*, Part 35 Experts and Assessors, Rule 35.5(1)
24 *Civil Procedure Rules*, Rule 1
25 *Civil Procedure Rules*, Part 35 Experts and Assessors, Rule 35.7
26 *Civil Procedure Rules*, Part 35 Experts and Assessors, Rule 35.12

17

Malingering and Litigation Stress in Motor Vehicle Accident Victims

WILLIAM J. KOCH, Ph.D., ABPP

Vancouver Hospital & Health Sciences Centre, Vancouver, British Columbia, Canada

REGAN SHERCLIFFE, M.A.

Simon Fraser University, Burnaby, British Columbia, Canada

INGRID FEDOROFF, Ph.D., GRANT L. IVERSON, Ph.D. and STEVEN TAYLOR, Ph.D.

University of British Columbia, Vancouver, British Columbia, Canada

Most health conditions occur without reference to others' negligent actions. Posttraumatic Stress Disorder (PTSD; APA, 1994) and other health conditions that can result from motor vehicle accidents (MVAs) are unique in that PTSD requires, as part of its diagnostic criteria, a precipitating event, and MVAs are alleged precipitants. Thus, compensation for health care payments, lost wages, and/or pain and suffering may become the responsibility of a third party.

A number of implications arise from this unique situation. For example, people other than the injured party have a vested interest in the assessment and rehabilitation of the patient. As well, some parties have a vested interest in doubting the veracity of the patient's health problems. The effect of these vested interests can be seen in the skepticism frequently attached to diagnoses of PTSD, while diagnoses of Major Depression (MDE, APA, 1994) outside the context of litigation are accepted with less skepticism. The upshot of these vested interests and skepticism is that plaintiffs with alleged psychological problems arising from MVAs will be subjected to more intensive, frequent, and possibly hostile assessment of their health problems. Thus, an individual seeking relief for symptoms of depression and anxiety while in litigation will experience a very different health care environment than will the person seeking such relief outside the context of litigation.

What is Litigation Stress?

We have recently begun to investigate this phenomenon, which has been briefly described by Weissman (1990).

> "*Involvement in litigation renders plaintiffs susceptible to stressors* and to influences that *may lead to increased impairment*, *biased reportage*, and *retarded recovery*. Underlying personality patterns play a critical role in defining and shaping reactions to trauma, to the stress of litigation, and to treatment interventions. Protracted litigation creates conditions that promote mnemonic and *attitudinal distortions*, as well as conscious and unconscious *motivations for secondary gain*." (Weissman, 1990, p. 67, emphases added).

What is apparent from this quote is Weissman's perception that litigation produces negative effects on the plaintiff's mental state through multiple pathways, including greater stressor susceptibility, attitude change, motivational change, and biases in self-report of difficulties. Conceptually, understanding litigation stress involves determining just what aspects of the litigation process are stressful for plaintiffs, and then the relative contributions of litigation stress to their psychological difficulties, as well as to biases in disclosure of these difficulties.

We recently surveyed 50 personal injury lawyers and 50 psychologists (mainly forensic psychologists) concerning their perceptions of litigation stress. First, we asked them for their personal definitions of "litigation stress" and subsequently categorized those personal descriptions. There were essentially 4 main categories of response from both lawyers and psychologists: stress resulting from the litigation process alone (e.g., court procedures, depositions), stress secondary to financial difficulties (e.g., loss of income, legal fees), stress from a combination of the initial trauma (e.g., MVA)

Table 1. Percentages of respondents who rated the following factors as moderate or major contributors to litigation stress. Scale included Major, Moderate, Minimal, None.

Sources of Litigation Stress	Lawyers (n = 50)	Psychologists (n = 50)
Uncertainty about physical/emotional recovery	96%	84%
Post-injury financial hardship	86%	82%
Home/work role changes	82%	68%
Adjuster/plaintiff conflict	76%	68%
Pre-existing personality vulnerabilities	72%	72%
Health professional disagreement (unreliability)	60%	60%
Conflict with family/friends	58%	54%
Insurance company policies	54%	56%
Too many health care appointments	34%	36%
Secondary gain	32%	64%
Lawyer/lawyer conflict	26%	46%

and litigation process, and stress due to uncertainty in the plaintiff's life (e.g., end of litigation, return to work). The most commonly given definition of litigation stress was that due to the litigation process alone.

How Forensic Psychologists and Personal Injury Lawyers View Litigation Stress. In the same survey mentioned above, we asked lawyers and psychologists to rate different sources of litigation stress according to their relative influence. These data are shown in Table 1. While there are some predictable differences between these two professional groups (psychologists are about twice as likely to blame litigation stress on conflict between lawyers and secondary gain as are lawyers), a relatively clear picture emerges from these data. Both professional groups see the primary sources of litigation stress as uncertainty about recovery, financial hardship, post-injury role changes, adjuster/plaintiff conflict, and pre-existing personality vulnerabilities.

Next, what do these professionals see as the causes of personal injury plaintiffs' psychological distress? The same samples of lawyers and psychologists rated whether the variables shown in Table 2 had a major, moderate, minimal, or no effect on the psychological problems of plaintiffs.

In this case, there are more substantive differences between the professional groups. Those possible causes that were rated significantly differently by lawyers and psychologists are described below. First, psychologists are twice as likely as lawyers to see secondary gain as having at least a moderate effect on plaintiffs' symptoms. They are also more likely to believe that iatrogenic effects of poor health care might cause psychological problems than do

Table 2. Percentages of personal injury lawyers' and forensic psychologists' ratings of variables having moderate to major effects on the psychological states of personal injury plaintiffs.

Putative Causes	Lawyers (n = 50)	Psychologists (n = 50)	Chi Square (p)
Severity of initial physical injury	81%	98%	6.8 (.009)
Pre-existing personality or psychiatric problems	90%	93.5%	.42 (.52)
Secondary gain	31%	73%	17.1 (.001)
Litigation stress	57%	80%	5.6 (.018)
Iatrogenic effects of poor treatment	44%	67%	4.5 (.034)
Chronicity of physical injury	86%	98%	4.4 (.036)
Frightening nature of trauma	62.5%	85%	6.0 (.015)

lawyers. Psychologists are more likely than lawyers to see litigation stress to have untoward effects on the mental health of litigants. Psychologists are also more likely to see the frightening nature of the trauma, severity of initial physical injury, as well as the chronicity of physical injury to have at least moderate effects on the plaintiff's psychological status. In short, forensic psychologists are much more sensitized to the influences of secondary gain and iatrogenic factors on psychological symptoms than are lawyers, as well as more attentive to PTSD criterion A (severity of traumatic event). The majority of psychologists and about half the lawyers view litigation stress as having a moderate to major role in the cause of psychological problems in personal injury litigants.

Predictors of Psychological Distress after Traumatic Injury. Predictors of PTSD can be roughly categorized by their temporal relationship to the trauma. Victim characteristics preceding the trauma, which we will call *predisposing factors*, include prior mental health history. Characteristics of the traumatic event (including the victim's immediate subjective response to the trauma, objective severity of the trauma, and severity of physical injuries caused by the trauma) may be called *event factors*. Finally, those *post-event* factors, such as victim coping characteristics and post-injury stresses may also influence the victim's adjustment. We will discuss here only those post-event factors related to psychological adjustment.

With respect to post-event factors, slow recovery from physical injuries appears to predict worse psychological status (Blanchard et al. 1997; Ehlers et al., 1998). Litigation or compensation status is another post-event variable that has been shown to predict psychological disturbance by some authors (Blanchard et al., 1996; Bryant & Harvey, 1995, Ehlers et al., 1998). Delahanty et al. (1997) have data suggesting that the injured party's perception of other people being responsible for their injury predicts psychological distress. It is intuitively plausible that this responsibility perception will be related to the probability of litigation and to related attitudinal changes by the victims concerning their injuries.

Avoidant coping style has also been associated with poorer recovery from trauma and with post-traumatic psychological distress (Bryant & Harvey, 1995; Wolfe et al., 1993). Ehlers et al. (1998) found that a number of psychological variables were related to PTSD status after MVAs. Rumination about the accident, negative interpretations of intrusive memories, and attempts to suppress these memories of the MVA all predicted PTSD status. Therefore, coping style is one post-event variable that predicts psychological distress following accidental injury. In addition to coping style, low social support (Perry et al., 1992) and maladaptive emotions such as guilt or anger (e.g., Riggs et al., 1992; Ehlers et al., 1998) have frequently been linked to increased psychological distress or poor treatment response for PTSD.

In short, there are a number of variables following traumatic events such as MVAs that predict psychological distress or PTSD status. In particular, post-event variables that have been associated with psychological disturbance include: litigation/compensation status, slow recovery from physical injuries, post-trauma pain severity, avoidant coping style, low social support, maladaptive emotions such as guilt or anger, and recent trauma to family members.

Litigation Stress Predictors of Psychological Treatment Outcome. Litigation stress is relevant to MVA victims because many of them have some relationship with an insurance company during their symptomatic period. In our treatment outcome study at UBC, approximately 65% of our subjects were in litigation. From our perspective, the following variables may constitute domains of litigation stress: (a) problematic physical recovery, (b) conflict with adjuster or insurer, (c) disagreement among health providers about the best diagnosis or treatment, (d) too much health care, (e) conflict with family and friends concerning diminished role functioning or symptoms, and (f) financial hardship.

Table 4. Sample items from the Litigation Stress Scale (Koch, Iverson, Taylor, & Fedoroff, 1997).

Item Number	Examples of Litigation Stress Scale Items
4	How often have health care providers disagreed among themselves about the diagnosis of your.....
8	How optimistic are you right now that you will recover fully from your physical injuries?
13	Before you had your accident, how fairly did you expect to be treated by the insurance company?
16	How fairly have you been treated by health care professionals hired by the insurance company?
27	Has your insurance adjuster disagreed with any of the advice given to you by any of your health care providers?
30	Since your accident, how many times have you been warned by anyone that you may not get a fair assessment.....

To assess the degree to which patients varied in their experience with litigation and other post-MVA stressors, we constructed the Litigation Stress Scale (LSS), a questionnaire intended to measure the self-reported stressful experiences of litigants that may be associated with personal injury litigation for physical and mental injuries. Sample items from our Litigation Stress Scale are shown in Table 4.

Our preliminary data suggest that some of these items are related to treatment outcome. For the first 28 subjects completing treatment in our treatment outcome study, we have computed correlations between total PTSD symptom change and a large number of variables that were assessed prior to treatment. The following Litigation Stress Scale (LSS) variables all predicted poor treatment outcome: slow physical recovery, subjects' pessimism about physical recovery, self-reported number of health care appointments, and self-reported number of hours worked per week prior to MVA. These findings are presented in Table 5.

The first two of these items may reflect what has been shown by Blanchard and his colleagues, that slow physical recovery is a predictor of PTSD status and continued psychological distress. The second item, pessimism about physical recovery, may reflect the attitudinal changes referred to by Weisman (1990).

In addition, self-reported number of health care appointments is negatively related to treatment outcome in our study. This confirms a common observation of forensic psychologists, who frequently comment that MVA litigants are over-assessed and receive too many concurrent treatments without benefit. The upshot of this is that such litigants frequently devote an undue amount of their time and energy to attending health professional appointments, which

Table 5. Pre-treatment Litigation Stress Scale correlates of treatment response of group cognitive-behavioural treatment for 28 subjects. *P ≤ .05, **P < .01

Litigation Stress Scale Item	Penn PTSD Scale	Posttraumatic Stress Scale-Self Report Version	Mean PTSD
Slow physical recovery	–.34	–.38*	–.38*
Optimism about recovery	–.37	–.36	–.39*
# of health care appts.	–.39*	–.35	–.39*
Pre-MVA hours worked	–.54**	–.31	–.45*

interferes with their daily functioning. If replicated, this finding may have ramifications for insurance policy with respect to assessment and rehabilitation of MVA victims, and suggests that more health care is not necessarily good for the patient.

Finally, the number of hours worked prior to the MVA is significantly associated with treatment outcome. This likely reflects the patients' unsatisfactory role changes since the MVA (i.e., changing from being fully employed to being unemployed in many cases).

It is notable that of those possible sources of litigation stress endorsed by lawyers and psychologists, uncertainty about recovery and negative role changes were endorsed by more than two-thirds of both professional groups. We have here some data to confirm their suspicions.

We think the most important conclusion from the research literature as a whole, and our preliminary data with respect to litigation stress in particular, is the prominence of post-event variables in predicting ongoing psychological distress. This runs counter to both the traditional diagnostic view that event variables (e.g., severity of injury, severity of trauma) are most important, and to an alternative skeptical view that pre-disposing variables (e.g., prior mental health or personality problems) are most important. Rather, our interpretation of the literature and our own data suggest that multiple post-MVA stressors influence the psychological recovery of these patients. They appear to have independent effects on outcome, over and above pre--disposing and event variables.

Assessment of Malingered PTSD

Models of Malingering. According to Rogers (1997), there are three explanatory models of malingering; pathogenic, criminological, and adaptational. The most relevant model for the current discussion is the adaptational model of malingering. According to Rogers, malingering is more likely to occur when the context of the health care assessment is seen by the patient to be adversarial, when the personal stakes to the patient are high, and when other alternatives do not appear to be available. Thus, in the case of personal litigation regarding psychological problems, malingering is more likely to occur when the patient views him/herself to have an adversarial relationship with the health professional, insurance company, or adjuster. It is also more likely to occur when the patient senses a significant personal loss attached to his psychological problems, and a method for obtaining compensation for this loss. Finally, it is more likely to occur under conditions of limited personal options (e.g., poor job skills, limited financial resources, treatment or rehabilitation resources not easily available).

Thus, within compensation or torts liability settings that may be stressful to claimants, the constructs of litigation stress and malingering may be interconnected. Individuals with stress-related mental health symptoms may be encouraged to exaggerate these symptoms because of the adversarial litigation context and their desire to be heard. Alternatively, when exposed to other losses or stresses, litigating patients may be biased in their attribution of cause as well as in their retrospective recall of symptoms.

Estimated Base Rates of Malingering. There is no "gold standard" for diagnosing malingering (i.e., a concrete criterion against which diagnosticians can test their tests and diagnostic decisions). Therefore, it is not surprising that estimates of the prevalence of malingering are highly variable. In his work on the forensic evaluation of personal injury claimants, Lees-Haley claims a substantial incidence of malingering. For example, he recently reported on the MMPI-2 profiles of 492 personal injury plaintiffs (Lees-Haley, 1997). His interpretation of these data suggested that between 20 and 30 percent of his subjects showed some evidence of malingering. In contrast, a large auto insurance company estimates malingering at only 3 percent of cases (G. Lee, personal communication, October 1998). The insurance company perspective is more likely to represent the suspected number of cases of blatant fraud. As the reader can discern, there is little certainty about the actual base rate of malingering in MVA claims.

Best Methods. The best researched scales of symptom over-endorsement or exaggeration applicable to this population are the validity scales of the Minnesota Multiphasic Personality Inventory: Second Edition (MMPI-2), which have not changed substantially from those in the original version of the MMPI. The malingering/exaggeration indices of the original MMPI have been studied extensively. Berry et al. (1991) published a meta-analysis

Table 6. Mean effect size by nature of contrast, adapted from Berry, Baer & Harris (1991).

Contrast (N)	Mean Effect Size (d)
Normals standard vs. fake bad instructions (21)	2.66
Normals faking bad vs. psychiatric patients (14)	1.86
Psychiatric Patients standard vs. fake bad instructions (3)	1.48

of 28 studies assessing exaggerating response style via the MMPI. They found that F-scale was the best measure of malingering with an average effect size of 2.34. Effect sizes for discriminating different groups using the F-scale are shown in Table 6. While effect sizes for discriminating these different groups with respect to symptom over-endorsement are impressive, what is apparent is the shrinkage of the effect size as one uses contrasting groups that are closer to the contrasts necessary in actual forensic practice. Thus, when comparing normal subjects some of whom respond under normal instructions and some of whom are asked to "fake bad", it is easy to tell these two groups apart because their mean scores on the F-scale are more than two and one-half standard deviations apart. However, as one makes more ecologically valid comparisons of psychiatric patients under standard versus fake bad instructions, it is much harder to tell the groups apart because their mean scores on the F-scale are only about one and one-half standard deviations apart.

Rogers and colleagues (1994), in their meta-analysis of the MMPI-2 determined that F, F-K, and the obvious versus subtle score demonstrated the greatest effect sizes for both normal controls and psychiatric comparison groups. Cutoff scores for suspecting biased responding were provided (Rogers, et al, 1994), and the use of these cutoff scores for malingering has been described by Franzen and Iverson (1998).

Since multiple other variables can mediate the exaggeration of health symptoms, one caveat is suggested in the assessment of malingering in MVA litigants. Depression can mediate symptom exaggeration. For example, among combat-related PTSD subjects, the presence of depression was more associated with symptom exaggeration as measured by the MMPI-2 F-K index of exaggeration than was financial compensation (Smith & Frueh, 1996).

Examples of exaggerated recall of symptoms include retrospective recall of vomiting from gastric bypass patients (Stunkard et al., 1985), and biased recollections of physical and affective menstrual symptoms (McFarland et al., 1989). The latter study was particularly instructive in that the authors showed that strength of belief in an affective model of menstrual distress predicted exaggerated negative symptoms during the subjects' last menstrual period. Thus, the personal model a subject has for understanding some aspect of his/her physical and emotional status may lead to exaggerated recall of specific symptoms. This is particularly important in the case of MVA plaintiffs who are often assessed years after the trauma.

These findings about various influences on symptom exaggeration are important for understanding the diversity of influences operating on MVA-PTSD patients' symptom descriptions. Over 40 percent of PTSD (Kessler et al., 1995) and over 50 percent of MVA-PTSD patients (Blanchard & Hickling, 1996) have comorbid depression. It is therefore likely that such comorbidity will negatively affect the reliability of such patients' self report of symptoms, irrespective of financial incentives to exaggerate.

Related to this problem is a problem with the item content of the MMPI infrequency scale (F). The infrequency scale has been criticized for over-diagnosing symptom exaggeration because many of its items measure legitimate symptoms of mental disorders. To alleviate this problem, Arbisi & Ben-Porath (1995) developed a scale referred to as the infrequency-psychopathology scale F(p), in which items were retained based on lowered correlations with the basic clinical scales of the MMPI-2. This new scale has promise because it should decrease the diagnosis of malingering in some individuals who are highly distressed.

Arbisi & Ben-Porath (1998) recently assessed the ability of F(p) to differentiate psychiatric inpatients under standard versus malingering instructions. This is seen as an ecologically more relevant comparison because of the high rate of previous and concurrent mental health conditions among personal injury plaintiffs. They showed that F(p) improved discrimination between the honest and malingered profiles.

Comparison of MVA Litigants versus Psychiatric Inpatients. Because one of the best predictors of PTSD status following MVAs is a prior history of depression, a more ecologically valid comparison of MVA litigants may be with respect to non-litigating individuals known to have serious psychological distress. Therefore, we contrasted 31 MVA litigants (MVA) assessed for medical-legal purposes with varied diagnoses of MVA-PTSD, Accident Phobia, Major Depressive Episode, traumatically-induced Body Dismorphic Disorder, and Malingering (only 2 of the 31 earned the diagnosis of malingering), with two psychiatric inpatient samples. Because the former patients were assessed during the litigation process, they would have both financial incentives to exaggerate their mental health symptoms and a potentially adversarial relationship with the assessment process.

The inpatient samples were obtained from teaching hospital records and excluded diagnoses of Schizophrenia, Organic Brain Syndrome, Bipolar Affective Disorder, other psychotic disorders, or cases where a personality disorder was the primary diagnosis. This left 131 patients with diagnoses of PTSD, MDE, OCD, Panic Disorder, Adjustment Disorder, and GAD. Fifteen of these inpatients were either in litigation or receiving financial compensation for mental health reasons (inpatients in litigation – PIL), while the rest had no litigation (inpatients not in litigation – PNIL). The PNIL group had no financial incentive for symptom exaggeration, nor were they in an adversarial assessment context. The PIL group had some financial incentive for symptom exaggeration, but because their assessment was done outside the context of litigation they did not have an adversarial relationship with the assessor.

In short, these three groups represent three different degrees of the Rogers' proposed contextual and incentive motivations for symptom exaggeration, and thus we should see three levels of symptom exaggeration, with the PNIL group showing the least symptom exaggeration and the MVA group showing the greatest symptom exaggeration. The means and standard deviations for each group on the MMPI-2 validity, clinical scales, as well as F(p) are presented in Table 7.

No significant differences were found between the MVA and the PNIL groups on Fp ($t=1.82$, $df=143$, $p \geq 0.05$) or on the L scale ($t=.143$, $df=143$, $p \geq 0.05$). The PNIL group had a significantly higher F score than did the MVA group ($t=3.08$, $df=143$, $p \leq 0.05$), which could be interpreted as reflecting their more diffuse psychopathology. The PIL group had significantly higher Fp ($t=3.43$, $df=41$, $p \leq 0.05$) and F ($t=2.57$, $df=41$, $p \leq 0.05$) scores than did the MVA group. In summary, these preliminary data show some support for the utility of F(p) in detecting symptom exaggeration, but suggest that MVA litigants may be no more prone to indiscriminately exaggerate psychological distress than are non-litigating psychiatric patients.

Summary

In this chapter, we have discussed evidence regarding variables arising after the MVA that negatively affect victims' mental health. These include slow physical recovery, patients' pessimism about their recovery, a seemingly iatrogenic effect of too much health care given to such patients, and negative role changes at work. To their credit, personal injury lawyers and forensic psychologists working with plaintiffs recognize some of these variables as contributing to psychological distress. The research literature more generally points to a number of variables occurring after traumatic MVAs, as well as the stresses of litigation, that exert strong influences on MVA victims' emotional recovery. These include the degree of social support and unrelated stressful life events, among other variables.

Table 7. Mean MMPI-2 Scale Scores for three groups of patients. Standard deviations appear in parentheses.

MMPI-2 Scale	MVA Litigants	Psychiatric Inpatients with No Litigation	Psychiatric Inpatients with Litigation
L	52.8 (12.6)	53.1 (9.7)	55.5 (10.1)
F	60.8 (14.5)	72.0 (18.66)	77.8 (28.6)
K	48.2 (11.4)	47.3 (10.2)	45.9 (10.4)
HS	74.8 (11.4)	68.5 (13.4)	82.8 (16.0)
D	73.2 (15.9)	82.4 (15.0)	87.2 (13.7)
HY	78.4 (13.7)	73.6 (15.0)	84.1 (14.9)
PD	61.0 (13.4)	69.0 (12.1)	66.5 (15.2)
MF	49.8 (10.0)	51.2 (10.3)	52.2 (10.4)
PA	62.3 (18.5)	69.6 (13.9)	81.3 (17.1)
PT	68.3 (14.2)	79.4 (13.3)	82.6 (16.4)
SC	67.0 (16.7)	77.5 (14.8)	82.3 (19.9)
MA	49.1 (9.7)	51.0 (12.8)	58.5 (13.6)
SI	54.9 (11.6)	63.6 (12.6)	65.0 (13.6)
Fp	52 (11.0)	57.1 (14.5)	69.6 (22.7)

Litigation stress and other losses involved with traumatic injury are intertwined with the motivation to exaggerate mental health symptoms as articulated in Rogers' (1997) model of adaptational malingering. However, research from diverse sources tells us that the causes of symptom exaggeration and biased recall of symptoms are multidimensional. These potential causes include negative influences of comorbidity as well as the more obvious influence of possible financial compensation. Our own preliminary data suggest that many MVA litigants may be no more likely to exaggerate their mental health symptoms than are non-litigating mental health patients with similar diagnoses.

References

American Psychiatric Association, (1994). *Diagnostic and Statistic Manual of Mental Disorders: Fourth Edition.* Author: Washington, D.C.

Arbisi, P. A. & Ben-Porath, Y. S. (1995). An MMPI-2 infrequent response scale for use with psychopathological populations. The Infrequency-Psychopathology Scale, F(p). *Psychological Assessment, 7*, 424–431.

Arbisi, P. A. & Ben-Porath, Y. S. (1998). The ability of Minnesota Multiphasic Personality Inventory-2 validity scales to detect fake-bad responses in psychiatric inpatients. *Psychological Assessment, 10*, 221–228.

Berry, D. T., Baer, R. A. & Harris, M. J. (1991). Detection of malingering on the MMPI: A meta-analysis. *Clinical Psychology Review, 11,* 585–598.

Blanchard, E. B. & Hickling, E. H. (1996). *After the Crash: Assessment and Treatment of Motor Vehicle Accident Survivors.* American Psychological Association: Washington, D.C.

Blanchard, E. B., Hickling, E. J., Barton, K. A., Taylor, A. E., Loos, W. R. & Jones-Alexander, J. (1996). One-year prospective follow-up of motor vehicle accident victims. *Behaviour Research and Therapy, 10*, 775–786.

Blanchard, E. B., Hickling, E. J., Forneris, C. A., Taylor, A. E., Buckley, T. C., Loos, W. R. & Jaccard, J. (1997). Prediction of remission of acute posttraumatic stress disorder in motor vehicle accident victims. *Journal of Traumatic Stress, 10*, 215–234.

Bryant, R. A. & Harvey, A. G. (1995). Avoidant coping style and post-traumatic stress following motor vehicle accidents. *Behaviour Research and Therapy, 33*, 631–635.

Delahanty, D. L., Herberman, H. B., Craig, K. J., Hayward, M. C., Fullerton, C. S., Ursano, R. J. & Baum, A. (1997). Acute and chronic distress and posttraumatic stress disorder as a function of responsibility for serious motor vehicle accidents. *Journal of Consulting and Clinical Psychology, 65*, 560–567.

Ehlers, A., Mayou, R. A. & Bryant, B. (1998). Psychological predictors of chronic posttraumatic stress disorder after motor vehicle accidents. *Journal of Abnormal Psychology, 107,* 508–519.

Franzen, M. D. & Iverson, G. L. (1998). Detecting negative response bias and diagnosing malingering: The dissimulation exam. In P. J. Snyder and P. D. Nussbaum (Eds.). *Clinical Neuropsychology: A Pocket Handbook for Assessment.* American Psychological Association: Washington, D.C.

Kessler, R. C., Sonnega, A., Bromet, E., Hughes, M. & Nelson, C. B. (1995). Posttraumatic stress disorder in the national comorbidity survey. *Archives of General Psychiatry, 52*, 1048–1060.

Koch, W. J., Iverson, G., Taylor, S. & Fedoroff, I. C. (1998). Litigation Stress Scale. Unpublished test, University of British Columbia.

Lees-Haley, P. R. (1997). MMPI-2 base rates for 492 personal injury plaintiffs: Implications and challenges for forensic assessment. *Journal of Clinical Psychology, 53*, 745–755.

McFarland, C., Ross, M. & DeCourville, N. (1989). Women's theories of menstruation and biases in recall of menstrual symptoms. *Journal of Personality and Social Psychology, 57*, 522–531.

Perry, S., Difede, J., Musngi, G., Frances, A. J. & Jacobsberg, L. (1992). Predictors of posttraumatic stress disorder after burn injury. *American Journal of Psychiatry, 149*, 931–935.

Riggs, D. S., Dancu, C. V., Gershuny, B. S., Greenberg, D. & Foa, E. B. (1992). Anger and post-traumatic stress disorder in female crime victims. *Journal of Traumatic Stress, 5*, 613–625.

Rogers, R. (1997, Ed.), *Clinical assessment of malingering and deception: Second Edition.* Guilford Press: New York.

Rogers, R., Sewell, K. W. & Salekin, R. T. (1994). A meta-analysis of malingering on the MMPI-2. *Assessment, 1*, 227–237.

Smith, D. W. & Frueh, B.C. (1996). Compensation seeking, comorbidity, and apparent exaggeration of PTSD symptoms among Vietnam combat veterans. *Psychological Assessment, 8*, 3–6.

Stunkard, A. J., Fostger, G., Glassman, G. & Rosato, E. (1985). Retrospective exaggeration of symptoms: Vomiting after gastric surgery for obesity. *Psychosomatic Medicine, 47*, 150–155.

Weissman, H. N. (1990). Distortions and deceptions in self presentation: Effects of protracted litigation on personal injury cases. *Behavioral Sciences and the Law, 8*, 67–74.

Wolfe, J., Keane, T. M., Kaloupek, D. G., Mora, C. A. & Wine, P. (1993). Patterns of positive readjustment in Vietnam combat veterans. *Journal of Traumatic Stress, 6*, 179–193.

18

Posttraumatic Stress Disorder Stemming From Motor Vehicle Accidents: Legal Issues in Canada and the United States

KEVIN S. DOUGLAS

Simon Fraser University, Burnaby, British Columbia, Canada

MATTHEW T. HUSS

University of Nebraska, Lincoln, Nebraska, United States

LYNDA L. MURDOCH

Simon Fraser University, Burnaby, British Columbia, Canada

DAVID O'NEIL WASHINGTON

University of Nebraska, Lincoln, Nebraska, United States

WILLIAM J. KOCH

Vancouver Hospital & Health Sciences Centre, Vancouver, British Columbia, Canada

Introduction

A number of the chapters in this text indicate that Posttraumatic Stress Disorder (PTSD; American Psychiatric Association, 1994) is very common following motor vehicle accidents (MVAs). Complicating this with respect to legal judgements of liability and damages, however, are a number of factors. First, many pre-MVA and post-MVA factors influence the extent to which MVA survivors will develop PTSD or other psychological injuries (Blanchard et. al.; Koch et. al.; Taylor et. al.; this book). Thus, expert evidence with respect to the causal contribution of the MVA versus other factors may be very complicated. This will result in a diversity of expert opinion, and subsequently a diversity of judicial judgements leading to legal precedents.

Second, treatments for PTSD until recently have been of marginal success and few longitudinal studies or rigorously controlled treatment trials for MVA-PTSD have been conducted. Thus, the prognosis for treated MVA-PTSD as well as the nature of appropriate treatments has been largely unknown. This leaves legal decision-makers at a loss for determining the future costs to the plaintiff. However, preliminary results from two controlled trials (Blanchard et. al.; Taylor et. al.), and one uncontrolled trial (Ehlers) described in this book, as well as a recently-completed dissertation (Fecteau, 1999), suggest that effective treatment is becoming more available. Third, although financial awards to MVA-PTSD plaintiffs have been quite variable, courts have become more willing to compensate plaintiffs for mental injuries over time, reflecting perhaps an evolving change in courts' opinions concerning the worth of mental health.

This chapter describes legal issues related to PTSD following MVAs. This generally is covered by the law of *negligence*.[1] As such, the organization of the chapter will follow the key elements of a negligence lawsuit. This chapter cannot summarize all existing case law. Rather, we will describe general legal principles that arise in PTSD/MVA litigation, and illustrate these with relevant case law. Both American and Canadian law will be discussed. Where differences between the two countries are evident, they will be drawn out. However, the elements of negligence law are quite similar in the two countries.

Negligence is one of two main areas of tort law, the other being *intentional torts*. A tort, generally, can be defined as a civil (opposed to criminal) wrong that the law will compensate (Linden, 1997). The word "tort" is derived from the Latin *tortus*, meaning "crooked," and the French word *tort*, meaning "wrong" (Klar, 1996). In essence, then, a tort is a wrong caused by one party to another for which the former party is legally at fault, and for which that party is legally responsible to compensate the victim. The key difference between intentional torts and negligence is the intent requirement. For intentional torts (such as battery), the wrongdoer or *tortfeasor* must "intend" the act that produces harm. In negligence, no intention is required. Rather, the tortfeasor is held at fault for acts that he or she reasonably *ought to have known* would cause harm. Although one may imagine that a MVA may give rise to an intentional tort action, the vast majority of civil actions for MVAs stem from behaviour that falls below a proscribed standard of care, and hence fall under negligence law.

In any negligence action, there are several main elements that have to be proved by the plaintiff, who is the person alleging the wrong-doing and injury. These elements are as follows: 1) duty of care; 2) standard of care; 3) breach of the duty of care; 4) injury (to person, property, etc) sustained by the plaintiff; 5) causal connection between the defendant's breach of the duty of care and the plaintiff's injury, and 6) that the plaintiff has suffered damages (Rest. 2d δ281, δ282). These elements are similar in Canada and the United States.

Overview of the Elements of Negligence

Duty of Care, Standard of Care, and Breach of Duty

Although duty, standard, and breach are important elements of negligence that must be proved in any negligence action, they are likely of less interest to mental health professionals than are the legal issues of injury, causation, and damages. As such, the discussion of these elements will be brief. Generally, all persons owe a *duty of care* to avoid foreseeable harm to others. In England, Canada, and other Commonwealth countries, this duty was first clearly expressed in the English House of Lords case of *Donoghue* v. *Stevenson* (1932), prior to which persons could only be held liable for damage caused to another person if there was a contractual or statutory duty to avoid such damage.[2] In American jurisprudence, there are two types of duties imposed upon a defendant: (1) the duty to conduct oneself as a reasonable person would under the same circumstances; or (2) a special duty imposed by a jurisdictional statute or case law.

A *standard of care* describes the basic level of behaviour that persons must attain. The duty of care is to meet this standard. The standard of care is usually expressed in "reasonable person" language, stating that a person has a duty to act as a reasonable person in similar circumstances (e.g., *Brown* v. *Kendall*, 1850; Rest. 2d δ283). In the case of MVAs, a driver has a duty to all motorists and pedestrians in his or her immediate zone of danger and to any bystander that may observe the injury of a close relative (e.g., *Mazzagatti* v. *Everingham*, 1986). Courts in both countries have construed this to mean that persons have a duty to drive vigilantly, prudently, and within the limits of the law and road conditions.

If a plaintiff is owed a duty, he/she must also prove that the defendant breached that duty thereby exposing the plaintiff to an unreasonable risk. Once there has been an act, a duty, and a breach of that duty a negligent act has occurred. Injury, causation, and damages must also be found to establish liability.

Injury

It is in regard to the injury or damages[3] element of negligence that PTSD has had an extensive legal history. In the present chapter, the injury of interest is PTSD. Legally, PTSD is considered to be an example of the generic category of injury known variously as *emotional shock*, *nervous shock*, *psychiatric damage*, or *emotional injury* (Linden, 1997). Historically, courts in both the United States and Canada were reticent to award damages for such "psychic injuries." As Linden (1997), a justice of the Federal Court of Canada, explains, "[t]ort law was slow to grant protection to the interest of mental tranquility" (p. 385). Reasons for this reluctance were fear of a "flood" of litigation, fear of "imaginary" claims, and difficulties with proof (Linden, 1997). This reluctance was also prevalent in the American development of the doctrine surrounding emotional or psychiatric injuries (Romeo, 1997).

In Canada and the United States, various legal requirements have restricted compensation for this type of injury. In Canada, plaintiffs were in the past required to sustain physical injury or at least impact from the negligent act in order to be compensated for psychiatric damage (Linden, 1997). Some jurisdictions in the United States require that plaintiffs suffer a physical injury or impact in order to recover for emotional injuries, and some require that plaintiffs be in a "zone of danger," meaning that they were at least in danger of suffering physical impact or injury (American Jurisprudence, 1968/1997b).

Canadian courts currently require either a physical manifestation of psychiatric damage, *or* the presence of a "recognizable" psychiatric disorder, as well as *reasonable foresight* of the psychiatric damage by the defendant (Linden, 1997). PTSD seems to fit the requirements of Canadian law, and case law supports this assertion. In the mid-twentieth century, jurisdictions in the United States began to remove the earlier restrictions placed on recoverable damages (i.e., physical impact; physical injury) by allowing for psychological damages independent of physical injuries (Brown, 1996). The recognition of mental or psychological injuries has slowly evolved as a distinct injury claim. The emergence of PTSD as an official diagnostic entity has helped to reduce the courts' reluctance to accept emotional or nervous shock cases as legitimate claims of action (Newman & Yehuda, 1997). A psychological disorder, such as PTSD, has been defined to occur when any medically determined non-permanent injury endures for 90 days or more and substantially limits the performance of daily activities (*Granowitz* v. *Vanwickle*, 1993; N.J. Superior Ct.). For example, in the New York case of *Quaglio* v. *Tomaselli* (1984), PTSD and other psychiatric ailments were accepted as sufficient evidence to conclude that the plaintiff sustained a serious psychiatric injury.

Many states now allow PTSD claims without an accompanying physical injury (Slovenko, 1994). Further, it has been stated that the diagnosis of PTSD has been especially relevant in the courts' recognition of the viability of psychological injuries (Pitman & Sparr, 1998), and PTSD has been identified as much of the foundation for emotional injuries in the law (Raifman, 1983; Slovenko, 1994). Others have gone so far as to fear for the erosion of traditional legal restrictions and barriers to recovery because of a flood of litigation from PTSD (Brown, 1996). Appeal courts have over-turned trial courts that have rejected expert testimony demonstrating PTSD (see, for example, *Koury* v. *Lanier Express, Inc.*, 1988; La. App. 3rd Cir.). In *Johnson* v. *May* (1992; Ill. App. Ct.), the court rejected an expert's position that PTSD was a "malingerer's disorder," and asserted that the validity of PTSD as a disorder is not open to serious question.

Proving PTSD: The Importance of Expert Evidence. Despite the emergence of PTSD as a diagnostic entity, and the importance of this in emotional injury cases, some jurisdictions have still expressed concern over PTSD as a "sure-fire" way to establish an emotional injury. Subjectivity in the diagnosis of PTSD has resulted in doubt being cast on the utility of PTSD as a "stand-alone" injury (Newman & Yehuda, 1997). Some courts have retained the historical requirement of physical injury or impact as necessary to uphold an action with PTSD involved (*Sullivan* v. *Boston Gas Company*, 1993; Sup. Jud. Ct. of Mass.). The introduction of the *Daubert* test for the admissibility of expert evidence, which is discussed below, may have the effect of introducing more objectivity into testimony on PTSD (Newman & Yehuda, 1997). The use of neurochemical and psychophysiological indicators of PTSD may be welcomed in court as providing objective evidence for the existence of the disorder, as well as evidence that symptoms are not malingered. The presence of neurochemical changes associated with PTSD also may satisfy the physical impact or injury requirements of some jurisdictions if such changes could be proved with respect to the individual plaintiff (Pitman, Saunders, & Orr, 1994).

Plaintiffs must prove, on a balance of probabilities, that they have PTSD. Inevitably, this is determined through the testimony of experts. Given the pivotal and critical nature of (1) the requirement of proving PTSD and (2) the necessity of recruiting experts to testify to the diagnosis and presence of PTSD, a brief discussion of the admissibility of expert testimony and evidence is necessary. There are specific legal tests that, depending on the jurisdiction, must be satisfied in order to allow expert testimony into evidence.

Tests for the Admissibility of Expert Evidence and Testimony. In North America, there are essentially three tests by which the potential admissibility of expert evidence will be adjudicated. First, in *Daubert* v. *Merrell Dow Pharmaceuticals* (1993), the United States Supreme Court ruled on the admissibility of expert evidence in jurisdictions that are governed by the Federal Rules of Evidence (FRE).[4] Although *Daubert* is binding in these jurisdictions only, many states have in fact adopted evidence codes that are analogous to the FRE (Goodman-Delahunty, 1997), and hence *Daubert* may have an influence in jurisdictions other than the federal one. The *Daubert* test has important implications for experts who testify about PTSD, and the research findings and assessment practices they rely upon in their testimony. In a case involving PTSD stemming from a MVA, psychological and other health professional testimony was scrutinized with the *Daubert* test (*Miramon* v. *Bradley*, 1997; La. App. 1st Cir.). Citing *Daubert*, the court noted that the "trial judge serves a 'gatekeeping' function to screen and exclude 'invalid' and irrelevant material" (p. 478–9).

The second test, in place in many United States jurisdictions, stems from the 1923 decision of *Frye* v. *United States* (U.S. S.Ct.).[5] This test has sometimes excluded evidence on PTSD (Goodman-Delahunty, 1997). Finally, the Supreme Court of Canada recently spelled out the criteria for the admissibility of expert evidence in R. v. *Mohan* (1994). The enumerated elements for admissibility of expert testimony in Canada are as follows: (1) relevance; (2) qualification of the expert; and, (3) necessity of the evidence.[6]

Causation

It may be proved successfully that (1) a person had a MVA and (2) a person has PTSD. However, recovery will only be permitted where it is proved that the MVA caused the PTSD. How do courts determine that PTSD was caused by a MVA? Causation in both Canada (*Athey* v. *Leonati*, 1996, S.C.C.) and the United States (*Chaney* v. *Smithkline Beckman Corp.*, 1985; U.S. 8th Circuit Ct.) is proved through use of the "but-for" test. This test asks, "but for the negligent act, would the injuries have resulted?" If it can be answered that, on a balance of probabilities, the injury would not have occurred *but for* the negligence of the defendant, then causation is made out. The legal issue in PTSD/MVA cases, then, is whether PTSD would have occurred but for the MVA.

Sometimes the but-for test is not appropriate. Courts have then employed a *material contribution* test. If the MVA can be viewed as a material contribution to the development of PTSD, despite the presence of other causal factors, then causation may be found. It should be pointed out that, at least in Canada, causation need not be proved with a high degree of scientific precision (*Snell* v. *Farrell*, 1990; S.C.C.).

To illustrate, in *Miramon*, the plaintiff suffered two car accidents roughly two years apart. One issue was whether the second accident caused any of the plaintiff's physical and emotional problems, including PTSD. The lower trial court held that it did not, because the second accident could not be isolated as the sole cause of the aggravation of psychological problems. The appellate court held that this was an error. It ruled that tortious conduct need not be the sole causal factor of a plaintiff's injury, as long as it is a "significant contributing factor" (p. 478).

Similarly, in a case in which the plaintiff experienced a very minor MVA and then alleged serious physical and psychological injuries, the court held that the plaintiff's condition would have existed despite the MVA, and that the MVA did not materially contribute to the symptoms (*West* v. *Zehir*, 1997; Alta. Ct. Queen's Bench). In this case, the plaintiff was held to have been exaggerating his symptoms, and this was confirmed in part by the rejection of PTSD by an expert.

In determining issues of causation, courts rely upon the inter-related concepts of *proximity*, *remoteness*, and *foreseeability*. In general, if a putative cause (e.g., MVA) is considered to be too remotely connected to the injury (e.g., PTSD), then it is not considered to be a proximate cause, and causation will not be made out (Epstein, 1995). Again, generally, if an injury is deemed to not have been foreseeable to the defendant, then causation may not be made out.[7] The establishment of proximate cause entails an examination of how far the defendant's liability should extend for the consequences of the negligent act (Epstein, 1995). Generally, the foreseeability of the injury is emphasized in this determination and again is especially suited to MVA-PTSD (Spaulding, 1988).

In the case of *Pokrifchak* v. *Weinstein* (1998; Wash. App. Div.), a woman was involved in a MVA, and suffered serious emotional reactions to the accident, including anxiety and nightmares (although it was not specified whether PTSD was diagnosed). During the course of treatment for her accident-related injuries, she claimed to have recalled that she was sexually abused as a child. She attempted to receive damages not only for the emotional and physical injuries that flowed directly from the MVA, but also for the serious emotional trauma that arose from her recollection of sexual abuse. Under the but-for test, causation for the physical and emotional injuries stemming from the MVA was conceded. The judge, however, held that the MVA was not a proximate cause of the emotional injury stemming from the recollected memories. This injury was considered too remote or far-removed from the putative cause. This case also illustrates the concept of "cause-in-fact," to be determined through use of the but-for test, and "legal cause," which involves policy considerations of proximity and how far the liability of the defendant should extend.

In some cases, there are multiple possible causes of a plaintiff's injuries. This issue is important in terms of both assessment (i.e., to determine which of several possible causes actually led to the development of PTSD) and legal causation. This situation may arise in cases involving a pre-existing condition, or in cases where other traumas may have caused the PTSD (e.g., different MVA; assault; traumatic illness). The presence of multiple possible causes of PTSD will be a major focus of litigation, for it represents to the defence an opportunity to negate liability. As Brown (1996) states, "causation *must* be attacked." (p. 57; emphasis in original).

The Supreme Court of Canada recently visited the issue of multiple causal factors in the case of *Athey* v. *Leonati* (1996), in which a plaintiff with a pre-existing back condition was injured in two successive motor vehicle accidents. He then sustained a disc herniation during a stretching exercise. Applying the but-for causal test discussed above, the Supreme Court held that the proper practice under Canadian law is to determine whether the injury would have occurred "but for" the MVA, despite the presence of other possible causes.

Thin Skulls, Crumbling Skulls, and Eggshell Psyches. The legal constructs of *thin skulls*, *crumbling skulls*, and *eggshell psyches* or personalities all have implications for determining causation. These issues arise when a pre-existing condition of the plaintiff is material to the MVA-related injuries. Where a plaintiff was predisposed to develop some particular injury, but was asymptomatic prior to the accident, the "thin skull" doctrine applies. In short, tortfeasors take their victims as they find them (*Athey* v. *Leonati*, 1996). This doctrine has been expanded to cover predisposition to psychological injury, under the unflattering term of the "eggshell personality" doctrine (*Janiak* v. *Ippolito*, 1985).

Jurisdictions in the United States vary in the degree to which pre-existing sensitivity to emotional injuries precludes a claim for negligent infliction of emotional distress. In Texas, it would appear that courts are willing to compensate persons with "eggshell psyches" (*Padget* v. *Gray*, 1987; Tex. Ct. App.), whereas in other jurisdictions, courts are reluctant to compensate persons who are more than ordinarily sensitive (*Theriault* v. *Swan*, 1987; Maine Sup. Jud. Ct.).

If, on the other hand, a plaintiff was experiencing symptoms that were worsened or aggravated by an accident, the "crumbling skull" doctrine applies. The tortfeasor is still liable for causing the injuries, but a reduction in the award will be made. These doctrines have evolved from the principle that the plaintiff ought to be returned to the position he or she would have been in if the accident had not occurred (Waddams, 1997), and hence the defendant ought not be made to compensate that person as if he or she were in perfect health.

To illustrate some of these concepts dealing with pre-existing conditions and multiple causal factors, we discuss again the case of *Miramon*, a decision of the Louisiana Court of Appeal. Complicating this case was an earlier MVA, in addition to the plaintiff's pre-existing psychological problems. After the first accident, the plaintiff was described as having difficulties with an eating disorder, as well as difficulty managing stress. She sought treatment from a multi-disciplinary team comprised of various health and mental health professionals. The second (less objectively severe) accident occurred in the midst of her treatment program for the first accident. Her treatment team agreed that the second accident led to depression, increased anxiety, fear of driving, and setbacks in treatment progress. Further complicating matters, there were additional stressful events occurring in the plaintiff's life that also affected her psychological health. About a year after the second accident, the plaintiff was diagnosed with PTSD stemming from her involvement in both accidents.

At trial and on appeal, only the second accident was being litigated. Issues included whether the second accident caused an aggravation of the plaintiff's pre-existing psychological problems, whether the second accident was, or was required to be, the sole cause of the plaintiff's injuries, and the damages that the plaintiff was entitled to. The experts were unable to attribute the plaintiff's psychological problems to one or the other accident. The appeal court over-ruled the trial court (which had held that the plaintiff could not recover compensation), and held that "if a defendant's tortious conduct aggravates a pre-existing condition, the defendant is liable to the extent of the aggravation" (p. 478). The subject MVA need not be the sole cause of the aggravation, and the presence of pre-existing psychological weaknesses does not preclude recovery for aggravation of those weaknesses. Other cases have struggled with the issues of pre-existing conditions and multiple causes that manifest themselves in somewhat different form.[8]

Third-Party PTSD. In most cases, plaintiffs who seek damages for PTSD were directly involved in the MVA and also suffered physical injuries. However, there are more legally complex situations in which persons may suffer damages for emotional injuries that arise from the physical injuries *of others*. This is commonly known as the *bystander problem*. If Person A observes Person B get hit by Person C, and A then develops PTSD, can he or she sue C? There are circumstances that would allow for recovery, and there are those that would preclude recovery. A central point of this debate is over the issue of causation.

This area of negligence law has a long and tumultuous history. A cross-sectional representation of this area of law reveals that various legal tests are employed and limiting factors endorsed, depending on the jurisdiction.[9] This issue is illustrated in the California Supreme Court case of *Dillon* v. *Legg* (1968). In *Dillon*, a mother was standing some distance from her daughter, and observed her being run over and killed. The mother was not struck, nor was she in danger. The mother brought an action for emotional or psychological injuries. The Court held for the plaintiff (the mother). In its ruling, the court limited recovery to those who were near the MVA, those who observed it (rather than learning about it later), and to those who were closely related to the primary accident victim.

Subsequent jurisprudence, in both California and other states, has modified this ruling, either tightening or loosening its requirements. There has been a general trend to permit recovery for severe emotional injury in the absence of physical impact (Marrs, 1992). Part of this stems from the recognition by some courts of an increased sophistication of medical and psychological science and research, hence making proof of emotional injury more objective and reliable than in the past (*James* v. *Lieb*, 1985; Neb. S. Ct.). The degree of proximity between the plaintiff and the accident that is alleged to have given rise to the psychological injuries differs by state (American Jurisprudence, 1968/1997b, c, d), with some requiring physical impact, others requiring presence in the "zone of danger," others requiring that the accident is directly witnessed, and finally some requiring a close (familial) relationship to the primary accident victim (e.g., spouse, parent, child, sibling).

Damages

The plaintiff must show actual damages or injuries in order to prove legal liability and be compensated (Epstein, 1995). Many intentional torts, such as battery, are "actionable per se," meaning that injury or damage need not be shown in order to establish a successful tort action (although the quantum of damages obviously would be nominal if there were no or slight injury). Negligence actions are not actionable per se, and require proof of injury or damages.

In negligence cases the basic function of awarding damages is to compensate the victim for his or her injuries. The general theory of damages in tort law is to return the plaintiff from the "injured position" to the "original position," in so far as monetary compensation can accomplish that goal

(Waddams, 1997). Both American and Canadian law recognize various "heads of damage" under which injured parties may recover. Various terminology has been used to categorize the heads of damage, including, but not limited to, compensatory and non-compensatory damages, general and special damages, pecuniary and non-pecuniary damages, punitive damages, and future damages. Although courts in Canada and the United States employ similar terminology with respect to damages, these terms do not always refer to identical concepts. Important differences will be highlighted as necessary.

As both Canadian and American tort systems are based on compensatory models, it is understandable that much of the law of damages for negligence comprises various forms of compensatory damages (as opposed to punitive damages which are intended to "punish" the tortfeasor for outrageous behaviour). A basic distinction within compensatory damages is between *general damages* and *special damages*. In the United States, "special damages" are those damages that arise from the injury, but do so in a manner that is peculiar or special to the case. They reflect natural and actual, though not necessary, results of the case, and may include any economic losses or expenses that have occurred as a result of the accident or that will accrue in the future (Rest. 2d δ671). *General damages* refer to more immediate, direct, and proximate results of the wrongdoing, and may consist of any form of direct economic loss such as medical bills, lost wages, property damage, and so forth (Rest. 2d δ670). *Pecuniary damages*, which can be either general or special, refer to losses that can be estimated financially and compensated with money. Plaintiffs can recover *future damages* for the future effects of an injury, including loss of capacity to work, future pain and suffering, and future medical expenses. In order to grant damages for future pain and suffering, there must be an evidentiary basis for such future pain and suffering. Speculative estimates of future pain and suffering will not attract damage awards (Zitter, 1997). In addition, injured parties can recover damages that are said to be inherent to the injury itself, such as pain and suffering, disabilities, or disfigurements.

In Canadian jurisprudence, valid heads of damages were laid down in the "trilogy" of personal injury cases decided by the Supreme Court of Canada in 1978, and which form the cornerstone of personal injury damage law in Canada (*Andrews* v. *Grand and Toy Alberta Ltd.*, 1978; *Arnold* v. *Teno*, 1978; *Thornton* v. *Prince George Board of Education*, 1978). Generally, in Canada, damages are assessed through comparison to similar cases. *General damages* in Canadian law refer to *non-pecuniary damages* (damages that are not quantifiable), and include pain and suffering (which itself subsumes "lost expectation of life" and "lost enjoyment of life"). *Special damages*, also called *pecuniary damages*, are those that can be quantified, and essentially include out-of-pocket expenses up to the time of trial (such as medical expenses, loss of earning capacity and past wages, and pretrial care). Other heads of damage in Canadian law include *cost of future care*, and *loss of future earning capacity*. As is evident, though there is common terminology between the countries, the meaning of terms differs.

It is not possible to say, in Canada, what a particular injury "is worth." For example, if a plaintiff suffered a fractured leg, a fractured rib, and PTSD in a MVA, the court would generally award one global amount for non-pecuniary loss without division of the amount amongst the injuries.

In all loss of earning capacity cases, the plaintiff must prove there was a "real possibility" of earning a particular income in the future and, due to the accident, the ability to earn that income has been compromised (Arnason, 1994; *Pallos* v. *ICBC*, 1995). A defendant is liable for the full cost of the plaintiff's future care, as well as the full amount of the damage claim, despite the existence of publicly funded health care in Canada. The defendant becomes indebted to the government.

An essential distinction between the countries in terms of the amount of awards for non-pecuniary damages is the ceiling set by the Supreme Court of Canada in the trilogy. With explicit reference to awards in the United States having "soared to dramatically high levels" recently (*Andrews* v. *Grand & Toy*, 1978, p. 261), the Supreme Court of Canada ruled that only in very rare cases should non-pecuniary damages in excess of $100,000 be awarded. In practice, the trilogy set the absolute ceiling for damages for pain and suffering. There is no maximum for any other head of damage. The limit is increased yearly to account for inflation and currently is approximately $275,000 CDN (Kerr, Kurtz, & Olivo, 1997). That amount would be awarded only in the most serious of cases, such as quadriplegia. An "excessive" award by a jury may be set aside by the trial judge or reversed on appeal (Waddams, 1997).

What appears evident is that the law of damages is complex and requires many determinations about the effects of an injury upon a person's life. Experts must estimate, and courts must decide, the extent to which PTSD and other injuries affect all realms of a plaintiff's past, present, and future life in terms of employment, physical and mental well-being, marital and other relationships, and so forth. Courts must decide the amount of monetary compensation that will adequately provide "solace" to plaintiffs for past and future pain and suffering. In terms of the latter, Mr. Justice Spence stated in *Arnold* v. *Teno* (1978; S.C.C.): "There is simply no equation between paralyzed limbs and/or injured brain and dollars. The award is not reparative: there can be no restoration of the lost function" (p. 332).

It does seem certain, however, that each case is very much decided on its own facts, as there are likely unique factual issues that arise in any case (*Joseph* v. *Ford Motor Company* (1986; La. 4th Cir.). This comment would seem to

Table 1. Sample PTSD Cases

American Cases

Chappetta v. *Bowman Transportation, Inc.*, (1982; La. App. 4th Cir.)
Tires of a tractor-trailer truck rolled over the hood and roof of the plaintiff's car. Although suffering no physical injuries at all, the court awarded damages for PTSD in the amount of $1000.

Parrilla-Lopez v. *United States* (1988; Puerto Rico CA1)
Appealed amount of damages for mental anguish stemming from PTSD. $16,500 not considered inadequate.

Koury v. *Lanier Express, Inc.* (1988; La. App. 3rd Cir.)
Woman suffered acute PTSD from MVA, and was deemed incapable of employment. Injury was aggravation of pre-existing psychological problems. $10,000 awarded specifically for PTSD.

Prevost v. *Cowan* (1983; La. App.)
Woman suffered substantial physical injuries, depression, and PTSD. Unable to return to pre-accident level of functioning. $25,000 general damages.

Breisch v. *New York* (1987; SD NY)
Plaintiff sustained serious physical injuries (collapsed lung; broken bone) and PTSD. Had residual pain, but returned to work. Unable to engage in sports as had previously. $100,000 awarded ($25,000 for present pain and suffering, $75,000 for future pain and suffering).

Joseph v. *Ford Motor Co.* (1986; La. App. 4th Cir.)
Man who suffered back injury, PTSD, and depression awarded $350,000 for mental anguish and pain and suffering. This amount was considered the highest reasonable amount for physical pain and suffering and mental anguish. Reduced from $1.7 million, which was considered excessive.

Arnold v. *Eastern Air Lines, Inc.* (1982; CA4 NC)
Man injured in *air* crash. Sustained serious physical injuries (burns and broken bones) as well as PTSD that resulted in total or permanent disability and inability to continue in his business. Awarded $1.14 million.

Kolwe v. *Taylor* (1987; La. App. 1st Cir.)
Husband and wife victims of MVA. Aggravation of pre-existing anxiety and depression from MVA that led to PTSD. Minor physical injuries. $20,000 to husband; $15,000 to wife.

Hawkinson v. *Geyer* (1984; Minn. App.)
Man was pinned against the wall of his house by a car that crashed through his outer wall and into his living room. Bruises, lacerations, strains, and back injury were suffered. Permanent PTSD for which medication was necessary. $72,000.

Weaver v. *Siegling* (1990; La. App. 4th Cir.).
Plaintiff suffered moderate physical injuries (lumbar sprain, lacerations) and PTSD that required treatment for one year. Damages reduced from $150,000 to $100,000 for pain and suffering.

Boudreaux v. *Farmer* (1992; La. App. 1st Cir.)
Plaintiff suffered permanent physical disability (prolapsed disc and subsequent spinal deformation) and PTSD following a MVA. Plaintiff was awarded $350,000 for past and future pain and suffering, and $250,000 for loss of enjoyment of life.

Fairchild v. *United States* (1991; U.S. Dist. Ct.)
A woman was seriously injured in a MVA with a United States cargo truck and brought an action under the Federal Tort Claims Act. In addition to brain injury and episodes of psychosis that were held to have resulted from the MVA, the woman suffered from PTSD. The PTSD contributed to the court's findings that the woman was unable to work in the future. She was awarded approximately $500,000 for loss of future wages, $150,000 for future medical care (including psychotherapy), general damages in the amount of $250,000, and roughly $85,000 for past medical care and lost wages.

Table 1. Continued.

Johnson v. *May* (1992; Ill. App. Ct.)
A man who developed PTSD from MVA was described in evidence as having been previously affectionate and considerate, but had become combative and disagreeable. In this case, the plaintiff was deemed permanently disabled because of his PTSD, which was described as very severe. The trial court granted damages under various heads, but gave no compensation for disability. Noting that other cases that have involved injuries comparable to those of the plaintiff had resulted in damage awards for non-economic losses of half a million dollars, the appeal court over-turned this decision and ordered a new trial for damages.

Canadian Cases

Anson v. *Koroway* (1997; B.C.S.C.)
Chronic PTSD following MVA worse after $4\frac{1}{2}$ years with various treatments; soft tissue injury; unrelenting pain. Damages: Non-pecuniary = \$105,000; Future income = \$586,610; Past income = \$100,222; Past pecuniary = \$46,547; Future care = \$217,845; Tax gross up = \$65,343.13.

Trapasso v. *Hendricks* (1996; B.C.S.C.)
Mild to moderate soft tissue injuries; PTSD with depression; possible post-concussive disorder, obesity and disfiguring stretch marks. Damages: Non-pecuniary = \$25,000; Past income = \$2,381; Future income = \$20,000; Past pecuniary = \$7,212.

Mazzon v. *Pribaz* (1993; B.C.S.C.)
Soft tissue injury to back and neck; lacerations and contusions; PTSD preventing return to work. Damages: Non-pecuniary = \$40,000; Past income = \$40,000; Future income = \$50,000.

Spencer v. *Davey* (1991; B.C.S.C.)
"Moderate whiplash;" PTSD (off work 24 weeks). Damages: Non-pecuniary = \$16,000; Past income = \$7,440.

Battilana v. *Korotana* (1990; B.C.S.C.)
Minor soft tissue injuries; "disabling PTSD" with anxiety, depression, sleeplessness and traffic phobia. Damages: Non-pecuniary = \$25,000; Past income = \$18,990; Future income = \$7,500.

Tully v. *Hassell* (1990; B.C.S.C.)
Soft tissue injury to back and neck, PTSD, depression, anxiety. Damages: Non-pecuniary = \$20,000; Reduction for failure to mitigate.

Lizotte v. *Rowe* (1997; B.C.S.C.)
In an unusual case, the court divided the award of general damages between a soft tissue injury and PTSD. In a total general damages award of \$70,000, the soft tissue injury was awarded \$50,000, while the PTSD was awarded \$20,000.

Rimmer v. *Alberta* (1996; Alta. Q.B.)
Court of Queen's Bench reviewed the case law on PTSD in terms of quantum of damages. The judge decided that, generally, the range of damages for PTSD is \$20,000 to \$30,000.

apply not only to damages, but also to other important issues such as causation and proof of PTSD. Because a single case usually has to deal with multiple heads of damages, it would be inefficient to discuss PTSD/MVA cases under each of the above-described areas of damages law, because each case may arise under numerous heads of damage. Rather, we provide in Table 1 a sample of relevant cases. This list is by no means exhaustive. Each case may include various issues.

Conclusion

Psychological or emotional injuries have a tumultuous history in tort law. Despite early skepticism by courts about the utility, veracity, and compensability of such injuries, contemporary jurisprudence permits recovery for certain types of psychological injuries, such as PTSD. Generally, compensation for MVA-PTSD is more straightforward and subject to fewer restrictions if a person was the primary victim of a MVA, rather than a third-party observer.

To receive compensation for MVA-PTSD, plaintiffs must prove, on a balance of probabilities, the elements of negligence. These include duty of care, standard of care, breach of duty of care, injury, causation of injury, and damages. The requirement of proof of PTSD often involves the testimony of expert mental health professionals. Depending on jurisdiction, this testimony and evidence is subject to the *Daubert* test, *Frye* test, or *Mohan* test. To prove that a MVA caused PTSD, the "but-for" or "material contribution" tests are used. These require the determination that the PTSD would not have developed but for the MVA, or that the MVA materially contributed to the PTSD. An important and complex issue arises when there are multiple possible causes of the PTSD, including other MVAs, stressors, or pre-existing psychological conditions. In such situations, it need not be established that the MVA was the sole cause of the PTSD. The concepts of thin skulls, crumbling skulls, and eggshell personalities or psyches are relevant to the issue of multiple causes.

Once it has been established that PTSD was caused by the MVA, compensation must be claimed under certain heads of damage. Of main relevance are compensatory damages, which themselves are divided into many sub-groups. Under these heads of damage plaintiffs with PTSD can recover for, among other things, past and future loss of earning capacity, past and future medical and other care costs, as well as past and future pain and suffering. Awards have ranged from $1,000 to half a million dollars for cases involving MVA-induced PTSD, depending on co-occurring physical injuries, the severity of injury, and the precise losses.

References

American Jurisprudence. (1968/1997a). Fright, shock, and mental disturbance, 38, s. 24.
American Jurisprudence. (1968/1997a). Fright, shock, and mental disturbance, 38, s. 36.
American Jurisprudence. (1968/1997a). Fright, shock, and mental disturbance, 38, s. 27.
American Jurisprudence. (1968/1997a). Fright, shock, and mental disturbance, 38, s. 25.
American Psychiatric Association. (1994). *Diagnostic and statistical manual of mental disorders* (4th ed.). Washington, DC: American Psychiatric Association.
Andrews v. *Grand and Toy Alberta, Ltd.*, 2 S.C.R. 229, 83 D.L.R. 3d 452 (1978).
Anson v. *Karoway*, [unreported], B.C.J. 2913, Vancouver Registry No. C932079 (B.C.S.C. December 31, 1997).
Arnason, T. B. (1994). Assessment of damages. In *Motor Vehicle Accident and Personal Injury Claims for Legal Assistants.* Vancouver, BC: Continuing Legal Education Society.
Arnold v. *Eastern Air Lines, Inc.*, 681 F.2d 186 (CA4 NC 1982)
Arnold v. *Teno,* 2 S.C.R. 297, 83 D.L.R. 3d 609 (1978).
Athey v. *Leonati*, 3 S.C.R. 458 (1996).
Battilana v. *Korotana*, [unreported], B.C.J. 1347, Vancouver Registry No. B884359 (B.C.S.C. June 12, 1990).
Boudreaux v. *Farmer,* 604 So.2d 641 (La. App. 1st Cir. 1992).
Breisch v. *New York*, 1987 WL 9443 (SD NY 1987).
Brown v. *Kendall,* 60 Mass. 292 (1850).
Brown, J. T. (1996). Avoiding litigation neurosis: A practitioner's guide to defending post traumatic stress disorder claims. *American Journal of Trial Advocacy, 20*, 29–41.
Chaney v. *Smithkline Beckman Corp.*, 764 F.2d 527 (8th Cir. 1985).
Chappetta v. *Bowman Transportation, Inc.*, 415 So.2d 1019 (La. App. 4th Cir. 1982).
Daubert v. *Merrell Dow Pharmaceuticals, Inc.*, 113 S.Ct. 2786 (1993).
Dillon v. *Legg*, 68 Cal.2d 728 (1968).
Donoghue v. *Stevenson, A.C.* 562 (HL 1932).
Epstein, R. A. (1995). Cases and material on torts. New York: Little, Brown, and Company.
Fairchild v. *United States of America*, 769 F.Supp. 964 (U.S. Dist. Ct. 1991).
Fecteau, G. W. (1999). *Treatment of Post-Traumatic Stress Reactions to Traffic Accidents.* Doctoral Dissertation, University of New Brunswick.
Frye v. *United States*, 293 F.Supp. 1013 (D.C. Cir. 1923).
Goodman-Delahunty, J. (1997). Forensic psychological expertise in the wake of Daubert. *Law and Human Behavior, 21*, 121–140.
Granowitz v. *Vanwickle*, 264 N. J.Super. 440, 624 A.2d 1047 (1983).
Hawkinson v. *Geyer*, 352 NW.2d 784 (Minn. App. 1984).
James v. *Lieb*, 375 N.W.2d 109 (Neb. S.Ct. 1985).
Janiak v. *Ippolito,* 1 S.C.R. 146 (1985).
Johnson v. *May,* 585 N.E.2d 224 (Ill. App. Ct. 1992)
Joseph v. *Ford Motor Co.*, 499 So.2d 428 (La. App. 4th Cir. 1986).
Kerr, M., Kurtz, J., & Olivo, L.M. (1997). *Canadian Tort Law in a Nutshell.* Toronto, Ont.: Carswell.
Klar, L. N. (1996). *Tort law* (2nd ed.). Scarborough, Ont.: Carswell.
Kolwe v. *Taylor*, 517 So.2d 236 (La. App. 1st Cir. 1987)
Koury v. *Lanier Express, Inc.*, 528 So.2d 734 (La. App. 3rd Cir. 1988).
Linden, A. M. (1997). *Canadian tort law* (6th ed.). Vancouver: Butterworths.

Lindsey, R. B. & Mussio, W. D. (1997). Athey and causation: Has the law changed perspective? In *Personal injury damages 1997 Update*. Vancouver, BC: Continuing Legal Education Society.

Lizotte v. *Rowe*, 32 B.C.L.R. 3d 192 (B.C.S.C. 1997).

Marrs, S. D. (1992). Mind over body: Trends regarding the physical injury requirement in negligent infliction of emotional distress and "fear of disease" cases. *Tort and Insurance Law Journal*, *28*, 1–39.

Mazzagatti v. *Everingham*, 512 Pa. 266, 516 A. 2d 672 (1986).

Mazzon v. *Pribaz*, [unreported], B.C.J. 2436, Vancouver Registry No. B913657 (B.C.S.C. November 26, 1993).

Miramon v. *Bradley*, 701 So.2d 475 (La. App. 1st Cir. 1997).

Newman, R. L., & Yehuda, R. (1997). PTSD in civil litigation: Recent scientific and legal developments. *Jurimetrics*, *37*, 257–267.

Padget v. *Gray*, 727 S.W.2d 706 (Tex. Ct. App. 1987).

Pallos v. *I.C.B.C.*, 100 B.C.L.R. 2d 260 (B.C.C.A. 1995).

Parrilla-Lopez v. *United States*, 841 F.2d. 16 (CA1 Puerto Rico 1988).

Pitman, R. K., Saunders, L. S., & Orr, S. P. (1994). Psychophysiologic testing for post-traumatic stress disorder. *Trial, 30* (4), 22–26.

Pitman, R. K. & Sparr, L. F. (1998). PTSD and the law. *PTSD Research Quarterly*, *9*, 1–8.

Pitman, R. K., Sparr, L. F., Saunders, L. S. & McFarlane, A. C. (1996). Legal issues in posttraumatic stress disorder. In B. A. van der Kolk, A. McFarlane, & L. Weisaeth (Eds.), *Traumatic stress: The effects of overwhelming experience on mind, body, and society* (pp. 378–397). New York: Guilford Press.

Pokrifchak v. *Weinstein*, 1998 W. L. 303732 (Wash. App. Div. 3 1998).

Prevost v. *Cowan*, 431 So.2d 1063 (La. App. 1983).

Quaglio v. *Tomaselli*, 99 A.D.2d 487, 470 N.Y.S.2d 427 (1984).

R. v. *Mohan*, 114 D.L.R. 4th 419 (S.C.C. 1994).

Raifman, L. J. (1983). Problems of diagnosis and legal causation in courtroom use of post-traumatic stress disorder. *Behavioral Sciences and the Law*, *1*, 115–130.

Restatement (Second) of Torts (1979). The American Law Institute: New York.

Rimmer v. *Alberta* (Motor Vehicle Accident Claims Act, administrator), [unreported] Alta. J. 250, Action No. 9203 05534 (Alta. Ct. Q.B. March 14, 1996).

Romeo, L. M. (1997). A case-by-case analysis: Connecticut adopts the foreseeability test for bystander emotional distress in Clohessy v. Bachelor. *Connecticut Law Review*, *30*, 325–341.

Slovenko, R. (1994). Legal aspects of post-traumatic stress disorder. *Psychiatric Clinics of North America*, *17*, 439–446.

Spencer v. *Davey*, [unreported], B.C.J. 2402, Vancouver Registry No. B900925 (B.C.S.C. July 22, 1991).

Snell v. *Farrell*, 2 S.C.R. 311 (1990).

Spaulding, W. J. (1988). Compensation for mental disability. In R. Michels (Ed.), *Psychiatry* (Vol. 3, pp. 1–27). Philadelphia: J.B. Lippincott.

Strain v. *Donesky*, [unreported] B.C.J. 350, New Westminster Registry C871072 (B.C.S.C. February 15, 1991).

Sullivan v. *Boston Gas Co.*, 605 N.E.2d 805 (Mass. Sup. Jud. Ct. 1993).

Theriault v. *Swan*, 558 A.2d 369 (Me. 1989).

Thornton v. *Prince George Board of Education*, 2 S.C.R. 267, 83 D.L.R. (3d) 480 (1978).

Trappaso (Guardian ad litem of) v. *Hendricks*, [unreported], B.C.J. 3160, Vancouver Registry No. B943944 (B.C.S.C. October 28, 1996).

Tully v. *Hassell*, [unreported], B.C.J. 550, Vancouver Registry No. B884083 (B.C.S.C. March 9, 1990).

Waddams, S. M. (1997). The Law of Damages (3rd ed.). Toronto, Ont: Canada Law Book.

Ward v. *West Jersey & Seashore Railroad.* 65 N.J.L. 383, 47 A. 561 (N.J. 1900).

Weaver v. *Siegling*, 569 So.2d 97 (La. App. 4th Cir. 1990).

West v. *Zehir*, [unreported] Alta. J. 818, Action No. 9001–14124 (Alta. Ct. Q.B. August 11, 1997).

Zitter, J. M. (1997). Excessiveness or adequacy of damages awarded for injuries causing mental or psychological damages. *American Law Reports (5th), 52*, 1 151.

Endnotes

1 Some MVA/PTSD cases could be covered under other legal frameworks, such as Workers Compensation.

2 In a quote commonly referred to as "Lord Atkin's famous neighbour principle," the House of Lords held as follows:

> You must take reasonable care to avoid acts or omissions which you can reasonably foresee would be likely to injure your neighbour. Who, then, in law is my neighbour? The answer seems to be persons who are so closely and directly affected by my act that I ought reasonably to have them in contemplation as being so affected when I am directing my mind to the acts or omissions which are called in question (p. 580).

3 It should be pointed out here that the term "damages" is often used in two ways. First, it may refer to the injuries sustained by a plaintiff. That is its use in the present section. Second, it may refer to concept of financial compensation, whereby persons are awarded "damages" for their injuries. A fuller discussion of this area of law is covered later in the chapter.

4 The basic elements of the *Daubert* test are *reliability*, *relevance*, and *legal sufficiency* of evidence. Together, these elements focus legal attention on the *quality of scientific evidence* (e.g., testable theoretical basis; peer-reviewed publication of data; acceptability of the assessment or research procedure in the field), the *relevance of testimony* (e.g., will admission of the evidence make a fact in issue more or less probable?), and the *legal sufficiency of expert evidence* (e.g., is the evidence more probative than prejudicial, as per FRE 403?).

5 This test, known as the "general acceptance" test, requires that scientific evidence or testimony be generally accepted in the particular field.

6 Under this test, expert testimony is admissible only when it makes the proof of some fact more or less probable, when the testimony is more probative than prejudicial, when the proposed expert has advanced or specialized knowledge in the field, and his or her testimony rests on an established body of knowledge. As well, the testimony must be necessary to assist the trier of fact, in that it must relate to issues that are beyond the understanding of the average layperson.

7 There is some controversy over this latter point, however, especially in regard to cases involving emotional injuries. Some authorities have held that a certain type of injury (i.e., psychological damage) need not be foreseeable to the defendant, as long as the negligent act remains the proximate cause of the injury (American Jurisprudence, 1968/1997a).

[8] In *Koury*, for example, the court held that the plaintiff's PTSD was caused by the MVA she had suffered, despite the fact that she had suffered a great many traumas in her life, including physical abuse, repeated sexual abuse, rape, the witness of a murder, and a miscarriage-inducing beating at the hands of her partner. In a different vein, the court in *West* accepted expert evidence that the plaintiff did not have PTSD, but rather had antisocial personality disorder (APD), and that this pre-existing psychological condition was consistent with the defence's argument that the plaintiff was exaggerating his difficulties. Finally, in *Strain* v. *Donesky* (191; B.C.S.C.), the judge, although accepting the "psychological thin skull' principle, also was of the view that the plaintiff's pre-existing anxious personality led him to establish his psychological difficulties (including PTSD). Although the MVA caused the PTSD, the pre-existing personality condition decreased damages.

[9] Jurisdictions in the United States subscribe to one of four tests: (1)The traditional rule that requires physical contact or injury for the recovery of an emotional injury (e.g., *Ward* v. *West Jersey & Seashore Railroad*, 1900); (2) A zone of danger rule that allows for recovery of emotional injuries without physical contact if the plaintiff is threatened with physical harm when witnessing harm to another (Rest. 2d δ313, δ436); (3) The bystander proximity rule allows for recovery if the plaintiff is not in the zone of danger if the plaintiff is physically near the scene of the accident, personally observes the accident, and is closely related to the victim (Rest. 2d. δ436); (4) Full recovery is allowed in instances in which a reasonable person would not have been able to cope with the emotional injury caused by the negligent circumstances. (Brown, 1996).

19

The Forensic Value of Psychophysiological Measures of Post-Traumatic Stress Disorder

LEIGH NEAL MRCPsych. MRCGP. DRCOG. Consultant Psychiatrist,
NICHOLAS HILL MRCPsych. Consultant Psychiatrist,
CHRISTOPHER FOX BSc. MRCPsych. Specialist Registrar

Psychological Injuries Unit, Duchess of Kent's Hospital, North Yorkshire, UK.

DAVID WATSON BSc.

Medeci Developments Ltd, 7 Southdown Road, Harpenden, Bedfordshire, UK.

Introduction

Biological tests hold the prospect of strengthening the forensic value of Post-Traumatic Stress Disorder (PTSD) by offering a more objective assessment for cases that find their way into the court room. Psychometric tests alone, reliant upon subjective evaluation, offer little protection against the mis-reporting of symptoms (Lees-Haley, 1990 and Perconte & Goreczny, 1990). The results from physiological tests may provide evidence helping to establish or refute the presence of the PTSD arousal criteria, as well as aiding the psychiatric expert in estimating the probability of the presence of PTSD in a given claimant (Pitman & Orr, 1993). Tests which have been assessed with this purpose in mind include measures of: brain electrical activity (Event Related Potentials), neuroendocrine hormone levels (noradrenaline and cortisol) and changes in electrodermal activity, muscle tension, heart rate and blood pressure.

There have been a number of studies of the diagnostic utility of Event Related Potentials (ERPs) in PTSD. Patients are presented with a stimulus such as a sound or a picture and the changes in the electrical activity over specified areas of the brain are recorded with electrodes during the milliseconds following the stimulus. Paige et al (1990) recorded ERPs 200 milliseconds after repeated presentation of a sound to 18 Vietnam veterans. Most of the veterans with PTSD showed a reduction in response as the sound was increased in intensity. With this method, 78% of the patients were correctly classified into those with and without PTSD and 17% were falsely classified as having PTSD. Attias et al (1996) measured ERPs in 40 Israeli combat veterans. These veterans were shown combat pictures and their ERPs were measured 300 milliseconds after presentation of the pictures. This method correctly classified 80% of the patients into those with and without PTSD and falsely classified 10% as having PTSD. However, a study by Metzger et al (1997) has indicated that the difference found in ERP responses between PTSD and non-PTSD patients may be better accounted for by co-existing symptoms of depression and anxiety rather than PTSD. As a forensic test in PTSD, ERP measurement is limited by the complexity of both the procedure and the interpretation of the waveforms.

The hypothalamus and other areas of the brain involved with emotional processing regulate the release of neuroendocrine hormones such as noradrenaline and cortisol. The levels of noradrenaline and cortisol can be measured in urine samples collected over a 24-hour period. A 24 hour urinary noraderenaline:cortisol (N:C) ratio measured in this way may be discriminatory in diagnosing PTSD. A study by Mason et al (1988) analysing the N:C ratio in PTSD patients in comparison to patients with other psychiatric disorders, correctly classified 86% into those with and without PTSD and falsely classified 11% as having PTSD. However, a subsequent study was unable to replicate these promising results (Pitman & Orr, 1990), but this may have been due to differences in the collection procedure. This technique requires further validation and replication before it could be accepted for forensic purposes. It is also limited by the complexity of the collection method which is critical to the correct measurement of the ratio.

Investigations of the activity of the peripheral nervous system in PTSD patients may show more promise for the development of measures with forensic utility. Friedman (199I) described physiological reactivity as "*the best and most specific biological diagnostic test for PTSD"* and Blanchard et al. (1991) described phasic arousal as one of the most *"robust features of PTSD"*. The main focus of enquiry has been the measurement of the DSM (American psychiatric Association, 1987, 1994), PTSD diagnostic criterion of *"physiological reactivity on exposure to reminders of the trauma"*. Physiological reactivity has been measured in terms of heart rate, blood pressure, muscle tension and electrodermal activity. Studies in combat veterans with PTSD (Pallmeyer et al, 1986; Orr, 1990, 1994; Pitman et al, 1990; Orr et al, 1993) have consistently found heightened physiological reactivity to combat related audiovisual and imaginal stimuli. Blanchard et al (1991) and Shalev et al (1993) have found similar results in non-combat related PTSD. However, the observation that different physiological measures are seldom highly correlated (Lacey 1959, 1967; Ohman 1987; Turpin 1990) reduces the possibility that any given psychophysiological measure is a definitive diagnostic tool. Lacey (1959) illustrates the fractionation of these measures by reviewing evidence that when subjects perform a task requiring them to attend to environmental stimuli, for example monitoring flashing lights, heart rate decreases whereas electrodermal activity increases.

Combinations of tests of physiological reactivity have been used to discriminate between veterans with PTSD and those without PTSD. The diagnostic accuracy of these combined tests has ranged from 75%–95% (Keane & Kaloupek, 1998), with incorrect classification of 0%–20% patients as having PTSD (Orr & Kaloupek, 1997). Of the available physiological parameters, electrodermal activity has been identified as one of the least susceptible to conscious manipulation (Orr & Pitman, 1993).

Biological tests of physiological reactivity on exposure to reminders of the trauma may have the potential for the forensic evaluation of this DSM criterion in PTSD. They are non-invasive, safe, can be conducted on outpatients, show some evidence of reliability, have been replicated and are not easy to fake. So far these experiments have mostly been limited to environmentally controlled laboratories with Vietnam veterans.

We describe an evaluation of the forensic utility of a non-laboratory measure of physiological reactivity in trauma patients during provocation with script driven imagery. This is based on the assessment of new technology applied to the assessment of Skin Resistance Response (SSR) in PTSD, which may confer technical and practical advantages over previous methods.

Data are presented from a prospective study of cases referred for assessment at the UK Defence Services Psychological Injuries Unit. Test validity and re-test reliability are examined, as well as the influence of variations in temperature and humidity.

The Measurement of Skin Resistance Response

Whilst skin conductance has been adopted as a standard in the measurement of electrodermal activity, the choice between units of conductance or resistance for exosomatic electrodermal activity appears largely academic, with insufficient empirical evidence favouring one over the other (Bouscein, 1992). Therefore, the measure of resistance used in this study, is scientifically supportable. Whereas the reciprocal of skin resistance level (SRL) approximates closely to skin conductance level (SCL), the same is not true of SRR and skin conductance response (SCR).

SRR was measured with Ultramind's Relaxplus Professional System (Ultramind Ltd., 1993). The RelaxPlus system comprises a sensor with an infrared biotelemetry transmitter, and a remote infrared receiver which communicates with computer software. The system employs changes in skin resistance to control the visual output of a personal computer (PC). If incorporating a lap-top PC, the apparatus is sufficiently compact to fit into a briefcase and is thus readily portable.

Direct current is applied through 12mm diameter, stainless steel, dry contact electrodes to cleansed skin. Skin resistance measurements with dry contact electrodes strongly correlate with changes in sweat gland activity (Thomas & Korr, 1957). Electrodes are attached with velcro fasteners to the volar aspect of the distal phalanges of the middle and index fingers of the left hand. Resistance values are measured through resistive source circuitry contained within matchbox-sized housing. The circuitry utilizes a 0 – 2 imposed voltage to yield a near logarithmic output ideal for highly accurate telemetry and a wide range of parametric discrimination. Skin resistance is sampled ten times per second. Signal post-processing converts the relatively wide physiological range of resistance values to those that can be transmitted within an infrared bandwidth. Physical separation of the subject from the computer is achieved through the use of an infrared communications system: an output pulse representing skin resistance value activates a transistor driver in the transmitter, which feeds infrared emitting diodes. The receiver is mounted in a small plastic box adjacent to the PC. Pulses of infrared radiation emitted by the transmitter are detected by a reverse biased large area PIN photoelectrode. Photocurrent from the detector diode is fed to the input of an infrared pre-amplifier integrated circuit, which incorporates a pass-band designed to reject signals from all other infrared sources (e.g. sunlight or lighting fixtures). Logarithmically compressed data is then passed via the serial port into the PC. The micro-controller operating program incorporates measures designed to maintain low noise levels despite subject movement. The software then utilizes the modified pulses to generate a smooth, real time, graphical representation of skin resistance a visual analogue of one parameter of arousal.

Procedure

The study sample comprised consecutive serving and ex-Service personnel, with a history of traumatic experience, referred from primary care for evaluation at the Defence Medical Services PTSD Unit. One investigator (LAN) conducted preliminary screening interviews, formulating Axis I diagnoses according to DSM-III-R criteria.

Initial screening excluded subjects taking psychotropic or other medication with potentially confounding autonomic effects. Subjects reporting the use of non-prescribed substances, other than alcohol, within the last two months were excluded from the trial. Subjects with alcohol dependence were also excluded.

The presence or otherwise of PTSD was assessed using the Structured Clinical Interview for DSM-III-R (SCID) PTSD module (Spitzer et al, 1989). Subjects were further assessed with the Impact of Event Scale (IES) (Horowitz et al, 1979), a self report measure with a total scale range of 0–75 comprising subscales measuring the severity of symptoms of Intrusion (range 0–35), and Avoidance (range 0–40). The IES has been validated in a similar mixed group of combat veterans and civilians (Neal et al, 1994).

A sub-sample of consecutive subjects with SCID diagnosed PTSD was subject to a short interval (1 hour) test-retest reliability study. The influence of temperature and humidity on SRR was also assessed in this sample during the first of these tests.

Provocation testing utilizes a modification of the technique of script driven imagery, originally defined by Lang (1985) and first applied to PTSD by Pitman et al (1987). Under the guidance of a specifically trained Registered Mental Nurse a subject prepares three, thirty second scripts. The scripts detail 3 events: the traumatic event, a self-selected happy event, an event with neutral emotional associations and they are presented in the second person present tense. The subject is informed that scripts will be read aloud by the investigator in random order. He (she) is instructed to attempt to re-live the content of each script in imagination, and stay with any emotions generated for 30 secs after the script has ended (thus "re-living" for one minute). In practice, only the neutral and traumatic scripts are presented, and the ordering is always neutral script followed by traumatic script. Such ordering ensures standardization between patients, and within an individual across time. The role of the "happy" script is to represent a theoretical third option that preserves uncertainty about the identity of the second script until reading.

The subject is seated in a sound attenuated room in which temperature and humidity are monitored with an independent ETI 8703 thermo-hygrometer (ETI Ltd.). Electrodes are attached. Following orientation and adaptation to the setting, the subject receives guided relaxation. Resistance measurements commence 3 minutes before the end of the initial relaxation period. After the initial relaxation the investigator reads out the neutral script. There follows a second, 3 minute period of guided relaxation, following which the traumatic script is presented. Resistance recording is terminated 30 seconds after completion of the traumatic script.

The 3 minute inter-trial period has a precedent in the study of Pitman et al (1987), and in pilot studies we found this sufficient to allow return of skin resistance to within 5% of pre-stimulus baseline following neutral script exposure. In contrast, pilot studies measuring the duration of persisting arousal following exposure to the traumatic script found that subjects remained symptomatic for up to 30 minutes.

Measurements are taken from the continuous computer graphical representation of changing SR, at the lowest recorded reading for each script's 1 minute imagery period. Pilot studies found a closer correlation between the Intrusion sub-scale of the IES and SRR with this method than when SR measurements were averaged during the imagery periods. This is a unique advantage of this technology. Values are converted to actual resistance in kilo-Ohm (kΩ). The difference between the resistance of the two scripts has face validity as representing the magnitude of SRR attributable to imaginal re-exposure to the traumatic event.

Analysis

Significant positive skew was corrected with a log transformation of the SRR variables resulting in near normal distribution of all data. Pearson's Product Moment Correlation Coefficient and Spearman's Rho were used to calculate bivariate correlations for normally and non-normally distributed data. The Kappa coefficient (Cohen, 1960) was used as a measure of chance corrected agreement.

Results

Sixty six subjects were assessed for the study and following application of the exclusion criteria, 55 subjects remained. The subjects comprised 53 (98%) males, 44 (80%) were currently in Service and 11 (20%) were ex-Service. The age range was 19 to 58 years; mean age was 31.9 years with a standard deviation of 9.5. Traumas were discreet events from both military and non-military situations, and are summarized in Table 1.

Table 1. Distribution of traumatic experiences (N = 55)

Category	N (%)
Combat related	41 (74)
Assault (sexual, physical)	7 (13)
Accident	7 (13)

Table 2. Distribution of IES scores and Skin Resistance Response (SRR), (N = 55)

Measure	Range	Mean (S.D.)
IES (Total)	0, +71	+38.09 (24.43)
IES (Intrusion)	0, +36	+19.56 (12.36)
IES (Avoidance)	0, +38	+18.51 (12.91)
SRR (kΩ)	−10, +332	+25.81 (56.46)

Using the SCID, 35 subjects (64%) met DSM-III-R criteria for PTSD. Clinical interview identified 28 subjects (51%) fulfilling DSM-III-R criteria for current major depressive disorder, and 8 subjects (15%) with DSM-III-R panic disorder. No other DSM-III-R Axis I disorders were detected.

Table 2 illustrates the means, standard deviations and ranges of the SRR and IES scores for the 55 subjects.

Table 3 presents the means, standard deviations and ranges of temperature, humidity and SRR for the subgroup of 16 patients subject to test re-retest analysis.

Individual SRR scores for subjects with and without PTSD are illustrated in Figure 1. The maximum Kappa coefficient of reliability is obtained with an SRR cut-off score set at 25/26 kΩ (Kappa = 0.20), (95% C.I. 0.06,0.34) ($p < 0.05$). This give a diagnostic hit rate of 52%, a specificity of 100% (95% CI 87,100) and a sensitivity of 26% (95% C.I. 15,37).

SRR values demonstrated a significant positive skew (skew = 3.90). Following the elimination of negative SRR scores by adding a constant (+20) to all SRR scores, log transformations of SRR values were computed, the transformed values approximating to a normal distribution (skew = 1.62). Bivariate correlations (Pearson's Product Moment) were calculated between the SRR and IES (total) ($r = 0.43$; 95% C.I. 0.19, 0.62; $p < 0.01$); the SRR and the IES Avoidance sub-scale ($r = 0.35$; 95% C.I. 0.09, 0.56;

Table 3. Age, humidity, temperature and Skin Resistance Response (SRR) at times 1 and 2, (N = 20).

	Range	Mean (S.D.)
Age (years)	19.0, 58.0	31.9 (9.5)
Humidity ^{1}(% sat)	24.5, 48.6	38.2 (7.8)
Temperature ^{1} (°C)	19.0, 27.0	23.5 (2.1)
SRR^1 (kΩ)	4.0, 332.0	61.7 (93.1)
SRR^2 (kΩ)	4.0, 283.0	54.3 (79.3)

^{1}Time 1
^{2}Time 2 (Test retest interval = 1 hour)

$p < 0.01$); and the SRR and the IES Intrusion sub-scale ($r = 0.47$; 95% C.I. 0.23, 0.65; $p < 0.001$) (Figure 2). The adjusted shared variance between SRR and the IES Intrusion sub-scale was 20%.

Short interval (one hour) test re-test reliability analysis (Pearson's r) on a sub-sample of 20 patients with PTSD was conducted after log transformation of all SRR results to reduce positive skew [$r = 0.73$; (95% C.I. 0.42, 0.87); $p < 0.001$].

Temperature and humidity were non-normally distributed. In the same sub-sample of 20 subjects, the rank order correlation coefficient (Spearman's rho) between temperature and SRR $= -0.18$, $p = 0.44$ and between humidity and SRR $= 0.03$, $p = 0.91$; indicating no significant association between temperature, humidity and SRR across the measured ranges (Table 3).

Discussion

This study aimed to evaluate the application of new technology to the quantification of SRR on imaginal exposure to a traumatic event as a tool for forensic evaluation.

The apparatus employed conferred a number of advantages over traditional technology. These include ready portability; reliability in the clinic environment and the generation of a clean curve (representative of SRR) negating the need to rely upon mean scores taken across specified time fields.

The optimum cut-off SRR determined in this study (25/26 kΩ) gave a PTSD diagnostic "hit rate" of 52% and a Kappa coefficient of agreement of 0.20. Which is classed as poor agreement. However, an SRR above 25 kΩ did not give any false positive diagnoses of PTSD (specificity = 100%). This indicates that a positive result with this test provides a strong indication that

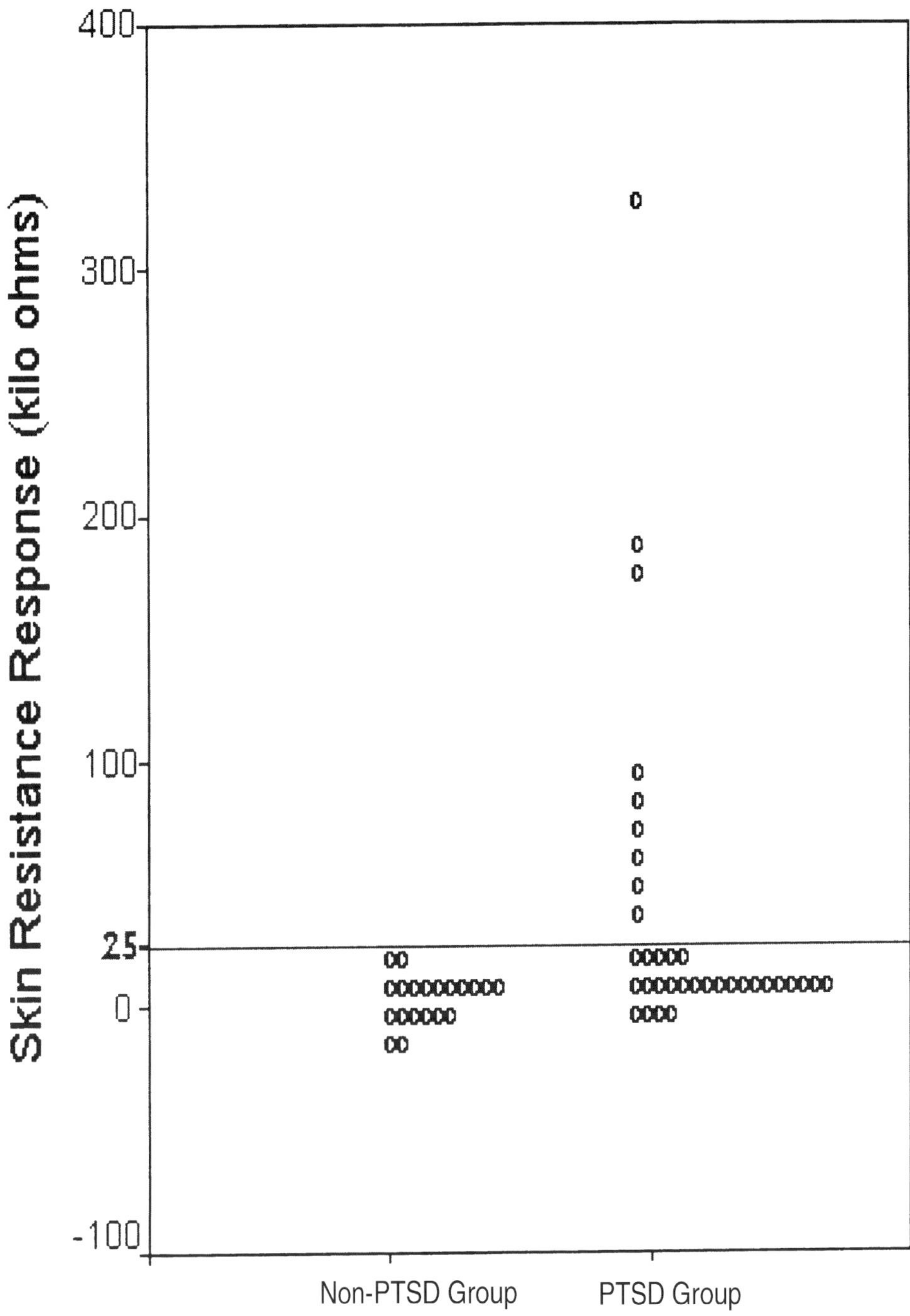

Figure 1. Dotplot of SRR against subjects with PTSD and subjects without PTSD.

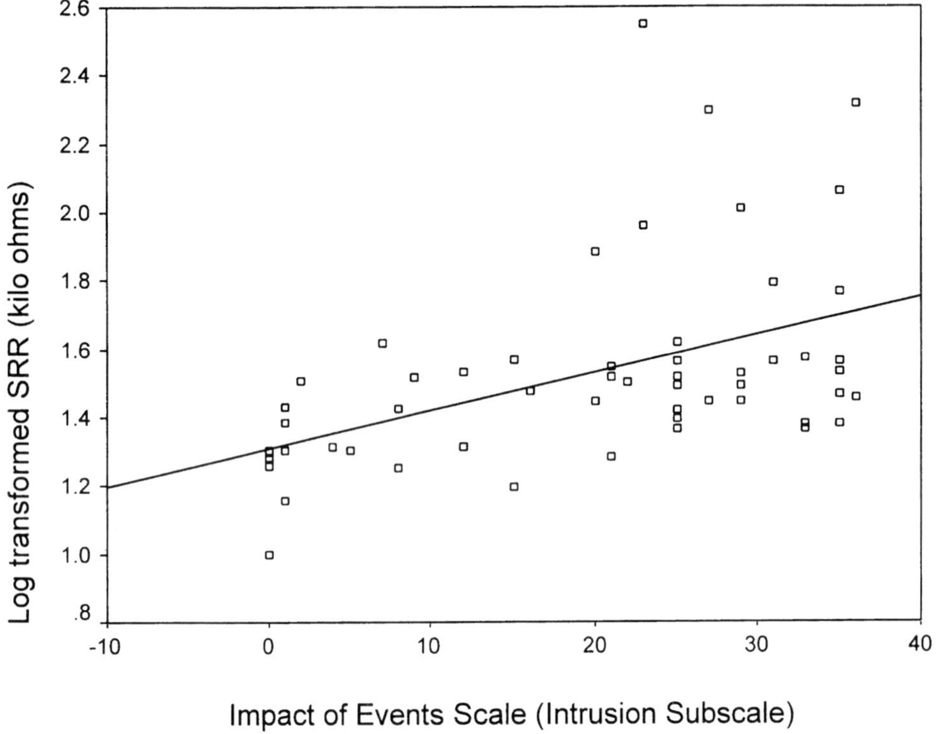

Figure 2. Scattergram of Log transformed skin resistance response and the Intrusion subscale of the IES in 55 subjects presenting with psychological reactions to trauma.

PTSD is present. An SRR of above 25 kΩ may also mark the point at which SRR becomes characteristic of those PTSD patients suffering from significant physiological reactivity.

The finding of significant shared variance (20%) between SRR on script provocation, and the Intrusion sub-scale of the IES, supports the concurrent validity of this method as one measure of some of the variance in symptoms of intrusion (re-experiencing) in PTSD.

The interpretation of this test for clinical practice must be carefully based on the demonstrable test properties in relation to PTSD. A positive result (> 25 kΩ) is strongly indicative of PTSD, but a negative result (< 26 kΩ) gives no indication of whether the patient has PTSD or not. Although the level of SRR is related to the severity of PTSD, 80% of the variance in the severity of PTSD is accounted for by other factors and so it is not particularly useful as a severity measure in practice.

It is traditional for electrodermal studies in PTSD to control environmental temperature and humidity within laboratory conditions. However, literature on the effects of temperature and humidity on SRR is sparse and inconclusive (Bouscein, 1992). Our results fail to lend empirical support to the hypothesis that SRR results are significantly affected by these environmental influences within the ranges encountered in our study; although the sample size was small and this finding may thus represent a type II error.

The results suggest adequate test-retest reliability (r = 0.73). This finding requires replication with a larger sample size.

The study did not control for order effects in script presentation. However, the long duration of SRR in some subjects following traumatic script exposure, evident in our pilot studies, precluded a paradigm dependent upon a prompt return of SRR to baseline levels.

It has been shown that the menstrual cycle may contribute to gender differences in electrodermal activity (Edelberg, 1972). The population from which our sample was drawn led to an under-representation of females and therefore this limits generalisation of the results to other populations.

The test re-test interval employed was shorter than described in most psychometric studies of test re-test reliability. However, the practice and memory effects that confound short interval psychometric studies of test re-test reliability are less important in this test. Inter-rater reliability studies would be of relevance, although the audio scripts have the potential to be standardized as digitized speech.

Put in perspective, this test quantifies only one parameter of physiological reactivity and enhanced arousal upon exposure to reminders of trauma which is neither necessary nor sufficient to qualify for the diagnosis of PTSD; its measurement can do little more than help quantify a single DSM criterion of PTSD. The quantification of global physiological reactivity requires a synthesis of different measurement parameters (e.g. heart rate, muscle tension and blood pressure) and this has most utility in a multi-method assessment of PTSD, relying upon converging evidence from different measurement sources (Malloy et al, 1983).

If tests measuring physiological changes in PTSD are to be used in the medico-legal assessment of psychiatric injury, they must have sufficient validity and reliability to with-stand forensic cross-examination. In fact, it does not yet appear that any single test is sufficiently robust to cope with the in-depth legal probing required of expert testimony. However, the so called gold standard of clinical assessment by "experts", which presently holds sway in court, also has questionable validity.

The fair distribution of disability compensation among claimants would benefit considerably from the objectivity of appropriately developed and tested biological markers. Although SRR is a long way from being an adequate single measure of PTSD, it may have a limited place as a "user friendly" physiological measure in a comprehensive multi-method forensic PTSD assessment protocol.

References

American Psychiatric Association (1987). *Diagnostic and Statistical Manual of Mental Disorders* (3rd edn – Revised). American Psychiatric Press: Washington, DC.

American Psychiatric Association (1994). *Diagnostic and Statistical Manual of Mental Disorders* (4th edn). American Psychiatric Press: Washington, DC.

Attias, J., Bleich, A. & Gilat, S. (1996) Classification of veterans with PTSD using visual brain evoked P3s to traumatic stimuli. *British Journal of Psychiatry, 168*, 110–115.

Blanchard, E. B., Kolb, L. C., Pallmeyer, T. P. & Gerardi, R. J. (1982). A psychophysiological study of posttraumatic stress disorder in Vietnam veterans. *Psychiatric Quarterly, 54*, 220–229.

Blanchard, E. B., Hickling, E. J. & Taylor, A. E. (1991). The psychophysiology of motor vehicle accident related posttraumatic stress disorder. *Biofeedback and Self Regulation, 16*, 449–458.

Boucsein, W. (1992). *Electrodermal Activity*. Plenum Press: New York.

Cohen, J. (1960). A coefficient of agreement for nominal scales. *Educational and Psychological Measurement, 20*, 37–46.

Edelberg, R. (1972). Electrical activity of the skin: Its measurement and uses in psychophysiology. In Greenfield, N. S. & Sternbach, R. A. (Ed.), *Handbook of Psychophysiology* (pp. 367–418). Holt, Rinehart and Winston: New York.

Friedman, M. J. (1991). Biological approaches to the diagnosis and treatment of posttraumatic stress disorder. *Journal of Traumatic Stress, 4*, 67–91.

Horowitz M. J., Wilner N. & Alvarez W. (1979) Impact of events scale: a measure of subjective stress. *Psychosomatic Medicine, 41*, 209–218.

Keane, T. M. & Kaloupek, D. G. (1998). VA cooperative study #334:I, Summary of findings on the psychophysiological assessment of PTSD. *PTSD Research Quarterly:* Winter Issue.

Lacey, J. I. (1959). Psychophysiological approaches to the evaluation of psychotherapeutic process and outcome. In Rubinstein, E. A. & Parloff, M. B. (Ed.), *Research in Psychotherapy*, 1, 160–208. American Psychiatric Association: Washington, DC.

Lacey, J. I. (1967). Somatic response patterning and stress: Some revisions of the activation theory. In Appleby, M. H. & Trumbull, R. (Ed.), *Psychological stress: Issues in Research*, Appleton-Century-Crofts: New York.

Lang, P. J. (1985). The cognitive psychophysiology of emotion: Fear and anxiety. In Tuma, A. H. & Maser, J. D. (Ed.), *Anxiety and the Anxiety Disorders* (pp. 131–170). Erlbaum: Hillsdale, New Jersey.

Lees-Haley, P. R. (1990). Malingering mental disorder on the Impact of Event Scale (IES): Toxic exposure and cancerphobia. *Journal of Traumatic Stress, 3*, 315–321.

Malloy, P. F., Fairbank, J. A. & Keane, T. M. (1983). Validation of a multimethod assessment of posttraumatic stress disorder in Vietnam veterans. *Journal of Consulting and Clinical Psychology, 51*, 488–494.

Mason, J. W., Giller E. L. & Kosten, T. R. (1988). Elevation of urinary norepinephrine/cortisol ratio in PTSD. *Journal of Nervous and Mental Diseases, 176*, 498–502.

Metzger L. J., Orr S. P., Lasko N. B. & Ritman, R. (1997) Auditory event-related potentials to tone stimuli in combat related PTSD. *Biological Psychiatry, 42*, 1006–1015.

Neal, L. A., Busuttil, W., Rollins, J., Herepath, R., Strike, P. & Turnbull, G. (1994). Convergent Validity of measures of PTSD in a mixed military and civilian population. *Journal of Traumatic Stress, 7*, 447–450.

Ohman, A. (1987). Psychophysiology of emotion: An evolutionary-cognitive perspective. In Ackles P. K., Jennings J. R. & Coles M.G.H. (Ed.), Advances in Psychophysiology, *2,* 79–127. JAI Press: Greenwich, CT.

Orr, S. P. (1990). Psychophysiologic studies of post-traumatic stress disorder. In Giller, E. L. (Ed.), *Biological Assessment and Treatment of Post Traumatic Stress Disorder*, American Psychiatric Press Inc.: Washington, DC.

Orr, S. P. & Kaloupek, D. G. (1997) Psychophysiological assessment of PTSD. In Wilson J. P.& Keane T. M. (Ed.), *Assessing psychological trauma and PTSD: a handbook for practitioners* (pp 69–97). New York, Guildford.

Orr, S. P. (1994). An overview of psychophysiological studies of PTSD. *PTSD Research Quarterly, 5*, 1–7.

Orr, S. P. & Pitman R. K. (1993). Psychophysiologic assessment of attempts to simulate posttraumatic stress disorder. *Biological Psychiatry, 33*, 127–129.

Orr, S. P., Pitman, R. K., Lasko, N. B. & Herz, L. R. (1993). Psychophysiological assessment of posttraumatic stress disorder imagery in World War II and Korean combat veterans. *Journal of Abnormal Psychology, 102,* 152–159.

Orr, S. P., Meyerhoff, J. L., Edwards, J. V. & Pitman, R. K. (1998). Heart rate and blood pressure resting levels and responses to generic stressors in Vietnam veterans with PTSD. *Journal of Traumatic Stress, 11*, 155–164.

Paige S. R., Reid G. M. & Allen M. G. (1990) Psychophysiological correlates of PTSD in Vietnam veterans. *Biological Psychiatry, 27*, 419–430.

Pallmeyer, T. P., Blanchard, E. B. & Kolb, L. C. (1986). The psychophysiology of combat induced posttraumatic stress disorder in Vietnam Veterans. *Behavioural Research and Therapy 24*, 645–652.

Perconte, S. T. & Goreczny, A. J. (1990). Failure to detect fabricated posttraumatic stress disorder with the use of the MMPI in a clinical population. *American Journal of Psychiatry, 147*, 1057–1060.

Pitman, R. K. & Orr, S. P. (1993). Psychophysiologic testing for posttraumatic stress disorder: Forensic psychiatric application. *Bulletin of the American Academy of Psychiatry and Law, 21*, 37–52.

Pitman R. K. & Orr S. P. (1990). Twenty four hour urinary cortisol and catecholamine excretion in combat related PTSD. *Biological Psychiatry, 27*, 245–7.

Pitman, R. K., Orr, P. S., Forgue, D. F., Altman, B., de Jong, J. B. & Herz, L. R. (1990). Physiologic responses to combat imagery of Vietnam veterans with posttraumatic stress disorder versus other anxiety disorders. *Journal of Abnormal Psychology, 99*, 49–54.

Pitman, R. K., Orr S. P., Forgue, D. F., de Jong, J. B. & Clairborn, J. M. (1987). Psychophysiologic assessment of posttraumatic stress disorder imagery in Vietnam combat veterans. *Archives of General Psychiatry, 44*, 970–975.

Shalev, A. Y., Orr, S. P. & Pitman, R. K. (1993). Psychophysiological assessment of traumatic imagery in Israeli civilian patients with posttraumatic stress disorder. *American Journal of Psychiatry, 150*, 620–624.

Spitzer, R. L., Williams, J. B. W., Gibbon, M. & First, M. B. (1989). *The Structured Clinical Interview for DSM-III-R*. Biometrics Research Department, New York State Psychiatric Institute, New York.

Thomas, P. E. & Korr, I. M. (1957). Relationship between sweat gland activity and electrical resistance of the skin. *Journal of Applied Physiology, 10*, 505–510.

Turpin, G. (1990). Psychophysiology and behavioural assessment: Is there scope for theoretical frameworks? In Martin, P. (Ed.), *Handbook of Behaviour Therapy and Psychological Science: An Integrative Approach*, Pergamon Press: New York.

Ultramind Ltd. (1993) Relaxplus. Ultramind Ltd, 99 Charter House Street, London EC1M 6HQ.

20

Simulation of Motor Vehicle Accident-Related PTSD: Effects of Coaching with DSM-IV Criteria

EDWARD, J. HICKLING

Capital Psychological Associates, University at Albany, SUNY

ANN E. TAYLOR

The Sage Colleges, University at Albany, SUNY

EDWARD B. BLANCHARD and TRISHUL DEVINENI

Center for Stress and Anxiety Disorders, University at Albany, SUNY

An issue of much concern in motor vehicle accident (MVA) civil litigation is the extent to which MVA survivors may be dissimulating or faking psychological symptoms, especially the symptoms of Posttraumatic Stress Disorder (PTSD). This study investigated how training in the diagnostic criteria of PTSD and Major Depression would affect the simulation performance of community dwelling adults and college students asked to simulate how they thought a MVA survivor would respond on a number of standard psychological tests frequently used to assess MVA survivors for PTSD; namely responses on the BDI, STAI, IES, and PTSD Checklist (PCL). The two simulation groups (trained and naive) were also compared to the responses of a group of MVA survivors with PTSD. Mean test scores were higher on every measure for the trained versus the naive simulators. When the trained simulators were compared to the genuine MVA-PTSD survivor group, the simulators were significantly higher on the BDI and IES scales, and significantly lower on STAI. The study supports the notion that training in diagnostic criteria can aid an individual wishing to simulate PTSD; however, the pattern of scores on commonly used psychological tests can aid in detection of dissimulation.

Simulation of Motor Vehicle Accident-Related PTSD: Effects of Coaching with DSM-IV Criteria

The exaggerating or faking of psychological symptoms for an external incentive is a recognized but controversial phenomenon in clinical and legal settings (Resnick, 1997). Due to the causal link between a traumatic event and a subsequent psychological disorder such as Posttraumatic Stress Disorder (PTSD), those who have sought legal recourse and compensation for emotional disorders following accident or injury are often suspected of being motivated by potential financial gains rather than true psychological distress. Trimble (1981) reports how prior to the concept of traumatic neuroses, personal injury cases were based solely upon observable, objective evidence that an injury had occurred. Miller (1961) has added to the notion of "accident neurosis", with his work reporting on an extremely high incidence of patients recovering fully, within two years after the claim had been settled. His work is often cited as evidence that patients will improve, not with treatment, but rather with the cessation and settlement of litigation.

There have been a large number of empirical studies that, in fact, challenge Miller's assertion. For example, Thompson (1965) found that financial settlement had little effect on symptoms of litigants diagnosed with posttraumatic neurosis, and Mendleson (1981, 1982) has reported that even after receiving compensation, the majority of patients do not return to work.

No one knows the incidence of malingered psychological symptoms following personal injury. There are a wide variety of estimates, ranging from 1% (Keiser, 1968) to over 50% (Miller & Cartlidge, 1972). Estimates of malingering by forensic evaluators have ranged from 15.7% of forensic cases to 7.4% of non-forensic cases. Rogers (1997a) attributes the relatively high non-forensic case estimate of malingering to the likelihood that forensic experts are asked more often to consult on more adversarial evaluations than most clinical psychologists or psychiatrists. Rogers (1997a; 1997b) comments that prevalence rates for non-forensic evaluations are, in fact, surprisingly absent. While most argue that malingering of symptoms is infrequent in post-traumatic cases, exaggeration of symptoms is thought to occur frequently (e.g.,Trimble, 1981). Scrignar (1996) has argued that the occurrence of malingering is extremely rare in personal injury litigants, due to the heightened scrutiny that litigants undergo from attorneys, private investigators, physicians, and mental health professionals. He believes fraud is more common in large governmental bureaucracies where the potential of compensation and low probability of discovery with little penalty for cheating can motivate people to malinger psychiatric illnesses.

As Resnick (1997) points out, the primary motivation for malingering a disorder such as PTSD is financial gain. The very act of litigation, however, may alter the patient's attitudes and the course of their illness. The plaintiff's attorney may over-dramatize the client's impairment, while defense attorneys may adopt an attitude of disbelief and imply that the individual is not suffering from any genuine psychiatric symptoms. Resnick comments how in the patient's perspective, a comparable attitude may also occur among evaluating clinicians, affecting the clinician's participation and presentation of assessment findings in expert testimony.

The ability to detect malingering or dissimulation has received considerable attention over the past decade (e.g., Rogers, 1997b; Weissman, 1990). Davidson (1965) believes that a person who has historically been responsible and honest is not likely to malinger. The malingerer tends to have an inconsistent history of employment, a prior history of injuries and extensive absences from work. They may also present themselves in extremely complimentary terms prior to their injuries (Layden, 1966). Contradictions in their presentation may be found, such as the ability to engage in recreational activities, but not in strenuous physical work. True PTSD sufferers are reported to withdraw from recreational as well as employment situations (Davidson, 1965). Nightmares may also be less varied or not reported at all, in comparison to individuals with genuine symptomatology (Garfield, 1987). As Resnick (1994) points out, the detection of a malingered mental disorder is sometimes quite difficult. He asserts that clinicians bear a heavy responsibility to assist society in differentiating genuine psychiatric illness from malingered madness.

Psychological tests have become increasingly used to aid in the detection of malingered psychological disorders (for a recent review of this area see Greene, 1997). However, they have often been criticized as susceptible to response styles (Rogers, 1997a). Psychological tests that have been shown to be vulnerable to malingering and defensiveness have included such testing mainstays as the MMPI-2 (Rogers, Sewell, & Salekin, 1994; Wetter & Deitsch, 1996), and the Wechsler Adult Intelligence Scale-Revised (Mittenberg,

Theroux-Fichera, Zielinski & Heilbronner, 1995), among others. This has led some investigators to develop specific inventories to detect malingerers such as the M Test (Beaber, Marston, Michelli & Mills, 1985), the Malingering Scale (Schretlen & Arkowitz, 1990), and the SIMS (Smith & Burger, 1997). While encouraging, these tests have not yet become common in clinical practice, leaving most clinicians to utilize standard inventories developed for a non-forensic evaluation, where malingering is frequently not as pressing a concern as adequate diagnosis and treatment.

Historically, the investigation of malingered PTSD has largely been conducted on Vietnam Veterans (e.g., Resnick, 1984, 1988; Fairbank, McCaffrey & Keane, 1985; Perconte & Goreczny, 1990). The motivation for veterans to fake symptoms has been summarized by Resnick (1997) to include (a) compensation, (b) to be admitted to a hospital, (c) to gain the retrospective glamour of combat, and (d) to reduce punishment for criminal conduct. It is unclear how relevant these concerns are to individuals involved in personal injury or civilian trauma situations.

When malingering has been studied experimentally, one method commonly used is the simulation design. This design involves providing varied information to the simulators and seeing the effect this information has on the scores of the instrument(s) of interest. The simulators are typically college students or community adults volunteering for the research. Rogers (1984) has pointed out that he sees no further need for research to demonstrate once again that nearly all instruments are susceptible to malingering and defensiveness. He argues that the studies should instead be focused upon constructive approaches to the assessment of dissimulation under conditions similar to those faced by clinicians. He then outlines that dissimulation research should investigate how the instructions, preparation of subjects, standardization of measures and incentives might impact the results.

One key variable outlined later by Rogers (1997b) is the impact of coaching on dissimulation. He argues that the assumption that persons being evaluated will not prepare and will remain naive to the purposes of testing is untenable for two reasons. The first reason is that they must give informed consent to the purposes of the evaluation, and secondly, that they may well have access to reference materials that describe psychological disorders and detection techniques. He argues that, if even the brief overview of detection strategies and information that investigators give subjects about a disorder are enough to lower the validity of the technique, how can we ever feel safe in using them? He goes on to state how the accessibility of information about psychological disorders continues to grow exponentially and is unlikely to be curtailed, especially when the stakes for dissimulation are so high. Recent articles have, in fact, reported on the coaching of clients by their lawyer in how to fake symptoms for a psychological evaluation (Youngjohn, 1995).

The present study investigated the role that coaching of diagnostic criteria for PTSD and of typical psychological responses to the trauma of a personal injury MVA would have on an individual's ability to simulate psychological injury on widely used self-report assessment instruments. It was hypothesized that increasing the knowledge of a dissimulator would enhance their ability to respond as if they suffered from PTSD and related clinical disorders such as Major Depression. It was further hypothesized that individuals who, in fact, had suffered a serious motor vehicle accident, but did not present with a clinical diagnosis of PTSD in a standard interview, would be more capable of faking PTSD symptoms than individuals who had not experienced a serious motor vehicle accident. Lastly, it was hypothesized that individuals believed to be presenting with true PTSD symptoms following a personal injury motor vehicle accident would have a unique pattern of test scores in comparison to trained simulators that would allow clinicians to discriminate between individuals suspected of malingering in a standard, non-forensic evaluation.

Method

Participants

Participants in the study included 130 community-dwelling adults and students (mean age = 29.3; 58.3% female, 41.7% male). Subjects were paid a small honorarium for their participation, which involved listening to the instructions for the study and completing a short battery of standard psychological tests that took less than 30 minutes. A clinical comparison sample was comprised of PTSD-positive participants recruited for an ongoing MVA survivor research project (n = 56; mean age = 36.5; 76.8% female, 23.2% male).

Experimental Conditions

Participants were randomly assigned to one of the two simulation groups (trained or naive; N = 130). Those in the trained condition (n = 64; 48.4% female, 51.6% male) were coached in the DSM-IV (American Psychiatric Association, 1994) criteria for Major Depressive Disorder (MDD) and Posttraumatic Stress Disorder (PTSD). They initially were provided an overview of the incidence of MVAs occurring in the United States, and a context for the study noting our current lack of knowledge of how someone faking psychological disturbance following an MVA would respond to these questionnaires. They were then given a narrative description of a typical personal injury MVA, and provided handouts of the DSM-IV criteria for PTSD and MDD. The MVA description was constructed from a composite of case material (with identifying details removed or altered) taken from various descriptions provided by MVA survivors in our previous assessment studies. Each symptom was reviewed and typical responses of MVA survivors shared (Blanchard & Hickling, 1997). Participants were then instructed to complete a series of questionnaires in the manner they thought a distressed MVA victim would respond, based upon the information they had been given.

Participants in the Untrained (naive) condition ($n = 66$; mean age = 26.3; 53% female, 47% male) were instructed to simulate or fake how they thought an accident victim might respond without any explicit training or specific information about any psychological disorders or examples of typical responses being provided. They were read a description of a motor vehicle accident (the same as provided the trained participants), but were then simply asked to complete the questionnaires as they thought someone experiencing this accident and having a significant subsequent psychological disorder might react.

A portion of the simulators had been solicited from an ongoing MVA survivor research project. These participants were assessed thoroughly by structured interview and found to be negative for PTSD and MDD. Thirty two percent of the simulators had been involved in a prior serious motor vehicle accident (51.2% trained, 48.8% untrained). A "serious" MVA was defined for the purpose of this study as one in which either the participant or someone else involved in the MVA sought medical attention due to physical injury resulting from the MVA. This definition is consistent with the inclusion criteria for our ongoing MVA survivor research projects. Having a history of a previous serious MVA was examined to see what the effect this might have on faking of symptoms.

The diagnoses for the PTSD-positive group was established by extensive structured clinical interview. These subjects had been entered into ongoing clinical investigations and were diagnosed as having PTSD on the basis of the Clinician-Administered PTSD Scale (CAPS; Blake et al., 1990). Participants' symptoms had been assessed 6 to 24 months post-MVA. An elaboration of the methods for diagnosis can be found in Blanchard & Hickling (1997). Sixty one percent ($n = 34$) of the PTSD-positive patients were involved in litigation at the time of their assessment.

Procedure

Participants were run in groups ranging in size from 1 to 10. All participants received the same experimental protocol, regardless of group size. The participants in the two simulation conditions were presented a standard description of an MVA survivor's experience. Both groups of simulators were instructed to respond to the same self-report inventories as if they were suffering from PTSD and Major Depression as a result of the MVA. Scores of the PTSD-positive group were then compared with the scores from both simulation groups.

Dependent Measures

The measures used included the following: The PTSD Checklist (PCL) is a 17-item, self-report inventory developed by Weathers, Litz, Herman, Huska & Keane (1994) that describes how much a PTSD symptom has been occurring and how bothersome it was over the past month. It has good reliability and correlates well with structured interview assessments (CAPS), (Blanchard, Jones-Alexander, Buckley and Forneris, 1996).

The Beck Depression Inventory (BDI; Beck, Ward, Mendelson, Mock & Erbaugh, 1961): a 21-item self-report measure of depressive symptoms with well-established reliability and validity (Beck, Steer & Garbin, 1988).

The State-Trait Anxiety Inventory (STAI; Spielberger, Gorsuch, & Lushene, 1970): a 40-item self-report measure that provides values for current state and general trait anxiety levels. Both the state and trait forms have good reliability and validity (Kleinknecht, 1986).

The Impact of Event Scale (IES; Horowitz, Wilmer & Alvarez, 1979): a 15-item scale which has been widely used in PTSD research. It yields two subscale scores for intrusion or reexperiencing symptoms and avoidance symptoms which are summed for a total score. The IES has demonstrated acceptable reliability and validity with various trauma populations including MVA survivors (Blanchard & Hickling, 1997).

Results

Effects of DSM-IV Training

In Table 1 are the scores on all 4 psychological measures, tabulated by experimental condition (Trained versus Naive simulators and PTSD positive MVA survivors) by gender, and by whether the participant had previously been involved in a serious MVA.

Table 1. Mean Scores on Psychological Tests for Simulation and PTSD-positive Groups by Diagnostic Training, Gender, and Previous MVA Experience

	Simulation sample (N = 130)				PTSD-positive sample (N = 56)	
Condition	Informed		Naive			
MVA experience	Males	Females	Males	Females	Males	Females
MVA						
n	12	9	8	12	13	43
Age (years)	28.3	34.9	31.1	36.3	37.5	36.2
BDI	29.9	40.6	21.0	13.5	29.5	28.6
State Anxiety	55.3	56.8	50.5	45.7	61.8	60.7
Trait Anxiety	51.8	56.6	49.6	45.4	61.4	59.8
IES Total	51.3	57.7	47.0	44.3	43.2	43.2
IES Avoidance	24.4	30.2	25.4	22.4	21.4	22.7
IES Intrusion	26.9	27.4	21.6	21.8	21.8	20.6
PCL	60.3	69.9	45.0	43.0	61.5	60.5

Condition	Informed		Naive	
MVA experience	Males	Females	Males	Females
Non-MVA				
n	21	22	23	23
Age (years)	23.0	24.4	22.6	23.1
BDI	33.6	39.7	15.7	21.7
State Anxiety	57.3	49.8	46.4	47.0
Trait Anxiety	58.6	50.4	47.8	47.1
IES Total	53.3	54.8	38.7	48.3
IES Avoidance	26.9	27.9	20.1	24.6
IES Intrusion	26.4	26.9	18.7	23.7
PCL	60.6	64.9	45.3	51.8

Note. BDI = Beck Depression Inventory; IES = Impact of Event Scale; PCL = PTSD Checklist.

The data from the simulators was initially subjected to a 2 (Training versus Naive) X 2 (Male versus Female) X 2 (prior MVA or no prior MVA) ANOVAs. There were no main effects of gender or prior MVA experience nor any interactions of either of these two variables with each other or the Training variable for any dependent variable.

An alpha level of .05 was used for all statistical analyses. The main effect of DSM-IV training was statistically significant for all dependent measures yielding the following the F ratios with $df = (1, 126)$ for each of the psychological measures: for BDI, $F = 38.07$, $p < .001$; for PCL, $F = 33.80$, $p < .001$; for State Anxiety, $F = 12.05$, $p < .01$; for Trait Anxiety, $F = 9.83$, $p < .01$; for overall IES, $F = 12.80$, $p < .001$; for the IES Intrusion subscale, $F = 18.82$, $p < .001$; and for the IES Avoidance subscale, $F = 7.59$, $p < .01$.

Table 2. Means and Turkey HSD Comparisons for Psychological Tests by Trained and Naive Simulators and PTSD-Positive Patients.

	Simulators		PTSD-positive
	Trained	Naive	patients
Measure			
PCL	63.3[a]	47.1[b]	60.7[a]
IES	54.1[a]	44.1[b]	43.2[b]
IES-Avoidance	27.3[a]	22.7[b]	22.4[b]
IES-Intrusion	26.8[a]	21.3[b]	20.8[b]
BDI	35.9[a]	18.1[b]	28.8[c]
State Anxiety	54.3[a]	46.9[b]	60.9[c]
Trait Anxiety	54.3[a]	47.4[b]	60.2[c]

Note. Means in the same row that do not share superscripts differ at $p < .05$ by Tukey HSD procedure.

The pattern of cell means was such that the mean scores for the DSM-IV trained groups were significantly higher on all of the psychological scales compared to the untrained (naive) groups.

DSM-IV trained simulators versus PTSD-positive patients

Given that one of the primary purposes of this study was to examine the impact of training or coaching on simulation of PTSD and related psychological disturbance, theoretically driven pairwise comparisons were conducted on the mean scores for all dependent variables between trained and naive simulators and a group of PTSD-positive patients. Because multiple comparisons were performed, the probability of a Type I error was maintained at the overall alpha level of .05 by Tukey's honestly significant difference (HSD) procedure. The mean scores on the BDI, IES, and IES Intrusion and Avoidance subscales were significantly greater for trained simulators compared to the PTSD-positive patient group and significantly lower on the State and Trait Anxiety scales. Mean scores for the two groups did not differ on the PCL. The relevant means and standard errors for each pairwise comparison along with the associated Tukey HSD statistic can be found in Table 2.

An item analysis was conducted comparing the mean scores for individual PCL items (that is, the 17 PTSD symptoms) between the trained simulators and PTSD-positive patient group. A Tukey HSD procedure was used to hold the probability of a Type I error in the set of multiple comparisons at the overall alpha level of .05. Trained simulators' mean scores were significantly higher on PCL item number 8 (dissociative amnesia) and marginally higher for item number 7 (behavioral/situational avoidance) ($p < .10$) compared to the PTSD-positive patients and significantly lower on PCL item numbers 9 (anhedonia) and 10 (emotional detachment/estrangement). Mean scores for the two groups did not differ significantly on any of the other PTSD symptoms.

Data for the two theoretically relevant groups were examined further. Trained simulators' scores on the dependent measures did not significantly differ as a function of age, gender, or previous MVA experience. The potential moderating role of litigation status on symptom presentation was examined to roughly assess the extent to which "true" (non-malingered) cases of PTSD were represented in the patient sample. Litigation status was defined as either the presence or absence of litigation that was expected or underway as a result of the MVA at the time of the assessment interview. PTSD-positive patients' scores on the dependent measures was not related to age, gender, or litigation status. Moreover, when compared to the trained simulators, PTSD-positive litigants ($n = 34$) did not appear significantly different from non-litigants ($n = 22$) or the overall PTSD-positive sample on any of the psychological tests. Trained simulators did have significantly more years of education ($M = 14.98$, $SD = 1.72$) than PTSD-positive patients ($M = 13.61$, $SD = 2.48$; $t\ (113) = 3.50$, $p = .001$). However, psychological test scores were not significantly correlated with years of education for either the trained simulator or PTSD-positive patient groups.

Discriminant Analyses

Discriminant analyses were conducted to determine whether the following five predictors (psychological test scores) – BDI, PCL, IES, State and Trait Anxiety (STAI) – could reliably distinguish among the trained simulator and PTSD-positive patient groups. For all analyses, predictor variables were entered simultaneously into the discriminant function. The discriminant loading of the PCL on the classification function indicated that it was a poor discriminator. This interpretation was supported by the lack of difference between the group means, $F\ (1, 116) = 1.02$, $p = .314$. To examine the possible suppression of significant relations of certain PCL items with the classification function by use of an aggregate of mostly poor discriminators in computation of the overall PCL score, further discriminant analyses were performed substituting individual PCL items for the overall PCL score. Items showing significant mean differences between the groups with Tukey t-tests did not differ from each other or with other items in their discriminative power. Items were examined in separate analyses to avoid likely problems of high multicollinearity among the variables. The results of these discriminant analyses indicated that the aggregate PCL's low discriminating value was not due to the suppression of item-level discriminators. In addition, when examined in separate discriminant analyses, the differences among the discriminating values of the IES, and the IES Avoidance and Intrusion subscales were found to be negligible. Thus, the overall IES was used in the final discriminant function. The discriminant function yielded an eigenvalue of .54 and canonical correlation of .59, indicating that 35% of the variability of the scores for the function were accounted for by differences between the two groups. The overall Wilks' lambda was significant, $\Lambda = .65$, $\chi^2 = (5, N = 118) = 48.8$, $p < .001$, indicating that overall the predictors differentiated significantly among the two groups. Because these tests were significant, it was appropriate to proceed with interpretation of the discriminant function.

The observed discrepancy between the relative size of the discriminant coefficients and the structure correlations may be attributable to multicollinearity among the predictor variables. However, the pattern of coefficients was not dramatically different and thus was not problematic for interpretation of the overall function.

In Table 3, are presented the within-groups correlations (discriminant loadings) between the predictors and the discriminant function as well as the standardized weights (canonical discriminant coefficients). The dis-

Table 3. Standardized Coefficients and Correlations of Predictor Variables with the Discriminant Function (Summary of Interpretative Measures for the Discriminant Analysis)

	Standardized coefficient	Structure correlation
Predictor variable		
IES Total	.89	.57
BDI	.80	.39
State Anxiety	−.29	−.37
Trait Anxiety	−.50	−.36
PCL Total	−.75	.13

Note. Structure correlation (discriminant loading) refers to the simple linear correlation between each predictor variable and the discriminant function. Standardized coefficients refers to the standardized discriminant weight assigned to each variable in computing the discriminant function. Variables are listed in rank order of their relative discriminating power in the model based on the absolute size of the structure correlations. By convention, a variable exhibiting loadings ± .30 or higher is considered significant.

criminant function was interpreted as representing a pattern of responses characteristic of a simulating response style distinguishable from the pattern demonstrated in the "true" PTSD-positive patients. BDI and IES had relatively large positive coefficients, while State and Trait Anxiety had a notable negative relationship.

The means on the discriminant function were consistent with this interpretation. The means for BDI and IES tended to be significantly larger for the trained simulators relative to the PTSD-positive patients. Conversely, the means for State and Trait Anxiety tended to be smaller compared to the trained simulator group. Based on the discriminant loadings, the IES had the highest discriminative power and the PCL the least. The results can be taken to mean that DSM-IV trained simulators instructed to adopt a "malingering response style" for PTSD are more likely to have significantly *higher* scores on the BDI and IES and more likely to have *lower* scores on State and Trait Anxiety compared to PTSD-positive patients.

In terms of predicting group membership, we were able to correctly classify 76.3 % (72 % with cross-validation) of individuals in our samples when assuming homogeneity of covariance matrices and 74.6 % not assuming homogeneity. The corresponding value of kappa (k), an index that corrects for chance agreements, was .53 and .50, respectively. By convention, these kappas indicate a moderate rate of accuracy in prediction of group membership.

Discussion

This study supports the notion that explicit training in diagnostic criteria can aid an individual wishing to simulate a clinical disorder such as PTSD. It further clarifies that the dissimulation results in a discernible pattern of responses that, across a small battery of self report inventories, allows one with fair reliability to distinguish trained simulators from individuals who had been determined to be genuine PTSD patients. The extent to which these trained simulators may represent a "true" malinger or exaggerator of symptoms in unknown. However, it is argued that this pattern of responding may be useful in the detection of suspected malingering of psychological injury secondary to motor vehicle accidents. Given that MVAs are one of the most frequent traumas occurring in western civilizations (Norris, 1992) and are commonly the basis of personal injury litigation, this may be an aid to clinicians concerned with detecting dissimulation as part of their clinical evaluation. One clear implication of these results is that when malingering needs to be considered in the clinical evaluation, a cautious and skeptical attitude may need to be adopted when employing these commonly used self-report measures. Norms for these tests, as answered by MVA survivors, are available in Blanchard & Hickling, (1997). Patterns of improbable responding, while not definitive, may add useful information to the overall judgment of potential malingering. It can be speculated that this pattern of improbable responding may represent a particular "malingering response style" on these measures for persons attempting to fake psychological distress following an MVA. Further systematic research is needed to investigate this possibility.

While this study appears to meet the earlier requests of Rogers (1984) for subsequent research to provide needed information of how instructional sets influence responses, and how coaching may impact assessments in a clinical setting, he has recently raised concerns about how the assessment of malingering with simulation designs are threatened by factors of external validity (Rogers & Cruise, 1998). Rogers & Cruise (1998) caution that the paradox of asking otherwise truthful persons to comply with instructions to fake (i.e., simulators), in order to study persons who fake when asked to comply with instructions be truthful (i.e., malingerers), place different demand characteristics upon the respondents which complicate the interpretation of any results. These authors state that patterns of responding on instruments, which may provide good discrimination among simulators and clinical patients, may not work well when tested in a known group comparison (i.e., actual malingerers). They further argue that sampling of simulators vs. personal injury claimants may lead to over-reporting of symptoms of mental disorders by the simulators, due to the differing contingencies thought to be operating upon simulators and malingerers.

The present study addresses these concerns in several aspects of its design. First, the simulators included not just uninjured , simulating students, but also included MVA survivors who had been carefully assessed not to have a clinical disorder. They were, however, known to have had a comparable traumatic event within the same time period. It was also believed that for most of the participants, the scenario of being in a MVA is not that far removed from the realm of experience for most adults, and arguably could be identifiable to many of the simulators. Thus, the present simulation task is probably more realistic than asking simulators to fake psychotic symptoms or some other mental disorder with which they may have had little or no experience.

The context of a car crash provided the participant with a familiar and applicable scenario for the simulation. The clinical group of most interest is an uninjured claimant trying to appear as if he/she has a psychological disorder following an accident. The group of MVA accident victims who did not have a diagnosed psychological disorder did not simulate any better than the group who had not been in a serious accident. The presence of ongoing litigation did not seen to lead to any difference between the groups diagnosed with PTSD or any simulating condition. It is, of course, possible that those individuals who would try to fake PTSD are quite different than either of our simulator comparison groups. The fact that we have had only a very small number of individuals in the ongoing MVA survivor research project even considered to be exaggerating symptoms may speak to the rarity of this event, the sampling of those individuals willing to undergo extensive evaluation as part of a large grant-funded assessment and treatment study, or to the insensitivity of methods available to date in the detection of these individuals.

It is agreed that future studies are needed that include a known-groups comparison with identified malingerers. To date we have carefully assessed over 300 MVA survivors, with no known malingerers being identified. Until we find a sample where more suspected malingerers can be obtained, this design appears difficult to fulfill. At this time, it does appear fruitful to examine in further studies the potential effects of the type of incentive, instructions on relevance of the research, varied types of coaching, and whether instruments designed to specifically assess malingering might add to the discrimination of simulators from true clinical cases. It is also thought that the addition of psychophysiological and biological indices such as cortisol assays, as well as examination of inconsistencies in clinical interviews may eventually lead to better capability to accurately assess the presence of PTSD in a clinical and forensic setting.

References

American Psychiatric Association. (1994). *Diagnostic and statistical manual of mental disorders* (4th ed.). Washington, DC: Author.

Beaber, R. J., Marston, A., Michelli, J. & Mills, M. J. (1985). A brief test for measuring malingering in schizophrenic individuals. *American Journal of Psychiatry, 142*, 1478-1481.

Beck, A. T., Steer, R. A. & Garbin, N. G. (1988). Psychometric properties of the Beck Depression Inventory: Twenty-five years of evaluation. *Clinical Psychology Review, 8*, 77-100.

Beck, A. T., Ward, C. H., Mendelson, M., Mock, J. & Erbaugh, J. (1961). An inventory for measuring depression. *Archives of General Psychiatry, 5*, 561-571.

Blake, D., Weathers, F., Nagy, L., Kaloupek, D., Klauminzer, G., Charney, D. & Keane, T. (1990). *Clinician-Administered PTSD Scale (CAPS)*. Boston, MA: National Center for Post-Traumatic Stress Disorder, Behavioral Science Division.

Blanchard, E. B. & Hickling, E. J. (1997). *After the crash: Assessment and treatment of motor vehicle accident survivors.* Washington, DC: American Psychological Association.

Blanchard, E. B., Jones-Alexander, J., Buckley, T. C. & Forneris, C. A. (1996). Psychometric properties of the PTSD Checklist (PCL). *Behaviour Research and Therapy, 34*, 669–673.

Davidson, H. A. (1965). *Forensic Psychiatry* (2nd ed.). New York: Ronald Press.

Fairbank, J. A., McCaffrey, R. J. & Keane, T. M. (1985). Psychometric detection of fabricated symptoms of posttraumatic stress disorder. *American Journal of Psychiatry, 142*, 501–503.

Garfield, P. (1987). Nightmares in the sexually abused female teenager. *Psychiatric Journal of the University of Ottawa, 12*, 93–97.

Greene, R. L. (1997). Assessment of malingering and defensiveness by multi-scale inventories. In R. Rogers (Ed.), *Clinical assessment of malingering and deception*. New York: Guilford Press.

Horowitz, M. J., Wilmer, N. & Alvarez, N. (1979). Impact of Event Scale: A measure of subjective stress. *Psychosomatic Medicine, 41*, 209–218.

Layden, M. (1966). Symptoms separate hysteric malingerers. *Psychiatric Progress, 1*, 7.

Keiser, L. (1968). *The traumatic neurosis*. Philadelphia: J. B. Lippincott Press.

Kleinknecht, R. A. (1986). *The anxious self: Diagnosis and treatment of fears and phobias*. New York: Human Sciences Press.

Mendelson, G. (1981). Persistent work disability following settlement on compensation claimants. *Law Institute Journal (Melbourne), 55*, 342–345.

Mendelson, G. (1982). Not "cured by verdict". Effect of legal settlement on compensation claimants. *Medical Journal of Australia, 2*, 132–134.

Miller, H. (1961). Accident neurosis. *British Medical Journal, 1*, 919–925.

Miller, H. & Cartlidge, N. (1972). Simulation and malingering after injuries to the brain and spinal cord. *Lancet, 1*, 580–585.

Mittenberg, W., Theroux-Fichera, S., Zielinski, R. E. & Heilbronner, R. L. (1995). Identification of malingered head injury on the Wechsler Adult Intelligence Scale-Revised. *Professional Psychology: Research and Practice, 26*, 491–498.

National Highway Traffic Safety Administration. (1995, August). *Traffic safety facts 1994: A compilation of motor vehicle crash data from the fatal accident reporting system and general estimates system*. Washington, DC: U.S. Department of Transportation.

Norris, F. H. (1992). Epidemiology of trauma: Frequency and impact of different potentially traumatic events on different demographic groups. *Journal of Consulting and Clinical Psychology, 60,* 409–418.

Perconte, S. T. & Goreczny, A. J. (1990). Failure to detect fabricated posttraumatic stress disorder with the use of the MMPI in a clinical population. *American Journal of Psychiatry, 147*, 1057–1060.

Resnick, P. J. (1984). The detection of malingered mental illness. *Behavioral Sciences and the Law, 2*, 20–38.

Resnick, P. J. (1988). Malingered psychosis. In R. Roger (Ed.), *Clinical assessment of malingering and deception* (1st ed., pp. 34–53). New York: Guilford Press.

Resnick, P. J. (1994). Malingering. In R. Rosner (Ed.), *Principles and practice of forensic psychiatry* (pp. 417–426). New York: Chapman and Hall.

Resnick, P. J. (1997). Malingering of posttraumatic disorders. In R. Rogers (Ed.), *Clinical Assessment of Malingering and Deception* (pp. 130–152). New York: Guilford Press.

Rogers, R., Sewell, K. W. & Salekin, R. T. (1994). A meta-analysis of malingering on the MMPI-2. *Assessment, 1*, 227–237.

Rogers, R., Sewell K. W. & Goldstein, A. (1994). Explanatory models of malingering: A prototypical analysis. *Law and Human Behavior, 18*, 543–552.

Rogers, R. (1984). Towards an empirical model of malingering and deception. *Behavioral Sciences and the Law, 2*, 93–112.

Rogers, R. (1997a). Current status of clinical methods. In R. Rogers (Ed.), *Clinical assessment of malingering and deception*. New York: Guilford Press.

Rogers, R. (1997b). Researching dissimulation. In R. Rogers (Ed.) *Clinical assessment of malingering and deception*. New York: Guilford Press.

Rogers, R. & Cruise, K. (1998). Assessment of malingering with simulation designs: Threats to external validity. *Law and Human Behavior, 22*, 273–285.

Schretlen, D. & Arkowitz, H. (1990). A psychological test battery to detect prison inmates who fake insanity or mental retardation. *Behavioral Sciences and the Law, 8*, 782–786.

Scrignar, C. B. (1996). *Post-traumatic stress disorder: Diagnosis, treatment, and legal issues.* New Orleans, LA: Bruno Press.

Smith, G. P. & Burger, G. K. (1997). Detection of malingering: Validation of the SIMS. *Bulletin of the American Academy of Psychiatry and the Law*, *25*, 183–189.

Spielberger, C. D., Gorsuch, R. L. & Lushene, R. E. (1970). *Manual for the State-Trait Anxiety Inventory.* Palo Alto, CA: Consulting Psychologists Press.

Thompson, G. N. (1965). Post-traumatic psychoneurosis: A statistical survey. *American Journal of Psychiatry, 121*, 1043–1048.

Trimble, M. R. (1981). *Post-traumatic neurosis from railway spine to the whiplash.* New York: Wiley.

Weathers, F. W., Litz, B. T., Herman, D. S., Huska, J. A. & Keane, T. M. (1993, October). *The PTSD Checklist: Reliability, Validity, & Diagnostic Utility.* Paper presented at the annual meeting of the International Society for Traumatic Stress Studies, San Antonio, TX.

Weissman, H. N. (1990). Distortions and deception in self-presentation: Effects of protracted litigation in personal injury cases. *Behavioral Sciences and the Law, 8*, 67–74.

Wetter, M. W. & Deitsch, S. E. (1996). Faking specific disorders and temporal response consistency on the MMPI-2. *Psychological Assessment, 8*, 39–47.

Youngjohn, J. R. (1995). Confirmed attorney coaching prior to neuropsychological evaluation. *Assessment, 2*, 279–283.

Section 4: Psychological Treatment

21

The Psychological Treatment of Motor Vehicle Accident-Related Posttraumatic Stress Disorder: Conceptualization and Two Pilot Studies

EDWARD J. HICKLING

Capital Psychological Associates, The Sage Colleges

EDWARD B. BLANCHARD

Center for Stress and Anxiety Disorders, University at Albany, SUNY

The treatment of motor vehicle accident-related posttraumatic stress disorder (PTSD) has received an increasing amount of interest over the past decade. This chapter will primarily describe the Albany Motor Vehicle Accident Research Project's effort at the treatment of PTSD. The original research at the Albany Project involved the comprehensive psychological assessment and follow-up of motor vehicle accident (MVA) survivors. Those who had a psychological disorder as a result of their MVA were initially referred for psychological treatment within the community. As reported elsewhere (Hickling, Loos, Blanchard & Taylor, 1997) the project also began to investigate how psychological intervention can help the identified disorders. This led to the development of a systematic treatment protocol which has been the focus of the Albany MVA project for the past few years. This chapter will describe our conceptualization of PTSD as it relates to treatment and share the results of two small cohort studies that have been conducted to date. The majority of this chapter will draw upon the findings from these studies. Where treatment interventions have been published elsewhere, the reader will be referred to the original source. One of the more comprehensive reviews of treatment can be found within our recent text *After the Crash* (Blanchard & Hickling, 1997).

The Albany MVA Project's Conceptualization of Treatment

The DSM-III-R (American Psychiatric Association, 1987) and the DSM-IV (American Psychiatric Association, 1994) criteria for PTSD lists six criteria that are necessary for the diagnosis of PTSD. These criteria are Criterion A (the experience of a traumatic event, generally thought to be outside the range of usual experience and 3 symptom criterion); Criterion B (reexperiencing of the traumatic event), Criterion C (persistent avoidance of stimuli associated with the trauma and/or numbing or decreased responsiveness), and Criterion D (persistent symptoms of increased arousal that had not been present prior to the trauma). As we have discussed elsewhere (Hickling et al, 1997; Blanchard & Hickling, 1997) we have developed a treatment rationale that conceptualizes PTSD somewhat differently. In addition to experiencing the traumatic event, we have looked at four inter-related symptom clusters, that lead to a logical extension of psychological treatment methods. We have identified: (a) reexperiencing, (b) avoidance, (c) psychic numbing, and (d) hyperarousal as distinct foci for treatment for many of the survivors of MVAs. Recently, King et al (1998) in their factor analytic investigation of the Clinician-Administered PTSD Scale (CAPS), identified a four factor model of PTSD that supports an alternative to the DSM-IV representation of PTSD symptom clusters consistent with our treatment rationale. The four factors of the CAPS responses they found were identified as reexperiencing, effortful avoidance, emotional numbing and hyperarousal.

Reexperiencing symptoms or the presence of intrusive thoughts, recollections and dreams of the MVA are very common. Dissociation or flashback experiences are particularly graphic representations of reexperiencing. MVA survivors in the United States and Western Civilization are often faced with a number of driving situations, as well as cultural experiences, such as movies or television, where stimuli reminiscent of their MVA are present. Consistent with earlier research (Foa et al, 1989), vicarious exposure and enforced reexperiencing of trauma coupled with education, cognitive therapy, designed to reinterpret the events, are reasonable and accepted treatments for reexperiencing symptoms. An exposure intervention can include verbal discussions within treatment session as well as having the individual write a description of the MVA, tape record their MVA description, and play the recording on a daily basis. Cognitive therapy and education can help the survivor make sense and gain control of the various parts of the cognitive network related to their traumatic memories. We believe that a supportive therapeutic environment, with reinterpretation of the negative aspects of the exposure into a positive event, can be very helpful and instrumental to change.

Avoidance Symptoms

Avoidance is a common experience for MVA survivors both at the cognitive level (trying not to think about the MVA) and at the behavioral level (avoiding the accident site or even all driving). The behavioral intervention for reexperiencing, begins the work of limiting the avoidance that can occur following a traumatic event. There has been considerable evidence that, again, education, graded exposure homework, applied relaxation and cognitive techniques can help with the avoidance behaviors. A complete description of this aspect of intervention can be found in our earlier work (Blanchard & Hickling, 1997).

Psychic Numbing

The third symptom cluster addressed is psychic numbing and estrangement. We believe, as Litz (1992) has pointed out, that psychic numbing and estrangement are perhaps the least studied and most poorly understood cluster of symptoms that make up PTSD. We have conceptualized the cluster of symptoms making up psychic numbing, the inability to recall important aspects of the trauma, markedly diminished interest or participation in activities, feelings of detachment and estrangement from others, a restricted range of affect, and a sense of a foreshortened future as closely resembling depression. For instance, depression can have feelings of sadness or emptiness, decreased concentration, irritability, diminished interest or pleasure in all or most activities, feelings of worthlessness, recurrent thoughts of death, symptoms causing distress or impairment in social, occupational or other aspects of functioning. Here, we have applied a behavioral technique such as pleasant events scheduling (Lewinsohn & Libet, 1972). We have found that within the physical limits for any sustained injuries, that the encouragement of interpersonal involvement and pleasant activities has made a reasonable extension for a behavioral approach to the numbing and estrangement symptom. Secondly, the use of cognitive techniques to challenge underlying schema and irrational beliefs, again, made a logical application for this symptom group.

Hyperarousal

One of the hallmarks of PTSD is the physiological reactivity that is present in hyperarousal in both the general and specific response style. We have utilized relaxation techniques to counter the arousal symptoms as well as using the relaxation to allow the exposure and avoidance treatment to occur in a more positive fashion. Cognitive therapy, again, is applied to attend to any self-defeating or negative thoughts that would provoke anxiety symptoms and lead to subsequent avoidance and heightened anxiety.

Lastly, while not specifically related to symptoms of PTSD, we have found driving phobia to be a frequent occurrence following MVAs. In the USA it is difficult in many cities and settings to function at a high level without the use of motor vehicle transportation. Again, a specific intervention for driving phobia is often required as part of any systematic treatment intervention (see Blanchard & Hickling, 1997).

Treatment Protocol

As part of a grant funded investigation for psychological treatment, a treatment manual was developed. In an attempt to attend to the multiple presentations found within this diverse group of individuals, a somewhat flexible treatment protocol was utilized. A listing of treatment highlights can be found within Table 1. A complete breakdown of the 9–12-session treatment protocol can be found in found in Table 2.

In general, the first six sessions are fairly fixed in structure. This allows a consistent provision of psychological treatment for a cognitive-behavioral intervention. We designed latitude within the later treatment sessions to allow each treatment protocol to be individually tailored somewhat for the needs of the individual involved. As you will note, the initial sessions involve education about trauma and about PTSD, as well as cognitive-behavioral interventions outlined from our treatment rationale. Each individual received extensive training in relaxation techniques. Relaxation techniques are introduced using progressive muscle techniques (Bernstein & Borkovec, 1973) with a culmination in relaxation-by-recall or cued conditioned response.

Table 1. Treatment of MVA-related PTSD

9–12 Individual Sessions
Overall Cognitive-Behavioral Orientation

Components:
- Education about trauma and PTSD
- Relaxation training
- Exposure to written description of MVA
- Graded exposure to difficult travel situations
- Correction of self-talk
- Correction of faulty schema
- Re-engagement in pleasurable activities
- Anger management
- "Existential" issues
- Cognitive treatment for depression

Behavioral treatments include daily, repeated exposure to the written description of the MVA as well as *in vivo* exposure to difficult travel and/or MVA-related scenes. These will be systematically varied in a hierarchical fashion depending upon the needs of each patient. Cognitive intervention includes correction of self-talk, teaching self-coping statements and addressing faulty cognitive schema. We draw heavily from the work of Meichenbaum (1977, 1985) and Ellis (1977).

Several other issues related to MVAs have been found to be of great importance. These have included anger management which is rather common in individuals following their MVA. We have found that individuals are often very angry at the legal system, of litigation, where they are often asked to prove their injury and are treated more as a malingerer rather than a victim in the accident. These individuals often deal with irritating issues such as being blamed for their own condition, rather than being seen as the injured party. Cognitive-behavioral interventions have been applied to this area, and draw on the work of cognitive psychologists such as Novaco (1975).

Existential issues, outlined in Session 7, are meant to refer to issues of mortality and one's place within life. Very common themes of "who I am" and "what would have happened, had I died" are frequently experienced by MVA survivors. Within treatment sessions we allow individuals to discuss their reactions to try to help them make sense of their views of these issues.

Looking closely at Table 2, one will note how the first session is rather active. Frequently, we have already conducted a rather lengthy three to six hour psychological evaluation prior to the initiation of treatment. This evaluation is reviewed and all scores and statements made by the survivor are clarified. The CAPS is reviewed symptom-by-symptom and it is explained

Table 2. Intensive Treatment Regimen for MVA-PTSD

Session 1: Introduction; Diagnostics by T; Education-What is normal response to trauma; Overview of treatment: different procedures to help with different symptom clusters; Relaxation Training – 16 muscle group – instruction in home practice; Verbal description of MVA and reactions by patient – instruction to write it out in detail for next visit. *Patient expectancy questionnaire administered.*

Session 2: Read and elaborate description of MVA – instruction in home practice; Relaxation Training – 16 muscle group, continued home practice; Discussion of Avoidance and idea of hierarchy of tasks; enlist significant other for next visit.

Session 3: Read patient's description of MVA and reaction, discuss negative self-talk and begin substituting coping and mastery self-talk; Avoidance-hierarchy – need for graduated approach behavior in vivo – Significant other to assist – explain symptoms and treatments to spouse, partner. Relaxation (8 muscle group). Continue all homework.

Session 4: Reading exposure to MVA and consequences – add coping outcomes; Relaxation 5 muscle group; Approach behavior homework; check on self-talk and introduce coping and mastery self-dialogue.

Session 5: Reading exposure to MVA – with coping; Relaxation-by-Recall; Approach behavior homework.

Session 6: Reading exposure to MVA – Cue controlled relaxation as coping strategy; Approach behavior homework; Examination and correction of self-talk.

Session 7: Focus is on Psychic Numbing, Depression, and Existential Issues. Remind to continue all previous homework. How to ask for help (to counter mind reading); Pleasurable Activity Scheduling; Explore for depressive schema and faulty logics. Continue approach behavior homework and correction of self-talk.

Session 8: Pleasurable activity scheduling; Explore depressive schema and faulty logic – Cognitive Restructuring. Other home practice.

Session 9: Same as Session #8.

Session 10: Final Visit – Review procedures, remind to continue practice at home. Cognitive schema restructuring. Make assessment appointment and schedule follow-up visit.

how psychological interventions will be applied for these aspects of their reaction. There is a very strong emphasis made on trying to *normalize* the experience for the MVA survivor. Education includes how each of their symptoms fit in an understandable reaction to the MVA. MVA survivors are introduced to Keane's two-factor theory of PTSD and how avoidance and anxiety are commonly found following this type of trauma.

Within this first session they are asked to provide a written description of their accident. Foa & Rothbaum (1998) have developed a technique where rape survivors would speak into a tape-recorder for their exposure-based intervention. We have modified this technique for several reasons. First, the written description is very easy to use within session, easily stored within files and is easy to modify. For us, it also appears to take less time. Furthermore, by asking individuals to read the description aloud, they are again, asked to expose themselves to their fears, thoughts and intrusive recollections in an active fashion. The sessions allow the patient to elaborate the exposure within their written descriptions and provide instruction in cognitive and behavioral techniques.

Relaxation training begins with the 16-muscle group relaxation. Audiotapes of the relaxation induction are provided for home practice. The relaxation techniques are subsequently shortened from 8 to 4 muscle groups and then to cued controlled relaxation. Coping strategies for dealing with the intrusive thoughts and the memories of the trauma are provided throughout many of the treatment sessions. There is a very strong effort made to find fallacies in logic and to correct any distortions or irrational beliefs that can be found within underlying patterns of thinking. There is extensive use of handouts and homework between sessions.

During Session 3, a "significant other" when available is requested to attend. We have found this useful for several reasons. First, we like to enlist this individual as a cooperative participant in the treatment. As there is frequently extensive driving homework, it is important for the significant other to understand this aspect of the treatment and how this can relate to the symptoms that their partner is experiencing. We have also found it important for the MVA survivor to be a passenger in a car as well as the driver. We find it extremely helpful if the person who is driving the car (the significant other) knows what their partner is experiencing, has an appreciation for what PTSD is and how it presents. This engenders increased cooperation and helps reduce any negative interpersonal reactions that might have occurred as a result of the MVA and subsequent PTSD symptoms.

Homework is checked at the beginning of each session. Any difficulties in the reading, the relaxation or cognitive-behavioral techniques are explored. The application of self-talk and cognitive therapy takes significant effort and attention. Exposure is generally performed in a hierarchical fashion building from the easier to the more difficult feared situations. Individuals early on are asked to rank what they find most difficult and modify this each session.

As discussed earlier, later sessions allows one to discuss survival, and mortality as well as depression. Building upon cognitive techniques for PTSD, treatment of depression is readily initiated. Due to the brief therapy model, however, it is not reasonable to believe that depression can be fully treated within this limited timetable. However, clinical experience outside of the treatment protocols would support the idea that this can be a very natural progression, addressing a co-morbid depression as well as the PTSD with cognitive techniques. Within our treatment study, the therapist has flexibility. They have the ability to make decisions about what is most sensible within treatment and use the rapport that they have developed to change the course of treatment. We have also built in the flexibility to arrange between 9 to 12 sessions for treatment. As not all individuals progress at the same rate, this has allowed the treatment study to have some tailoring for each individuals needs, whether it is to end somewhat earlier or to extend treatment in order to complete exposure or cognitive interventions.

Cohort Study 1

The first pilot study included 12 subjects. A complete breakdown of age, gender, time since MVA, diagnoses, CAP scores, and physical injuries can be found in Table 3.

Half of the subjects were treated by EJH and half were treated by EBB. We had one subject drop out of treatment for each psychologist. As Table 3 depicts, subjects had fairly high symptomatic scores and a fairly high incidence of psychiatric co-morbidity. There also is a high incidence of continuing physical problems as noted in the brief description of their injuries. A complete description of this study can be found in Blanchard and Hickling (1997). Subjects were recruited from physician referral and advertisements in local newspapers. Following the subjects' telephone inquiries for possible treatment, a telephone screening for possible PTSD was performed resulting in the 12 participants agreeing to be treated with a manual-based intervention at no cost to the subject. One of the MVA survivors dropped out of treatment because of scheduling and transportation difficulties, while the other left because of being re-injured resulting in worsening physical condition and inability to attend treatment. The 10 MVA survivors treated included 9 females and 1 male, with the mean age of 45.6 years. All had been involved in a MVA more than 6 months earlier than the time of the initial evaluation and all had sought medical attention for injuries relating to the MVA within 72 hours of the accident. As we have discussed elsewhere (Blanchard, Hickling, Vollmer, Loos, Buckley & Jaccard, 1995) the rationale for treating survivors who continue to have symptoms 6 months after the accident was to attempt to account for the large percentage of survivors who have shown spontaneous improvement in PTSD symptoms up to that period of time. Our earlier study found that by 6 months approximately 50% of patients who had initially met criteria for PTSD no longer met full criteria at 6 months. However, those who continue to show symptoms after 6 months were very unlikely to show any spontaneous change from that point on.

Treatment change was primarily assessed using the CAPS (Blake et al, 1990). All therapeutic interviews were taped and reviewed. MVA survivors were diagnosed using DSM-IV (American Psychiatric Association, 1994) criteria. Each participant also completed several psychological tests including the Beck Depression Inventory (Beck et al, 1961), the State-Trait Anxiety Inventory (Spielberger et al, 1970), the Impact of Events Scale (Horowitz et al, 1979), and the PTSD Checklist (Weathers et al, 1993) as a self-report measure of symptoms of PTSD.

Treatment Results

As can be found in Table 4, the initial, post-treatment and 3-month follow-up CAPS can be found for each participant. Additionally, one can find initial and post-treatment primary and co-morbid diagnoses. The CAPS scores were analyzed using a 2 (therapist) by 3 (assessment) repeated measures ANOVA which resulted in a main effect of assessments, exact $F(2,7) = 10.4$, $p = .008$, (Pillais corrected), but no main effect for therapist or interaction of therapist and assessment.

The follow-up analyses for the main effect were performed with correlated *t*-tests, revealing a significant decrease in CAPS scores from pre-treatment to post-treatment, $t(8) = 4.68$, $p \leq .001$, effect size, Cohen's $d = 1.480$. There was no further significant improvement found from post-treatment to follow-up. An analysis of each score for PTSD symptoms did show significant reduction for each symptom cluster ($p \leq .003$ or greater). CAPS scores and clinical evaluations suggested that all 10 patients showed improvement by the end of treatment. Of the 8 participants who started with full PTSD, 5 were at a non-PTSD level by the conclusion of treatment. The remaining 3 MVA survivors who have initially had PTSD did demonstrate decreased symptoms sufficiently to be diagnosed for sub-syndromal PTSD. At the 3-month follow-up evaluation, 2 of those 3 had, in fact, improved to non-PTSD. One of the 2 survivors who began with a diagnosis of sub--syndromal PTSD was determined not to reach criteria for PTSD by the end of treatment.

The psychological tests were also administered for the 3 assessment periods. The data were analyzed using a one-way MANOVA followed by univariate ANOVAs and post hoc tests. The analysis of the psychological tests yielded a significant main effect for time, approximate $F(10,22) = 3.25$, $p \leq .01$, (Pillais corrected). Univariate analysis of variance revealed a significant

Table 3. Description of Cohort 1 Treatment Sample

Sub. #	Age	Sex	Weeks Since MVA	Primary Diagnosis	Co-Morbid Diagnoses	Initial CAPS	Physical Injuries
301	45	F	131	PTSD	MDE GAD	65	Continuing muscle pain in the cervical, upper and lower back region secondary to whiplash injury. Loss of ROM in right arm with diminished grip strength. Continuing sharp pains in both her wrists and ankles. In addition, she was suffering from TMJ secondary to her MVA related injuries.
302	36	F	36	PTSD	MDE	69	Continuing pain in her upper and lower back secondary to whiplash-type injury, which has also left her with continuing cervical pain. Parathesias in left hand and left foot. Lost grip strength in her left hand.
304	63	F	23	PTSD	Driving Phobia MDE GAD	85	Continuing neck, shoulder, and lower back pain from whiplash-type injury. She also suffers from a noticeable headache problem since the accident.
306	63	F	18	PTSD	MDE GAD	86	Continuing neck and shoulder pain, in addition to, chronic headaches.
310	30	F	16	Sub-PTSD	Driving Phobia	37	No continuing physical problems secondary to the accident.
311	46	M	76	PTSD	GAD	46	Exacerbation of existing headache problem since the accident. Cervical muscle stiffness. Traumatic arthritis in the right thumb joint results in unremitting pain. Loss of grip strength in the right hand. (May have done some cartilage damage.)

312	51	F	37	Sub-PTSD	MDE Specific Phobia	46	Loss of strength in right arm secondary to soft tissue damage. Continues to have chest pain secondary to a fractured sternum and headaches secondary to a concussion. (Did not suffer a blow to the head.)
313	36	F	16	PTSD	GAD	65	No physical problems currently related to the MVA.
316	54	F	85	PTSD	MDE	119	Two fractured vertebrate secondary to MVA (t-10, t-11) have left this subject with considerable loss of strength and unremitting pain on a daily basis. At the time of initial interview she had one back surgery which resulted in two supportive metal rods placed in her back to support her spine. Injuries were severe enough to keep her from returning to work.
324	32	F	82	PTSD	GAD	54	Continuing low back problems which result in significant pain and loss of ROM. Permanent deformity of her nose. Continuing dental restoration work. In addition, this subject is suffering from loss of ROM and muscle strength in her right arm secondary to soft tissue damage sustained during the accident. Combined with the back injuries, the injuries have been severe enough to keep this subject out of work.

Table 4. Results from Pilot Trial of Treatment of MVA Victims

Subject No.	Primary Diagnosis	Co-Morbid Diagnoses (Initial)	Initial CAPS	Post-CAPS	3-MO. FU CAPS	Primary Diagnosis	Co-Morbid Diagnoses (3 MO. FU)
301	PTSD	MDE GAD	65	25	28	Non-PTSD	MDE
302	PTSD	MDE	69	37	44	Non-PTSD	MDE
304	PTSD	Driving Phobia MDE GAD		40	15	Non-PTSD	None
306	PTSD	MDE GAD	86	7	2	Non-PTSD	None
310	Sub-PTSD	Driving Phobia	37	10	3	Non-PTSD	None
311	PTSD	GAD	46	29	15	Non-PTSD	None
312	Sub-PTSD	MDE Specific Phobia	46	23	31	Sub-PTSD	Specific Phobia
313	PTSD	GAD	65	31	33	Sub-PTSD	Specific Phobia
316	PTSD	MDE	119	0	3	Non-PTSD	None
324	PTSD	GAD	54	14	13	Non-PTSD	None
Overall Sample			67.2	21.6	18.4		

FU = Follow-up.
GAD – Generalized Anxiety Disorder.
MDE – Major Depressive Episode Adapted from Table 3, Hickling & Blanchard, "The Private Practice Psychologist and Manual-Based Treatments: Post-Traumatic Stress Disorder Secondary to Motor Vehicle Accidents", *Behaviour Research and Therapy*, 1997. Vol. 35, 1–13. Copyright 1997 Elsevier Science Ltd. Adapted by permission of the publisher and author.

Table 5. Summary of Psychological Distress Measures

Measure	Initial	Post-Treatment	3-Mo. Follow-up	$F(29)$	p
Beck Depression Inventory	16.9 (9.0)[a]	8.61 (5.6)[b]	5.9 (5.0)[b]	8.21	.004
State Anxiety	70.2 (21.4)[a]	57.1 (13.8)[b]	48.5 (10.5)[c]	9.86	.001
Trait Anxiety	67.3 (17.1)[a]	54.0 (13.9)[b]	47.9 (8.4)[b]	6.65	.008
Impact of Event Scale	41.9 (14.0)[a]	14.4 (13.3)[b]	10.2 (12.0)[b]	24.4	<.001
PTSD Checklist	56.0 (12.0)[a]	34.4 (10.1)[b]	32.7 (11.5)[b]	17.3	<.001

Means which share a superscript do not differ at .05 or greater

Adapted from Table 4, Hickling & Blanchard, "The Private Practice Psychologist and Manual-Based Treatments: Post-Traumatic Stress Disorder Secondary to Motor Vehicle Accidents", *Behaviour Research and Therapy*, 1997, Vol. 35, 1–13.

decrease in symptoms on all measures used ($p \leq .008$ or better). There is a significant decrease from pre-treatment to post-treatment for all psychological test measures. The State-Anxiety score continued to show an improvement from post-treatment to the 3-month evaluation.

The changes in the overall CAPS scores strongly suggested, that a manual-based treatment protocol can be effective in the reduction of symptoms of PTSD for survivors of MVAs. The study contained several limiting factors. The most significant limitation was that without a control group we cannot say definitively that the improvement was due to the treatment intervention. Our earlier study found that from 6 months to 12 months only 5% of individuals who had PTSD fully remitted by 12 months and only another 5% showed some partial improvement spontaneously. This study certainly demonstrated greater improvement than one would expect for spontaneous improvement. The results show promise but still require a controlled investigation.

Cohort Study 2

The second study investigated the effectiveness of a supportive psychotherapy treatment condition. As part of the preparation for a controlled treatment study, it was necessary to pilot the capability for rendering a supportive psychotherapy treatment that was believable and delivered by the same treating psychologists. It is important to understand that this was not a random assignment of subjects. Cohort Study 1 was completed as the treatment manual was developed to see whether or not it might be effective for potential grant submission. The supportive psychotherapy condition was developed as a second treatment condition to allow comparison between treatment for a controlled investigation. The supportive psychotherapy condition was conceptualized as essentially anything but what was offered in the cognitive-behavioral intervention. By this, we mean, we wanted to be supportive and encouraging to individuals over time but to avoid implementing any of the specific cognitive-behavioral procedures described earlier. Rather, the focus for 10 sessions of treatment, was to spend a great deal of time gathering history, (whether this is history of prior traumas, or losses an individual may have gone through) and explore how the individual might have dealt with these losses and the events that occurred. Sessions are thought of as supportive for not just the traumatic events, but also for any life events that the individual may wish to discuss. For the supportive psychotherapy condition, it was encouraged that a variety of topics be explored and discussed. The supportive psychotherapy was an effort to provide a similar amount of contact with the cognitive-behavioral therapeutic situation, to have an interested, caring individual listen and respond but not performing any activities that could be construed as behavioral, directed or cognitive in form. There was no suggestion for exposure, there was no relaxation training, and there was no attempt to correct logical fallacies. It was important that this be performed to demonstrate that cognitive-behavioral therapists would not fall back into old habits and, instead, could deliver a credible treatment alternative.

Subjects

Subjects, again, were solicited through physician referral network and newspaper advertisements. Mean age for the subjects was 36.87 years. There were 3 male and 5 female subjects. Primary Axis I and co-morbid diagnoses can be found within Table 6 as well as initial CAPS scores and a description of physical injuries.

As with Cohort 1, each of the 8 subjects were found to have chronic physical difficulties related to the MVA. Mean CAPS score was 57.3 which is roughly comparable to that of the cognitive-behavioral condition.

All research participants in the second Cohort study, again, were seen for an initial, post-treatment and 3-month follow-up evaluation. The follow-up evaluation included the CAPS, the Beck Depression Inventory, State-Trait Anxiety Inventory, Impact of Event Scale and the PCL Scale. Half of the participants were treated by each psychologist. There were no treatment drop-outs for this condition. Results can be found in Table 7.

The pre-treatment CAPS scores and co-morbid diagnoses were roughly comparable to the cognitive-behavioral treatment. The supportive psychotherapy condition showed a significant drop in CAPS scores at post-treatment evaluation. Therapist by assessment repeated measures ANOVA was performed yielding a main effect of time, exact $F(2,14) = 12.56$, $p \leq .001$ (Pillais corrected). There is no main effect for therapist nor interaction of therapist and assessment time. Analyses of each score of the 4 PTSD clusters showed significant reductions for each of the symptom clusters ($p \leq .03$ or better). Psychological test scores did not show significant change for the Beck Depression Inventory or the State-Trait Anxiety Inventory. Nearly significant changes were noted for the Impact of Event Scale and the PTSD Checklist on univariate ANOVAs. The analysis of the psychological tests yielded a significant main effect for time for the Impact of Event Scale, $F(2,14) = 3.48$, $p \leq .06$ and for the PTSD Checklist $F(2,14) = 3.51$, $p \leq .06$.

Summary

At this time, both of our pilot studies appeared to support the provision of psychological treatments that are effective for MVA victims. Both the cognitive-behavioral and the supportive psychotherapy conditions showed significant changes in CAPS scores following treatment. Based upon within group changes, we have calculated that we would have needed between 30 and 35 subjects to achieve a significant difference between the cognitive-behavioral and the supportive psychotherapy condition. The strength of supportive psychotherapy condition raised several important questions. Historically, the cognitive-behavioral interventions have been the treatment of choice for many trauma survivors who suffer PTSD. The provision of exposure-based intervention, attention to underlying cognitions and beliefs, and intervention for hyperarousal have been hallmarks of treatment for PTSD. The supportive psychotherapy condition results appears to challenge these presumptions. Clinically, we have often been presented with individuals who have failed at traditional psychotherapy and have responded to a more specific treatment intervention. Our current data suggest that non-specific therapeutic variables may be more potent than heretofore considered. The supportive psychotherapy condition, while an alternative to the cognitive-behavioral intervention for our controlled treatment study, has to our knowledge never been purported to be as effective an intervention as cognitive-behavioral intervention. The need to clarify what factors may be producing change within that condition are thought important whether they are therapist variables, patient expectation variables, or other related issues of psychotherapeutic change. It is hoped that a controlled investigation will provide clarity and validation of these preliminary findings.

Table 6. Description of Cohort 2 Treatment Sample

Subject #	Age	Sex	Weeks Since MVA	Primary Diagnosis	Co-Morbid Diagnoses	Initial CAPS	Physical Injuries
404	71	M	16	Sub-PTSD	None	20	Fractures to 2 neck vertebrate and 1 back vertebrate. Limited ROM/chronic pain in back and neck. Blow to head and loss of consciousness for 3–4 hours. Posttraumatic headaches since MVA
407	43	F	119	PTSD	Specific Phobia GAD MD	79	Soft tissue injury to lumbar region. Ongoing problems with pain and lack of ROM in lower back region.
408	26	M	131	PTSD	MD	58	Torn Tendons/ligaments in neck. Rotator cuff tear on right shoulder. Experiences parathesias in both arms and hands since MVA. Very limited ROM in right arm. Loss or ROM in neck and weakness in both arms. Posttraumatic headache activity.
410	42	F	32	PTSD	Binge Eating D/O Dysthymia	77	Soft tissue damage to neck and lower lumbar region. Restricted ROM in right shoulder. Right shoulder easily fatigued with strenuous demands.

412	25	F	34	PTSD	MD	43	Bruising of chest and legs. Friction burns from airbag at time of MVA. No continuing physical problems.
415	38	F	18	PTSD	Panic Disorder w/ Agoraphobia Hypochondriasis	57	Continuing lumbar region back pain and restricted ROM since the occurrence of the MVA
417	25	F	25	PTSD	MD GAD Binge Eating D/O	94	Exacerbation of pre-existing headache problem. Chronic pain problems in neck and shoulders subsequent to soft tissue injury (whiplash).
418	19	M	27	Sub- PTSD	None	30	Posttraumatic headaches on a near daily basis. Parasthesias through shoulders and thoracic region of back.

GAD = Generalized Anxiety Disorder.
MD = Major Depression.
ROM = Range of movement.
D/O = Disorder.

Table 7. Results from Pilot Trial of Supportive Psychotherapy Treatment of MVA Victims

Subject No.	Age	Sex	Primary Diagnosis	Co-Morbid Diagnoses	Initial CAPS	Post-CAPS	3-Month FU CAPS
404	71	M	Sub-PTSD	None	20	19	18
407	43	F	PTSD	GAD MD Specific Phobia	79	75	61
408	26	M	PTSD	MD	58	13	0
410	42	F	PTSD	Binge Eating D/O Dysthymia	77	37	2
412	25	F	PTSD	MD	73	13	14
415	38	F	PTSD	Panic Disorder w/Agoraphobia Hypochondriasis	57	35	39
417	25	F	PTSD	MD GAD Binge Eating D/O	94	41	36
418	19	M	Sub-PTSD	None	30	15	16
Overall Sample					57.25	31.00	23.25

$F(2,14) = 12.56, p = .001$

GAD = Generalized Anxiety Disorder.
MD = Major Depression.
FU = Follow-up.
D/O = Disorder.

Table 8. Summary of Psychological Distress Measures for Supportive Psychotherapy.

Measure	Initial	Post-Treatment	3-Month Follow-up	F (2,14)	p
Beck Depression Inventory	24.5(13.0)	18.6(12.3)	20.5(16.6)	1.32	ns
State Anxiety	49.0(15.2)	48.1(15.0)	44.9(18.9)	.373	ns
Trait Anxiety	54.9(10.0)	48.1(13.0)	49.5(16.4)	2.23	ns
Impact of Event Scale	37.0(19.1)	25.3(17.1)	17.9(21.2)	3.48	.06
PTSD Checklist	50.0(19.5)	40.0(15.9)	35.2(15.9)	3.51	.06

References

American Psychiatric Association. (1987). *Diagnostic and Statistical Manual of Mental Disorders* (3rd ed., rev.). Washington, DC: Author.

American Psychiatric Association (1994). *Diagnostic and Statistical Manual of Mental Disorders* (4th ed.) Washington, DC: Author.

Beck, A. T., Ward, C. H., Mendelson, M., Mock, J. & Erbaugh, J. (1961). An inventory for measuring depression. *Archives of General Psychiatry, 5*, 561–571.

Bernstein, D. A. & Borkovec, T. D. (1973). *Progressive relaxation training: A manual for the helping professions.* Chicago: Research Press.

Blake, D., Weathers, F., Nagy, L., Kaloupek, D., Klauminzer, G., Charney, D. & Keane, T. (1990). *Clinician-Administered PTSD Scale (CAPS).* Boston, National Center for Post-traumatic Stress Disorder, Behavioral Science Division.

Blanchard, E. B., Hickling, E. J., Vollmer, A. J., Loos, W. R., Buckley, T. C. & Jaccard, J. (1995). Short-term follow-up of post-traumatic stress symptoms in motor vehicle accident victims. *Behavior Therapy, 25*, 453–467.

Blanchard, E. B. & Hickling, E. J. (1997). *After the Crash: Assessment and treatment of motor vehicle accident survivors.* American Psychological Association, Washington, D.C.

Ellis, A. (1977). *How to live with and without anger.* New York: Readers' Digest Press.

Hickling, E. J. & Blanchard, E. B. (1997). The private practice psychologist and manual-based treatments: A case study in the treatment of post-traumatic stress disorder secondary to motor vehicle accidents. *Behaviour Research and Therapy, 35*, 191–203.

Hickling, E. J., Loos, W. R., Blanchard, E. B. & Taylor, A. E. (1997). Treatment of post-traumatic stress disorder (PTSD) after road accidents. In Margaret Mitchell (Ed.) *The Aftermath of Road Accidents: Psychological, social and legal consequences of an everyday trauma.* London, Routledge.

Foa, E. B., Steketee, G. & Rothbaum, B. O. (1989). Behavioral/cognitive conceptualizations of post-traumatic stress disorder. *Behavior Therapy, 20*, 155–176.

Foa, E. B. & Rothbaum, B. O. (1998). *Treating the trauma of rape: Cognitive-behavioral therapy for PTSD.* New York: Guilford Press.

Horowitz, M. J., Wilmer, N. & Alvarez, N. (1979). Impact of Events Scale: A measure of subjective stress. *Psychosomatic Medicine, 41*, 209–218.

King, D. W., Leskin, G. A., King, L. A. & Weathers, F. W. (1998). Confirmatory factor analysis of the clinician-administered PTSD Scale: Evidence for the dimensionality of posttraumatic stress disorder. *Psychological Assessment, 10*, 90–96.

Lewinsohn, P. M. & Libet, J. (1972). Pleasant Events Activity Schedule and depression. *Journal of Abnormal Psychology, 79*, 291–295.

Litz, B. T. (1992). Emotional numbing in combat-related post-traumatic stress disorder: A clinical review and reformulation. *Clinical Psychology Review, 12*, 417–432.

Meichenbaum, D. (1977). *Cognitive behavior modification: An integrative approach.* New York: Plenum Press.

Meichenbaum, D. (1985). *Stress inoculation training.* New York: Pergamon Press.

Novaco, R. W. (1975). *Anger control.* Lexington, MA: Lexington.

Spielberger, C. D., Gorsuch, R. L. & Lushene, R. E. (1970). *STAI Manual for the State-Trait Anxiety Inventory.* Palo Alto, CA: Consulting Psychologists Press.

Weathers, F. W., Litz, B. T., Herman, D. S., Huska, J. A. & Keane, T. M. (1993, October). *The PTSD Checklist: Reliability, Validity and Diagnostic Utility.* Paper presented at the annual meeting of the International Society for Traumatic Stress Studies, San Antonio, TX.

22

Psychological Approaches to the Treatment of Posttraumatic Stress Disorder

ALLISON G. HARVEY

Department of Experimental Psychology, University of Oxford, UK.

> "Historically, some of the most effective treatments for emotional disorders have been developed by constructing a model of the development and maintenance of the disorder and then devising a set of treatment procedures that focus on the core pathology and reverse the maintaining factors" (Clark, 1997, p. 121).

Theoretical accounts of posttraumatic stress disorder (PTSD) are crucial for the development of effective treatments to alleviate the potentially debilitating symptoms of PTSD. A theoretical model provides clues as to the factors maintaining the disorder and thus points to the areas in which intervention may effectively reverse the maintaining factors, thereby reducing the symptoms characteristic of the disorder. Consequently, in discussing psychological approaches to PTSD, this paper will begin by describing a theoretical model of the maintenance of PTSD and then describe the way treatments have been developed to reverse the maintaining factors.

At the outset, it is important to highlight the descriptive and explanatory value of various biological (Kolb, 1987; Krystal et al., 1995), psychodynamic (Horowitz, 1976; Kardiner, 1941), behavioural (Keane et al., 1985; Kilpatrick et al., 1985) and psychobiological (Jones & Barlow, 1990) theories of trauma response. Cognitive theories are the focus of this chapter, however, for three reasons. First, because of their potential to address the range of symptoms that constitute PTSD. Relatedly, it is generally agreed that cognitive theories, to date, have provided the most fully developed account of trauma symptoms (Brewin et al., 1996). Finally, cognitive theory has contributed to the development of cognitive behaviour therapy (CBT). CBT has not only attracted the most research attention of all of the psychological treatments for PTSD but, as will be discussed later in this chapter, is a highly effective treatment for PTSD (Foa & Meadows, 1997).

Cognitive Theories of PTSD

Cognitive theorists have explained PTSD primarily in terms of information processing and memory function (Chemtob et al., 1988; Creamer et al., 1992; Foa & Kozak, 1986; Foa et al., 1989; Litz & Keane, 1989). Cognitive theories are based on the work of Lang (1977, 1979) who proposed that emotions are stored in a propositional network in memory. He argued that this emotional memory network contains information about (1) stimuli that elicit the emotion, such as the physical details and valence, (2) responding, which includes the verbal, cognitive, physical, and behavioural responses elicited on exposure to the stimuli, and (3) the meaning of the stimuli and response (Lang, 1977). This position was extended in Foa and Kozak's (1986) seminal paper on the emotional processing of fear, and in the subsequent extensions of the position to PTSD (Foa et al., 1989; Litz & Keane, 1989). Foa et al. (1989) proposed that a fear network, the equivalent of Lang's propositional network, is formed following a traumatic event and stores information about what is threatening and what should be escaped or avoided. Cognitive theories predict that activation of the fear network results in intrusive recollections of the trauma, attentional bias toward threat, and accompanying physiological reactions (Chemtob et al., 1988; Creamer et al., 1992; Foa & Kozak, 1986). It is proposed that the heightened arousal associated with PTSD predisposes the network to be readily activated (Chemtob et al., 1988). Consequently, cognitive theory predicts that a traumatised individual is likely to have a lower threshold for interpreting stimuli as threatening, as well as a bias toward searching for and identifying threatening information. Recently, Brewin et al. (1996) extended cognitive theory by postulating that dual representations of the trauma are formed in memory. The first, termed verbally accessible memory (VAM), contains the conscious recollection of the trauma. The second memory representation, termed situationally accessible memory

(SAM), which cannot be deliberately accessed, is comprised of sensory, physiological, and motor aspects of the trauma in the form of codes that enable the reexperiencing of the original experience.

According to cognitive theory, intrusive memories may either assist in the processing and resolution of the disturbing material or prompt attempts to avoid (Creamer et al., 1992) or control (Ehlers & Steil, 1995) aversive memories of the trauma. Initial evidence suggests that the latter process will exacerbate the intrusions (Clohessy & Ehlers, 1997; Ehlers et al., 1997; Harvey & Bryant, 1998) and maintain the disorder (Bryant & Harvey, 1995; Solomon et al., 1988).

In terms of recovery, it is argued that activation and modification of all elements of the memory network (Foa et al., 1989; Litz & Keane, 1989) weakens stimulus-response connections and reduces the magnitude and intensity of the fear network (Foa & Kozak, 1986). The presence of high arousal has been argued to be a factor that may impede effective cognitive processing (Creamer et al., 1990). Further, the provision of new information that is incompatible with existing fear structures purportedly facilitates the formation of new memories with content opposite to that contained in the fear network (Foa & Kozak, 1986). Creamer et al. (1992) considered that another path to the resolution of traumatic memories includes exposure to reminders of the trauma in the form of conversing or thinking about the event, and therapeutic activation of the traumatic material. These strategies may be more therapeutic with a longer duration of exposure. Consistent with this position, Ehlers & Steil (1995) argued that cognitive strategies often employed to control intrusions, such as safety behaviours, dissociation, numbing, thought suppression, rumination, and alternate emotions (e.g., anger, guilt), may block successful processing of traumatic memories. Accordingly, cognitive theory predicts that avoidant strategies result in impaired activation of the fear network, and this in turn contributes to poor resolution of the trauma because of restricted opportunities to modify the threat-related schema (Creamer et al., 1992).

In summary, PTSD is thought to result from the inadequate processing of traumatic memories. Cognitive theory predicts that the prerequisites for recovery from PTSD are threefold; to reduce avoidance of the memory of the trauma, enhance engagement with the memories (ie. facilitate emotional processing), and provide new information (information about safety and control) that is incompatible with the existing fear structures to facilitate the formation of new memories incompatible with the fear network (Foa & Kozak, 1986). It should be noted that many trauma survivors achieve these prerequisites for recovery from PTSD without formal intervention. The theory predicts that individuals who adopt an avoidant or dissociative coping style may be more likely to go on to develop PTSD because it is these individuals who cut off from the traumatic memories thus precluding habituation of the memories and resolution of the symptoms.

Cognitive theory not only provides an account of the role and maintenance of each of the hallmark PTSD symptoms; reexperiencing, avoidance and arousal symptoms, it also highlights factors to consider when treating PTSD. Specifically, cognitive theory predicts that therapeutic methods which aim to (1) reduce avoidance, (2) enhance engagement with the traumatic material, and (3) facilitate integration of new information incompatible with the information contained in the fear network should be incorporated into any successful treatment for PTSD. While there are significant differences between trauma types, it is likely that the general principles of this theory, as well as the general principles of treatment which are derived from it, are likely to apply to motor vehicle accident (MVA) survivors equally as to survivors of other trauma types.

Treatment

General Principles of Therapy for PTSD

In accord with the predictions of cognitive theory, the major treatment components typical of CBT for PTSD are exposure, cognitive therapy and, more controversially, anxiety management. I will now describe each of these in turn; what they involve and the proposed mechanism by which they may lead to reduction in symptoms.

Exposure. Cognitive theory of PTSD predicts that the avoidance of traumatic memories will maintain PTSD. It is necessary, therefore, to activate the fear structure and process the traumatic memories in order for the trauma to be resolved (Foa & Meadows, 1997). Accordingly, the primary goal of exposure based therapy is to maintain the heightened state of anxiety that is experienced during proximity to the feared stimulus so as to facilitate habituation. It has been proposed that exposure leads to symptom reduction because the client learns that reminders of the trauma objectively do not harm him/her, there is habituation of the anxiety while the client remains in proximity to the feared stimuli, and the experience of anxiety does not result in the feared loss of control (Jaycox & Foa, 1996).

Exposing the individual to the traumatic memories to facilitate the processing and resolution of the fear network involves, in practice, any or all of the following exposure techniques.

1. Imaginal or prolonged exposure involves facilitating the individual with PTSD to imagine the trauma as vividly as possible. The client is encouraged to visualise the scene in all its detail and describe it out loud as they

imagine it. Emphasis is given to the recall of all sensory cues and to the repetition of the process several times within the session until the anxiety is reduced. This form of prolonged exposure typically requires the individual to maintain this focus for at least forty minutes, by which time it is assumed that habituation will have occurred. Sessions are generally tape recorded and clients are instructed to listen to the tapes at home at least once a day. Other methods involve asking clients to write down detailed descriptions of the experience focusing on all aspects of the experience; the physical, cognitive, behavioural, affective, sensory.
2. In vivo exposure involves live exposure to the phobic object and is usually conducted in a graded fashion, beginning with situations that elicit a small amount of anxiety and moving up the hierarchy of fears as the anxiety habituates and confidence increases.
3. Modelling involves the therapist encouraging the client to have contact with stimuli associated with the traumatic event by providing demonstrations of approaching and contacting the phobic stimulus.
4. Systematic desensitisation (Wolpe, 1958) relies on progressive muscle relaxation to manage the anxiety elicited during imaginal exposure to the phobic stimulus. That is, the client is first trained in relaxation and is then asked to imagine a series of anxiety provoking images while maintaining the incongruent relaxed state.

The common thread between these exposure techniques is that they bring the traumatic material into consciousness allowing the material to be integrated into the individual memory system and processed by the individual. Therapists should employ exposure techniques creatively, always aiming to enhance emotional engagement. Exposure is typically organised in a graded fashion and exposure is repeated so that learning can take place. The information which constitutes the hierarchy is obtained by asking the clients about the feared events and feared outcomes. This information is organised in a hierarchy from the least feared event to the most feared event. An example of a graded hierarchy, for a client in treatment for PTSD following an MVA, can be seen in Figure 1. For this individual, being a passenger is the least anxiety provoking accident-related situation (rated 10/100 on a scale from 0 "no anxiety/fear" to 100 "extreme anxiety/fear") and driving to work via the intersection where the accident occurred, at night, with a passenger was the most anxiety provoking situation (rated 100/100). Exposure starts with the situations at the bottom of the hierarchy. As confidence builds and anxiety habituates exposure to situations further up the hierarchy is introduced. In addition to grading the feared events and feared outcomes it is also possible to grade the level of exposure to the feared material by skipping the worst details initially, suggesting to the client that they keep their

1. Being passenger	10
2. Driving around the block near home	40
3. Driving around the block at night	40
4. Driving to shops	50
5. Driving to work via quiet roads	70
6. Driving to work via intersection	80
7. Driving to work via intersection at night	90
8. Driving to work via intersection at night with passenger	100

Note. Ratings made on a scale from 0 "no anxiety/fear" to 100 "extreme anxiety/fear".

Figure 1. Example of a Graded Hierarchy for an Individual in Treatment for PTSD Following an MVA.

eyes open (eyes closed is likely to increase the intensity), do the exposure in the past tense (the present tense is likely to increase the intensity), or distancing (eg. imaging the accident as if watching it on a screen, rather than seeing oneself in it).

Cognitive therapy. One of the prerequisites to the resolution of PTSD, according to cognitive theory, is that new information that is incompatible with the existing fear structures be integrated to facilitate the formation of new memories incompatible with the fear network. The first aim of cognitive therapy is to facilitate this process. Second and relatedly, the experience of trauma nearly always leaves the individual with shattered assumptions relating to themselves and the world. In terms of assumptions about the self, it is common for trauma survivors to have lost a sense of themselves as good, competent copers and in terms of the world they see it as a place which is dangerous and unpredictable. In accord, the second aim of cognitive therapy is to address these shattered assumptions and assist the individual to move toward a middle position; sometimes the world is safe and sometimes it is dangerous and sometimes I am a competent, strong and good at coping and sometimes I do not cope as well, but generally the world is safe and I am competent.

Cognitive therapy for PTSD is based on Beck's (1976) theory that distorted beliefs about one's self and the world lead to heightened anxiety and depressive reactions. In the context of PTSD, it is proposed that people may develop exaggerated beliefs about threats, vulnerability, or worthlessness following a trauma (Foa & Riggs, 1993). In addition, where the trauma involved intentional violation perpetrated by another person (as opposed to an accident or natural disaster), the individual will often describe a belief that nobody can be trusted. Cognitive therapy aims to identify the shattered assumptions and erroneous beliefs, and teach the individual to modify their thoughts within a more realistic framework.

Cognitive therapy is a dynamic process during which, through collaboration and dialogue, the therapist assists the individual to identify negative automatic thoughts, beliefs and assumptions about the world which are unrealistic. Through careful socratic questioning, clients are assisted to generate more realistic alternative views of their situation. The cognitive therapist aims to emphasize and demonstrate that emotions are produced by the individual interpretation of an event rather than by the event itself. There are several styles of cognitive therapy, each emphasizing different aspects of Beck's work. The approach taken by Barlow & Rapee (1997) is particularly accessible and highly applicable to a range of psychological disorders, including PTSD. Barlow and Rapee highlight two errors in thinking for which therapists should be watchful; the overestimation of how likely it is that an unpleasant event will happen (clients with PTSD generally overestimate the probability) and the overestimation of how bad the consequences will be if the event does happen (they also typically catastrophise the outcome). Barlow and Rapee (1997) suggest that the steps of realistic thinking are to (1) identify the thought behind the emotion, (2) look for the evidence for the thought and evaluate it making sure the errors just described are not made, (3) list alternative accounts of the event concerned (steers clients away from narrow focus and assists them to obtain a broader view of the situation), and (4) ask what is the worst thing that could happen? Generally, when clients ask themselves the latter question they find that the worst that could happen is not so bad after all. Consider the case of a male client who has survived a severe MVA and subsequently presents with PTSD for treatment. One of the most crippling aspects of his disturbance was his overwhelming concern for his wife's safety. Specifically, he experienced an extreme emotional reaction when he did not know the whereabouts of his wife. If his wife was more than five minutes late home from work he would become overwhelmed with fear for her safety. The main cognition associated with his distress was the conviction that she had been involved in a car accident. He estimated the probability of the anticipated accident being fatal to be 100%. Through a cognitive intervention the client was relieved to discover that he was overestimating the probability of an accident occurring and was overestimating how bad the consequences would be. He found it particularly helpful to generate alternative interpretations of his wife's lateness (e.g., held up in traffic, delayed due to talking to a colleague).

Anxiety Management Training

Anxiety management training aims to provide individuals with coping skills in order to assist them to gain a sense of mastery over their fear. In the context of PTSD, anxiety management training is adopted to control arousal levels and other distressing symptoms and assist the individual to engage in exposure to the traumatic memories. Typically, anxiety management involves teaching clients breathing techniques and deep muscle relaxation. However, it is important to be creative by being mindful of individual differences. For example, some clients find it very difficult to engage in and enjoy traditional relaxation methods. These individuals are often highly energetic and do much better at controlling their anxiety with some type of aerobic exercise such as attending exercise classes, or dance classes, jogging or cycling.

There is concern that teaching anxiety management may reduce emotional processing, as the techniques may facilitate avoidance of engagement with the traumatic memories. In that way, it is perhaps questionable as to whether anxiety management can be derived from cognitive theories of PTSD. However, for many clients, relaxation techniques seem to help during the initial stages of exposure but can be dropped as habituation to the traumatic material occurs. Given that our concern is not just with developing successful treatments, but also with the acceptability of the treatment to the client, anxiety management training (and also grading the fears into a hierarchy before exposure) may not be necessary for treatment effectiveness but rather, may be important for improving the acceptability of the treatment to clients. Acceptable treatments will increase commitment and compliance and reduce drop-out rates from treatment.

Summary. The three treatment components are presented here as distinct entities but in reality there is overlap and feedback from one treatment approach to another. During any one session a therapist may draw on all three of the treatment components. While doing prolonged exposure one often draws on cognitive therapy and anxiety management. A typical treatment for PTSD would contain all three of the components discussed and would typically be conducted over a period of 9–12 sessions (see Chapter 23, 25, and 29). It should be emphasized that therapy would only be conducted after a thorough assessment. A discussion relating to how to assess PTSD is beyond the scope of this chapter. However, an excellent book by Wilson & Keane, (1997) is highly recommended.

Efficacy of CBT in the Treatment of PTSD

To date, while there have been several case studies, few treatment outcome studies have been published to test the efficacy of CBT for PTSD following MVA (see Blanchard & Hickling, 1997 for review). It is therefore exciting to note that a number of treatment outcome trials for PTSD following a

MVA are currently underway (see Chapters 23, 25, and 29). In considering the applicability to MVA survivors of treatment outcome studies conducted with other trauma types, it needs to be remembered that differences between trauma types may mean the results obtained are not directly applicable to MVA survivors. Obviously, the degree of violation of an individual's assumptions of control and safety, the chronicity of the experience, and the level of threat and fear evoked are just a few of the factors which differ across trauma types. Having highlighted this general point I would like to turn to briefly describe three recent treatment outcome studies to illustrate the efficacy of CBT for PTSD (see Foa & Meadows, 1997 for comprehensive review).

A rigorous investigation of the efficacy of prolonged exposure was conducted by Foa and colleagues (1991). This study randomly assigned female victims of sexual or nonsexual assault to either prolonged exposure, stress inoculation training, supportive counseling, or a wait-list control group. In this study, stress inoculation training comprised education, breathing retraining and muscle relaxation, thought stopping, cognitive restructuring, modeling, and role-plays. This study provided participants with 9 twice-weekly sessions, and included blind assessments at post-treatment and 3-months follow-up. Whereas stress innoculation training resulted in greater gains than supportive counselling or wait-list control at posttreatment, the prolonged exposure condition led to greater reduction in PTSD symptoms at follow-up. Interpreting these results in terms of cognitive theory, the authors claimed that whereas stress innoculation training led to short-term symptom reduction, prolonged exposure resulted in longer-term benefits because the fear networks were activated and modified. These authors subsequently replicated this study in a design that compared prolonged exposure, stress innoculation training, the combination of prolonged exposure and stress innoculation training, and a wait-list control condition (cited in Foa & Meadows, 1997). Somewhat surprisingly, PTSD severity at follow-up assessment (mean = 10 months) was reduced by 66% after prolonged exposure, 52% after stress innoculation training, and 48% after the combined exposure and stress innoculation training program. This result has been attributed to the reduced prolonged exposure and stress innoculation training provided to participants in the combined treatment group relative to those who received only exposure and stress innoculation training (Foa & Meadows, 1997).

More recently, Marks and colleagues (1998) randomly assigned survivors of a variety of traumas (20% were MVAs) to one of four treatment conditions; prolonged exposure alone, cognitive restructuring alone, combined cognitive restructuring and prolonged exposure, or relaxation without prolonged exposure or cognitive restructuring. Ten sessions of treatment were provided and follow-ups were reported up to 6-months posttreatment. The results indicated that prolonged exposure alone, cognitive restructuring alone and the combined treatment produced similar outcomes. All were superior to relaxation. As for the Foa et al. study (in Foa & Meadows, 1996), the full benefit of the combined treatment may not have been realized as the session duration may have been too short to allow the clients to master both the cognitive approach and exposure.

Taken together, these studies indicate the utility of the cognitive behavioral approach; particularly prolonged exposure and cognitive restructuring. They also illustrate the standards that should be adhered to in conducting treatment outcome trials. All three studies comply with the majority of the "gold standards" for PTSD treatment outcome research set by Foa and Meadows (1997).

Conclusion

This chapter has highlighted some of the fundamental theoretical and conceptual issues in the treatment of PTSD. It has emphasized the importance of the link between theoretical models of the cause and maintenance of PTSD with treatment. It has described a basic outline of and rationale for the main components of CBT and illustrated the efficacy of prolonged exposure and cognitive restructuring. Treatment outcome studies are required with a range of trauma types, including MVAs. Further, there is room for improvement to current treatments for PTSD, even in what are perhaps the best controlled outcome studies, the proportion of clients returning to high end-state functioning is approximately 50% (Foa et al., 1991).

References

Barlow, D. H. & Rapee, R. M. (1997). *Mastering Stress: A lifestyle approach.* Sydney: Lifestyle Press.

Beck, A. T. (1976). *Cognitive Therapy and the emotional disorders.* New York: International Universities Press.

Blanchard, E. B. & Hickling, E. J. (1997). *After the crash: Assessment and treatment of motor vehicle accident survivors.* Washington, DC: American Psychiatric Association.

Brewin, C. R., Dalgleish, T. & Joseph, S. (1996). A dual representation theory of posttraumatic stress disorder. *Psychological Review, 103,* 670–686.

Bryant, R. A. & Harvey, A. G. (1995). Avoidant coping style and post-traumatic stress following motor vehicle accidents. *Behaviour Research and Therapy, 33,* 631–635.

Chemtob, C., Roitblat, H. L., Hamada, R. S., Carlson, J. G. & Twentyman, C. T. (1988). A cognitive action theory of post-traumatic stress disorder. *Journal of Anxiety Disorders, 2,* 253–275.

Clark, D. M. (1997). Panic disorder and social phobia. In D. M. Clark and C. G. Fairburn (Eds.) *Science and practice of cognitive behaviour therapy.* Oxford University Press: UK.

Clohessy, S. & Ehlers, A. (1997). *PTSD symptoms and coping in ambulance service workers.* Manuscript submitted for publication.

Creamer, M., Burgess, P. & Pattison, P. (1990). Cognitive processing in post-trauma reactions: Some preliminary findings. *Psychological Medicine, 20,* 597–604.

Creamer, M., Burgess, P. & Pattison, P. (1992). Reaction to trauma: A cognitive processing model. *Journal of Abnormal Psychology, 101,* 452–459.

Ehlers, A., Mayou, R. A. & Bryant, B. (1997). *Psychological predictors of chronic PTSD after motor vehicle accidents.* Manuscript submitted for publication.

Ehlers, A. & Steil, R. (1995). Maintenance of intrusive memories in posttraumatic stress disorder: A cognitive approach. *Behavioural and Cognitive Psychotherapy, 23,* 217–249.

Foa, E. B. & Kozak, M. J. (1986). Emotional processing of fear: Exposure to corrective information. *Psychological Bulletin, 99,* 20–35.

Foa, E. B. & Meadows, E. A. (1997). Psychosocial treatments for posttraumatic stress disorder: A critical review. *Annual Review of Psychology, 48,* 449–480.

Foa, E. B. & Riggs, D. S. (1993). Posttraumatic stress disorder in rape victims. In J. Oldham, M. B. Riba, & A. Tasman (Eds.), *American Psychiatric Press Review of Psychiatry, 12,* (pp. 273–303). Washington, DC: American Psychiatric Press.

Foa, E. B., Rothbaum, B. O., Riggs, D. S. & Murdock, T. B. (1991). Treatment of posttraumatic stress disorder in rape victims: A comparison between cognitive-behavioral procedures and counseling. *Journal of Consulting and Clinical Psychology, 59,* 715–723.

Foa, E. B., Steketee, G. & Rothbaum, B. O. (1989). Behavioral/cognitive conceptualizations of post-traumatic stress disorder. *Behavior Therapy, 20,* 155–176.

Harvey, A. G. & Bryant, R. A. (1998). The effect of attempted thought suppression in acute stress disorder. *Behavior Research and Therapy, 36,* 583–590.

Horowitz, M. J. (1976). *Stress response syndromes.* New Jersey: Jason Aronson.

Jaycox, L. H. & Foa, E. B. (1996). Obstacles in implementing exposure therapy for PTSD: Case discussions and practical solutions. *Clinical Psychology and Psychotherapy, 3,* 176–184.

Jones, J. C. & Barlow, D. H. (1990). The etiology of post-traumatic stress disorder. *Clinical Psychology Review, 10,* 299–328.

Kardiner, A. (1941). *The traumatic neuroses of war.* Washington, DC: National Research Council.

Keane, T. M., Zimering, R. T. & Caddell, R. T. (1985). A behavioral formulation of PTSD in Vietnam veterans. *The Behavior Therapist, 8,* 9–12.

Kilpatrick, D. G., Veronen, L. J. & Best, C. L. (1985). Factors predicting psychological distress among rape victims. In C. R. Figley (Ed.), *Trauma and its wake* (pp. 113–141). New York: Brunner/Mazel.

Kolb, L. C. (1987). A neuropsychological hypothesis explaining post-traumatic stress disorder. *American Journal of Psychiatry, 144,* 989–995.

Krystal, J. H., Southwick, S. M. & Charney, D. S. (1995). Post traumatic stress disorder: Psychobiological mechanisms of traumatic remembrance. In D. L. Schacter (Ed.), *Memory distortion: How minds, brains and societies construct the past* (pp. 150–172). Massachusetts: Harvard University Press.

Lang, P. J. (1977). Imagery in therapy: An information processing analysis of fear. *Behavior Therapy, 8,* 862–886.

Lang, P. J. (1979). A bioinformational theory of emotional imagery. *Psychophysiology, 16,* 495–512.

Litz, B. T. & Keane, T. M. (1989). Information processing in anxiety disorders: Application to the understanding of post-traumatic stress disorder. *Clinical Psychology Review, 9*, 243–257.

Marks, I., Lovell, K., Noshirvani, H., Livanou, M. & Thrasher, S. (1998). Treatment of posttraumatic stress disorder by exposure and/or cognitive restructuring: A controlled study. *Archives of General Psychiatry, 55*, 317–325.

Solomon, Z., Mikulincer, M. & Flum, H. (1988). Negative life events, coping responses, and combat-related psychopathology: A prospective study. *Journal of Abnormal Psychology, 97*, 302–307.

Wilson, J. P. & Keane, T. M. (1997). *Assessing Psychological Trauma and PTSD.* Guilford Press: London.

Wolpe, J. (1958). *Psychotherapy by reciprocal inhibition.* Stanford, CA: Stanford University Press.

23

Posttraumatic Stress Disorder Due to Motor Vehicle Accidents: Patterns and Predictors of Response to Cognitive-Behaviour Therapy

STEVEN TAYLOR, Ph.D., INGRID C. FEDOROFF, Ph.D.
Department of Psychiatry, University of British Columbia

WILLIAM J. KOCH, Ph.D.
Vancouver Hospital and Health Sciences Centre

Motor vehicle accidents (MVAs) are widespread causes of injury, disability, and suffering. To illustrate, in the Canadian province of British Columbia, which is where our research was conducted, in 1994 there were 177,734 MVAs involving 48,597 injuries, with health care costs exceeding $800 million (personal communication, February 27, 1995, K. Wong, Information Resource Coordinator at the Insurance Corporation of British Columbia). Statistics for other countries similarly indicate that MVAs are a major public health concern (e.g., Norris, 1992).

It has become increasingly apparent that MVAs can produce severe psychiatric disorders (Mayou et al., 1993; Norris, 1992; Taylor & Koch, 1995). Recent studies show that many MVA survivors are left with significant psychological problems, with one of the most serious being posttraumatic stress disorder (PTSD) (Blanchard et al., 1995; Kuch et al., 1994; Mayou et al., 1993; Norris, 1992).

PTSD is characterized by 3 clusters of symptoms, arising after a person is exposed to a traumatic stressor: (1) recurrent reexperiencing of the traumatic event (e.g., flashbacks, nightmares, intrusive thoughts), (2) avoidance of trauma-related stimuli and numbing of general responsiveness, and (3) persistent hyperarousal (e.g., hypervigilance, exaggerated startle response) (American Psychiatric Association, 1994). PTSD occurs in a substantial proportion of MVA survivors, with estimates ranging from 8 to 39% (Blanchard et al., 1995, 1996; Mayou et al., 1993; Norris, 1992). MVAs are traumatic when the victim experiences extreme fear, helplessness, or horror during or after the accident, and believes that serious injury or death could occur. Thus, even minor MVAs can produce PTSD (for illustrative cases see Koch & Taylor, 1995). PTSD is often chronic, persisting for over a year in at least 50% of cases (Davidson et al., 1996). With regard to associated symptoms, people with MVA-PTSD typically fear and avoid accident-related stimuli, including motor vehicle travel (Blanchard et al., 1995; Mayou et al., 1993). Depression and injury-related chronic pain also are commonly found in MVA-PTSD victims (Blanchard et al., 1995, 1996; Kuch et al., 1994; Mayou et al., 1993). Accordingly, there are compelling reasons for developing and evaluating treatments for MVA-PTSD.

Cognitive-Behaviour Therapy for MVA-PTSD

We recently completed a quantitative (meta-analytic) review of the relative efficacy of psychological and pharmacological treatments for PTSD (van Etten & Taylor, 1998). The main findings are summarized in Table 1. Here, CBT refers to a class of treatments, including in vivo and imaginal exposure to distressing but harmless trauma-related stimuli. Relaxation training and cognitive restructuring are also included in many CBT packages. In terms of attrition, CBT performed about as well or better than other treatments, suggesting that it is reasonably well-tolerated (Table 1). According to effect sizes computed for self-report and observer-rated scales, CBT is among the most effective treatments for PTSD. It is superior to waiting list controls in terms of reductions in global PTSD symptoms, general anxiety, and depression, with gains maintained at 3-month followup (van Etten & Taylor, 1998).

Table 1. Meta-analysis of treatments for posttraumatic stress disorder: Dropout proportions and mean effect sizes.

Condition	No. Trials	% Dropout		Effect Size for PTSD Symptoms			
				Self-Report		Observer-Rated	
		M	90%CI	M	90%CI	M	90%CI
Tricyclic antidepressants	6	26.4	14.4–38.4	0.54	0.34–0.74	0.86	0.75–0.97
Carbamazepine	1	9.0	– – –	0.93	– – –	1.45	– – –
Monoamine oxidase inhibitors	7	36.4	24.7–48.2	0.61	0.38–0.84	0.92	0.73–1.11
Selective serotonin reuptake inhibitors	4	36.0	6.5–65.5	1.38	1.02–1.74	1.43	1.19–1.67
Benzodiazepines	1	38.0	– – –	0.49	— - —	0.54	– – –
Drug treatments (overall)	19	31.9	25.4–38.4	0.69	0.55–0.83	1.05	0.91–1.19
Cognitive behaviour therapies	13	15.1	9.8–20.4	1.27	0.80–1.74	1.89	1.66–2.12
Eye movement desensitization & reprocessing (EMDR)	11	14.4	7.8–21.0	1.24	0.99–1.49	0.69	−0.06–1.44
Relaxation training	1	8.0	– – –	0.45	– – –	—	– – –
Hypnosis	1	11.0	– – –	0.94	– – –	—	– – –
Dynamic psychotherapy	1	11.0	– – –	0.90	– – –	—	– – –
Psychological treatments (overall)	27	14.0	10.8–17.2	1.17	0.99–1.35	1.51	1.17–1.85
Pill Placebo	4	23.0	6.6–39.4	0.51	0.29–0.73	0.77	0.63–0.91
Waiting list control	5	6.2	0.2–12.2	0.44	0.28–0.60	0.75	0.67–0.83
Supportive psychotherapy	5	20.5	8.5–32.5	0.34	0.01–0.67	0.92	– – –
No saccade control (for EMDR)	1	—	– – –	0.22	– – –	—	– – –
Controls (overall)	15	16.6	10.5–22.7	0.43	0.33–0.53	0.77	0.71–0.83

Effect size = $(M_{pre} - M_{post})/SD_{pooled}$, where $SD_{pooled} = \sqrt{[(SD_{pre}^2 + SD_{post}^2)/2]}$. All means are weighted by sample size. 90%CI = 90th percentile confidence interval around weighted mean. Note that "—" refers to data missing or not reported. For the 90%CIs, "– – –" appears when there was only one effect size.

Source: M. van Etten, & S. Taylor (1998). Comparative efficacy of treatments for posttraumatic stress disorder: A meta-analysis. *Clinical Psychology and Psychotherapy, 5*, 126–145. Reprinted by permission of John Wiley & Sons, Ltd.

Predictors of Treatment Response

The patients in our meta-analysis had PTSD arising from a variety of traumatic stressors, such as rape, assault, and combat. Comparatively few patients had PTSD due to MVAs. Given the prevalence and cost of MVA-PTSD, further studies of CBT for MVA-PTSD are needed to determine how best to treat this disorder. Case studies and recent clinical trials suggest that CBT is effective for MVA-PTSD (Hickling & Blanchard, 1997; Taylor, 1998; Taylor & Koch, 1995). In this chapter we report the preliminary results of an ongoing study of CBT for MVA-PTSD. The findings described here concern our attempts to identify pretreatment predictors of treatment response. Identification of predictors can aid clinicians in treatment planning, and can suggest ways of modifying existing treatment protocols.

There have been no published studies on predictors of treatment outcome for MVA-PTSD, and very few studies on predictors for other forms of PTSD (Frueh et al., 1995). We examined two forms of treatment outcome: whether or not the patient dropped out of treatment, and degree of treatment response for those patients completing treatment. For treatment completers, we sought to identify the major patterns of outcome from pre- to posttreatment (e.g., response, nonresponse, deterioration) and to identify predictors of these patterns.

Drawing from clinical experience and from the treatment outcome literature on other forms of PTSD (e.g., Pitman et al., 1991), we examined the predictive significance of the pretreatment variables described in Table 2. These variables fall into three classes: (1) demographic variables, (2) background variables (i.e., variables pertaining to the nature of the traumatic event(s), treatments, and patient context variables), and (3) symptom variables. A set of variables pertaining to events occurring during the course of therapy (Table 4) were also examined to further understand the patterns of treatment response.

Given the paucity of data on the prediction of treatment outcome, our investigation was largely exploratory in nature, and all findings should be regarded as tentative and in need of cross-validation. Clinical impressions and research accounts were used to select some of these variables. Their rationales are as follows:

It is a common clinical observation that chronic and severe PTSD is more difficult to treat that acute PTSD (e.g., Peterson et al., 1991). Accordingly, we tested the prediction that chronicity predicts poorer treatment response.

Chronic pain (e.g., related to "whiplash" injury) is a common complaint of MVA victims (e.g., Blanchard et al., 1995). Clinical case studies (e.g., Koch & Taylor, 1995) suggest that chronic pain can interfere with the patient's ability to engage in, and benefit from CBT for MVA-PTSD. Thus, we examined the relationship between chronic pain and treatment outcome.

Table 2. Comparison of patients who completed versus dropped out of treatment: Pretreatment assessment.

	Dropouts ($n=6$)		Completers ($n=28$)		t-test for unequal variances or χ^2	df
	M	SD	M	SD		
Demographics						
Age (years)	44.5	6.3	36.5	8.2	2.65*	9.03
Female (%)	100		61		3.48	1.00
Caucasian (%)	50		79		2.07	1.00
Single, separated, or divorced (%)	100		50		5.10*	1.00
Education level	4.2	1.3	5.3	1.8	1.76	9.23
Yearly family income	1.0	0.0	2.8	1.6	6.01**	26.00
Unemployed or on disability support (%)	60		39		0.75	1.00
Background variables						
Number of serious MVAs (i.e., someone injured)	1.8		2.2		0.99	11.63
Duration of PTSD (years)	2.3	0.9	3.0	3.7	0.88	31.48
Loss of consciousness in most severe MVA (%)	75		36		2.23	1.00
Current litigation for MVA (%)	67		64		0.01	1.00
Dissatisfaction with previous medical treatment	177.3	24.5	137.8	26.8	3.49**	8.15
Satisfaction with social support	24.7	8.5	29.2	7.2	1.20	6.71
Current antidepressant or anxiolytic medication (%)	33		29		0.05	1.00
Analgesics (%)	83		71		0.36	1.00
Symptom variables						
PTSD symptoms (Penn PTSD Scale)	52.7	13.4	38.3	14.0	2.38*	7.55
PTSD symptoms (PTSD Symptom Scale)	41.7	1.9	34.5	7.5	4.43**	30.96
Anxiety	37.0	13.1	22.5	13.0	2.46*	7.28
Depression	38.7	5.7	23.1	10.9	5.01**	14.31
Anger proneness (trait anger)	22.5	8.3	19.2	6.9	0.90	6.76
Anger about accident & aftermath	6.0	3.0	3.8	2.7	1.71	6.96
Guilt about accident & aftermath	16.3	3.8	10.4	4.9	3.19*	8.93
Pain severity	4.5	1.3	3.5	0.9	1.78	6.11
Frequency of pain-related bedrest	3.5	2.1	2.1	1.6	1.51	6.30
Perceived loss of control over life	5.0	0.9	2.7	1.8	4.60**	15.10
Stressfulness of insurance claim	11.0	2.7	6.2	3.4	3.81**	8.87

* $p < .05$, ** $p < .01$ (2-tailed). MVA = motor vehicle accident.

Major depression and MVA-PTSD frequently co-occur (Blanchard et al., 1995). Depression may reduce treatment motivation and compliance. Thus, pretreatment depression may predict poorer response to CBT for MVA-PTSD.

Pitman et al. (1991) found that anger about the trauma was associated with poorer outcome in exposure treatment for combat-related PTSD. Similarly, Foa et al. (1995) found that anger predicted poorer outcome for CBT for assault-related PTSD. The same may apply to CBT for MVA-PTSD. Pitman et al. (1991) also found that the presence of guilt was associated with poorer outcome in exposure treatment for PTSD combat veterans. Again, the same may apply to CBT for MVA-PTSD.

MVA-related litigation may interfere with treatment because (1) it is stressful, thereby exacerbating PTSD symptoms, and (2) patients may fail to comply with treatment if they believe that they should retain symptoms in order to maximize the prospects of a successful legal settlement (Koch & Taylor, 1995). Thus, the presence of concurrent litigation may predict poorer outcome of CBT for MVA-PTSD.

Identification of significant predictors will provide important information as to which patients are best suited for CBT, and how therapy could be refined or modified in order to enhance its efficacy for other patients. Patients in the present study were assessed before, during, and immediately after a 12 week program of group CBT.

Method

Patients

The sample consisted of 34 people seeking treatment for MVA-induced PTSD. These included people who had been in motor vehicle accidents as drivers or passengers, those struck while riding on bicycles or motorcycles, and pedestrians who were hit by vehicles. Patients were recruited from advertisements in the local media, and from physician referrals to our Traumatic Stress Clinic at the University of British Columbia, Canada. Inclusion criteria were (1) PTSD (diagnosed according to DSM-IV criteria) as the primary (most severe) presenting problem; (2) over 18 years of age and able to provide written informed consent; (4) fluency in written and spoken English; and (3) willingness to participate in a 12 week treatment program and to complete the required assessments. Exclusion criteria were (1) Any condition that precluded participation in 12 consecutive weeks of treatment; (2) concurrent psychological therapy; (3) commencement of psychotropic medication (including analgesics) within the past three months. Patients currently on psychotropic medication were accepted into the study providing they (and their treating physicians) agreed to keep their doses constant throughout the course of the study.

The mean age was 38 years (SD = 8 years). Most (94%) had graduated from high school, and 68% were female. Most (74%) were Caucasian, 18% were Asian, and the remainder were from other ethnic groups. A total of 38% were single, 41% were married or cohabiting, and 21% were separated or divorced. Almost half (47%) were employed full-time or part-time outside of the home, 3% were students, 6% were full-time homemakers, 12% were unemployed and seeking work, and 30% were supported by some form of disability payments.

Most (74%) were taking some form of analgesic medication (prescription medication or over-the-counter medications – not including "antidepressant" medications). A total of 29% were taking some form of antidepressant medication (e.g., tricyclic antidepressant or selective serotonin reuptake inhibitors) or an anxiolytic medication (e.g., benzodiazepines). Almost two-thirds (65%) were in litigation for their MVA. The mean PTSD duration was 2.9 years (SD = 3.4 years). Almost a half the sample (41%) reported that they had lost consciousness during the accident.

With regard to comorbid diagnoses, 41% of patients current major depression and 9% had dysthymia. Comorbid anxiety disorders were common: driving phobia (71%), other specific phobia (12%), panic disorder with or without agoraphobia (29%), social phobia (3%), obsessive-compulsive disorder (6%), generalized anxiety disorder (9%). A total of 9% of patients had some other disorder (e.g., body dysmorphic disorder). Patients had a mean of 1.9 disorders in addition to PTSD (SD = 1.2, range 0 to 6). Note that strictly speaking, DSM-IV does not permit one to diagnose driving phobia in addition to MVA-PTSD. Nevertheless, we included the diagnosis of driving phobia because it conveys clinically important information about the nature of the patient's problems (i.e., information about the nature and breadth of fear and avoidance) and is relevant to treatment planning (i.e., relevant to the development of exposure exercises). Given that one of the main purposes of diagnosis is to convey information relevant to symptom description and treatment planning, we therefore considered it appropriate to suspend the DSM-IV rule of not diagnosing driving phobia in the presence of MVA-PTSD.

Measures

Diagnostic interviews. Diagnosis of PTSD was made by the Clinician Administered PTSD Scale (CAPS: Blake et al., 1997). For purposes of sample description, the Structured Clinical Interview for DSM-IV (SCID-IV: First et al., 1996) was used to diagnose other Axis I disorders.

Demographics. A short questionnaire was developed to assess demographic features of the sample. The variables derived from this measure (see previous section and Table 2) are self-explanatory, with the exception of education level and income. Yearly family income (Canadian \$) was assessed on the following scale: less than \$15,000 (score = 1), \$15,000 – \$25,000 (score = 2), \$25,000 – \$45,000 (score = 3), \$45,000 – \$60,000 (score = 4), greater than \$60,000 (score = 5). Education level was rated according to the following scale: completed less than grade 7 (score = 1), completed between grades 7 and 12 (score = 2), graduated high school (score = 3), partial college education (score = 4), graduated 2-year college program (score = 5), graduated 4-year college program (score = 6), partial graduate or professional school (score = 7), and completed graduate or professional school (score = 8).

Background variables. These variables (Table 2) were assessed on a questionnaire designed for the present study, with the following exceptions. Dissatisfaction with previous medical treatment was assessed by the Patient Satisfaction Questionnaire (Marshall et al., 1993), and satisfaction with social support was assessed by the Social Support Questionnaire (Sarason et al., 1987).

Symptom variables. Symptoms were assessed with the following self-report measures. Severity of PTSD symptoms was assessed by the Penn Inventory for PTSD (Hammarberg, 1992) and by the PTSD Symptom Scale (Foa et al., 1993). General anxiety was assessed by the Beck Anxiety Inventory (Beck & Steer, 1990). Depression was measured by the Beck Depression Inventory (Beck & Steer, 1987). Anger proneness (trait anger) was assessed by the trait version of the State-Trait Anger Expression Inventory (Spielberger, 1988). Pain severity was assessed by the Multidimensional Pain Inventory (Kerns et al., 1985). This inventory was also used to assess how often the patient remained in bed because of pain (7-point scale: 0 = never, 6 = very often). We thought this variable may be relevant to treatment outcome because CBT for MVA-PTSD requires patients to be actively involved during in vivo exposure exercises (e.g., returning to the scene of the accident).

The following scales were developed for the purposes of the present study. Anger about the accident and its aftermath was assessed by a 4-item scale in which each item was rated on a 4-point scale (0 = not at all, 3 = very). Sample items include "How angry are you with other people involved in the accident?" and "How angry are you with your family physician or other health care providers?" For pretreatment data on the 34 patients entering the study, Cronbach's α for this scale was .77. A similar 3-item scale was developed to assess guilt about the accident and its aftermath ($\alpha = .79$). Perceived loss of control over one's life was assessed by a 2-item scale ($\alpha = .81$), with each item rated on a 4-point scale (0 = very much, 3 = not at all). The items were "How much do you feel you can influence your physical and emotional health?" and "Do you feel your life is out of control?" Perceived stressfulness of the patient's insurance claim was assessed by an 8-item scale ($\alpha = .75$), with each item rated on a 4-point scale. Sample items are "Since your accident, how fairly have you been treated by the insurance company?" (0 = very fairly, 3 = very unfairly) and "Over the past six months, how often have you been upset by the way the insurance company has responded to your claim"? (0 = almost never, 3 = almost always). (In British Columbia insurance claims are required in order to receive compensation for any MVA-related injuries and damages.)

Treatment related variables and stressors during the treatment period. Number of sessions attended and homework compliance were assessed by therapist ratings. Homework compliance was assessed on a 6-point scale (1 = the patient did not attempt the assigned homework, 6 = the patient did more of the assigned homework than was requested). The other variables in Table 4 were assessed during the CAPS interview. "Other stressful events during treatment" includes stressful events pertaining to work (e.g., being fired from a job), romantic relationships (e.g., ending a relationship), health problems (e.g., being diagnosed with cancer), financial stressors (e.g., bankruptcy), and so forth.

Treatment Protocol

The CBT treatment protocol was derived from three sources: (1) protocols used in previous studies of MVA-PTSD (e.g., Hickling & Blanchard, 1997), (2) protocols for treating related disorders (e.g., Foa et al., 1991), and (3) clinical experience (e.g., Koch & Taylor, 1995). Patients completed 12 office-based 2hr weekly sessions, conducted in groups of 4–6 patients. Treatment consisted of the following components, delivered in sequence over the course of the sessions:

1. *Education.* Patients received information about the nature and psychological sequelae of MVAs, along with a cognitive-behavioural account of PTSD (based on Foa et al., 1989). Treatment procedures were explained in detail to patients.
2. *Applied Relaxation.* Patients were trained in applied relaxation using an adaptation of Öst's (1987) protocol. Patients were informed that the relaxation exercises were coping strategies that could be used for several purposes; e.g., (1) to make it easier to complete exposure assignments,

(2) to reduce tension-induced pain (if applicable), and (3) to cope with stressful events (e.g., litigation). Applied relaxation exercises were completed in some of the sessions and as homework assignments.
3. *Cognitive restructuring.* Patients were trained in cognitive restructuring (Beck & Emery, 1985), with an emphasis on identifying and restructuring dysfunctional MVA-related thoughts and beliefs (see Koch & Taylor, 1995). Patients completed cognitive restructuring exercises in sessions and as homework assignments (i.e., monitoring and challenging negative automatic thoughts, and practicing coping statements).
4. *Imaginal exposure.* Patients completed graded imaginal exposure to MVA-related fear stimuli. This included writing out and reading narratives of their accidents.
5. *In vivo exposure.* Treatment sessions were used to construct hierarchies for in vivo exposure assignments, which were completed as homework exercises.

Treatment also involved other components, such as warm-up exercises in the first session to acquaint group members with one another, and a discussion of relapse-prevention strategies in the final session.

Therapists. There were two therapists per group, consisting of either two doctoral-level psychologists (pairwise combinations of the authors) or a doctoral-level psychologist and predoctoral intern (one of the authors plus an intern). Therapists followed a detailed treatment manual, and sessions were audiotaped to assess treatment fidelity.

Design and Procedure

Potential patients were screened for suitability during a short telephone interview, and selected patients were invited to the clinic for a diagnostic assessment. Each patient was assessed by one of two trained research assistants. Structured interviews (CAPS and SCID-IV) were audiotaped to assess interrater reliability. During the initial assessment patients were given a verbal and written description of the study, and written informed consent was obtained.

Patients meeting study criteria were then randomly allocated to 12 weeks of CBT or 12 weeks on a waiting list. Waiting-list patients then received 12 weeks of CBT. In the present chapter we present pre- and post-treatment data only for the CBT phase of the study (i.e., some of the patients in the present study had completed a 12 week waiting period before commencing CBT). At the time of writing there was insufficient data on three-month followup for discussion here. Pretreatment predictor variables were assessed just before the patient began CBT.

Statistical Procedures

Patients were classified as dropouts if they entered treatment (i.e., attended one or more sessions) but failed to complete the posttreatment assessment. Dropouts and completers were compared on the variables shown in Table 2 to identify variables that predicted who would drop out. To identify predictors of treatment response, we computed residual gain scores (i.e., residualized pre- to post-treatment changes in scores) on the Penn Inventory for PTSD, and on the PTSD Symptom Scale. The sign of the scores was reflected so that larger scores corresponded to greater reductions in symptoms. The two residual gain scores were then cluster analyzed using Ward's method with squared Euclidean distance. This was done in order to identify patterns (clusters) of treatment outcome. Clusters were then compared in terms of the pretreatment variables in an attempt to identify variables that predict cluster membership. To further characterize the clusters, we also compared them in terms of the treatment related variables and stressors during the treatment period.

A two-stage series of analyses was conducted to identify potentially useful predictors of dropouts or cluster membership. First, *t*-tests were conducted for each potential predictor (i.e., *t*-tests comparing dropouts vs. completers, and *t*-tests comparing clusters). Because the sample sizes and SDs often differed across groups, *t*-tests for unequal variances were computed, along with adjusted degrees of freedom. All tests were two-tailed. For the second stage of analyses, variables that significantly discriminated between groups were entered as predictors in discriminant function analyses. This was done in order to assess the potential utility of the variables in predicting group membership. Due to the exploratory nature of this study, along with the small sample size (and correspondingly low statistical power), the α level was set at .05 for all analyses.

Results

Preliminary Analyses: Overall Outcome

Six of the 34 patients (18%) dropped out of treatment. That is, they entered treatment, attended one or more sessions, but then discontinued contact with the clinic and failed to complete the post-treatment assessment. Our dropout rate is similar to mean attrition rate found in our meta-analysis of CBT treatments (15%). Patients completing treatment attended a mean of 9.3 sessions (SD = 2.6). For the 28 patients completing treatment, scores on the PTSD Symptom Scale significantly declined from pre- to post-treatment: pretreatment M = 35.3 (SD = 7.4), posttreatment M = 30.9 (SD = 11.0), t(df = 27.00) = 2.49, $p < .05$. Scores also tended to decline on the Penn PTSD Inventory, but the reduction was not significant: pretreatment M = 39.2 (SD = 14.7), posttreatment M = 37.2 (SD = 11.6), t(df = 27.00) < 1.

The pre-post effect size was 0.47 for the PTSD Symptom Scale, and 0.15 for the Penn PTSD Inventory (see footnote to Table 1 for the formula used to compute effect sizes). These values are considerably smaller than the mean CBT effect size for self-report measures of PTSD symptoms found in our meta-analysis (M = 1.27), despite the fact that the duration of CBT in the present study (12 weeks) was similar to the mean duration of CBT in our previous meta-analysis (M = 10 weeks: van Etten & Taylor, 1998). Most patients in the meta-analysis developed PTSD subsequent to combat, sexual assault, or traumata other than MVAs. It may be that MVA-PTSD is an especially difficult-to-treat form of PTSD. We will return to consider this possibility later.

For treatment completers, residual gain scores for the Penn PTSD Scale and the PTSD Symptom Scale were uncorrelated with whether or not the patient was in litigation at the time of treatment (respectively, rs = .14 and .20, ps > .1).

Completers versus Dropouts

Dropouts tended to have more comorbid diagnoses than completers, t(df = 18.92) = 2.16, $p < .05$. Dropouts M = 2.5 disorders in addition to PTSD (SD = 0.5); completers had a mean of 1.8 additional disorders (SD = 1.3). According to a series of χ^2 tests, dropouts and completers did not differ in terms of the prevalence of any particular comorbid diagnosis, ps > .05. Table 2 shows the comparison of dropouts and completers on the candidate predictor variables. Dropouts, compared to completers, were more likely to be older, single, and have a lower income. They expressed greater dissatisfaction with previous health care, experienced more distress about their MVA-related insurance claim, and perceived themselves as having less control over their lives. Dropouts and completers did not differ in terms of the likelihood of being in litigation or use of medications. Dropouts had more severe PTSD and were more anxious and depressed than treatment completers. Dropouts also had more guilt about the accident, but did not differ from completers on measures of anger or pain.

A discriminant function analysis was conducted to assess the extent to which these variables could predict who would drop out of treatment. To limit the number of predictor variables, only those that discriminated between groups at $p < .01$ were included (see Table 2). These six variables (income, dissatisfaction with previous medical care, score on the PTSD Symptom Scale, depression, perceived loss of control over life, and stressfulness of insurance claim) each had salient loadings on the discriminant function (absolute values of loadings were > .50). They generally performed satisfactorily in predicting who would drop out of treatment: hit rate = 91%, sensitivity = 67%, and specificity = 96%. Further research is needed to determine whether these results can be replicated on a new sample of patients with MVA-PTSD.

Clusters of Treatment Response

A cluster analysis of two variables – residual gain scores on the Penn PTSD Inventory and residual gains on the PTSD Symptom Scale – was conducted in order to identify the major patterns of treatment outcome. A two-cluster solution was obtained. For each cluster Figure 1 shows the mean scores on the PTSD scales before and after treatment. As the figure suggests, one cluster ($n = 15$) was characterized by a decline in PTSD, while the other cluster ($n = 13$) was defined by an increase in symptoms. These impressions were confirmed via statistical tests.

A 2 × 2 ANOVA was conducted for each PTSD scale (dependent variable). The independent variables were time (pre- and post-treatment) and cluster (two clusters). For the Penn PTSD Inventory, there was no significant main effect for cluster, $F(\text{df} = 1, 26) = 2.24$, $p > .1$, or time, $F(\text{df} = 1, 26) < 1$, but a significant cluster-by-time interaction, $F(\text{df} = 1, 26) = 23.92$, $p < .001$. Followup simple effect comparisons were conducted via *t*-tests for unequal variances. The clusters did not differ at pretreatment, $t(\text{df} = 25.97) < 1$, but did differ at post-treatment $t(\text{df} = 26.00) = 4.60$, $p < .001$. Repeated measures *t*-tests indicated that scores decreased for the cluster of 15 patients, $t(\text{df} = 14.00) = 3.98$, $p < .001$, and increased for the cluster of 13 patients, $t(\text{df} = 12.00) = 2.98$, $p < .05$.

A similar pattern of results was obtained for the PTSD Symptom Scale. There was a significant main effect for cluster, $F(\text{df} = 1, 26) = 8.14$, $p < .01$, and time, $F(\text{df} = 1, 26) = 11.94$, $p < .005$, and a significant cluster-by-time interaction, $F(\text{df} = 1, 26) = 40.71$, $p < .001$. Followup simple effect comparisons (*t*-tests for unequal variances) indicated that the

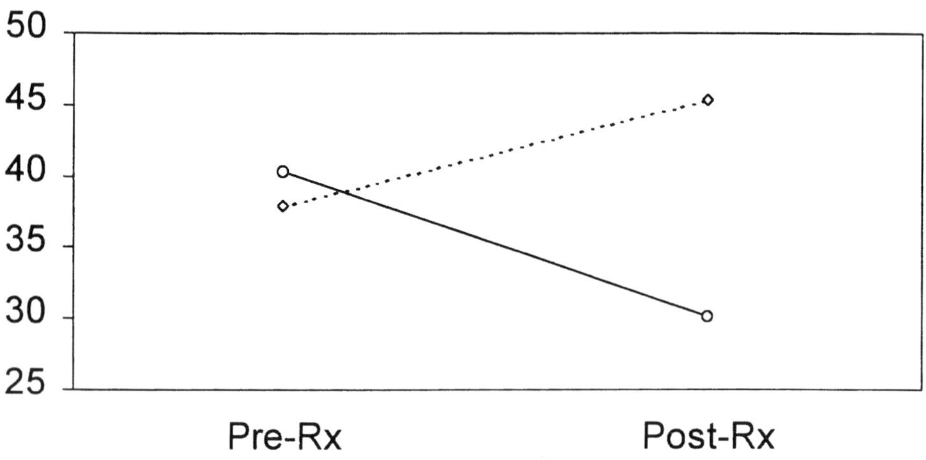

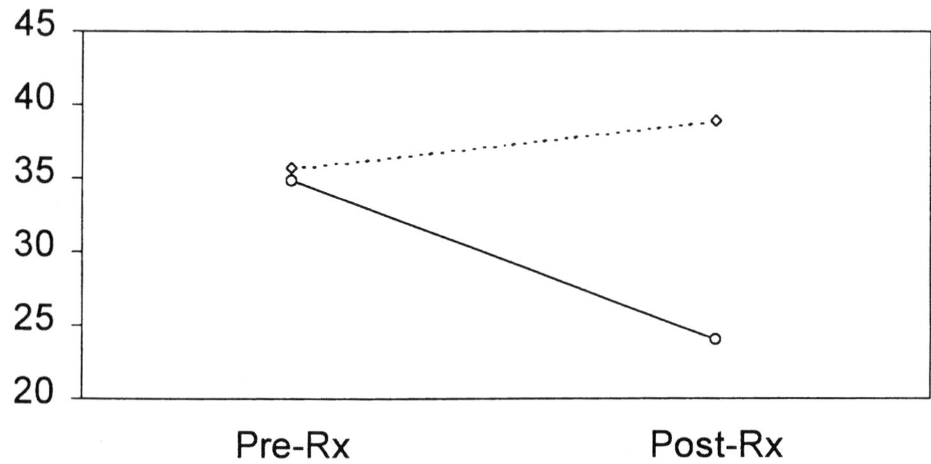

Figure 1. Scores on the Penn PTSD Inventory and PTSD Symptom Scale for the two-cluster solution. The panels show that one group of patients improved (solid lines; n = 15) while another group deteriorated (dotted lines; n = 13).

clusters did not differ at pretreatment, $t(\text{df} = 23.71) < 1$, but did differ at post-treatment $t(\text{df} = 44.91) = 25.98$, $p < .001$. Repeated measures *t*-tests indicated that scores decreased for the cluster of 15 patients, $t(\text{df} = 14.00) = 6.45$, $p < .001$, and increased for the cluster of 13 patients, $t(\text{df} = 12.00) = 2.38$, $p < .05$.

Predicting Improvement Versus Deterioration

The results of the cluster analysis raise two important questions. First, why did some patients improve while others deteriorated? Second, how well can we predict these patterns of treatment outcome? Patients who improved, compared to those who deteriorated, did not differ in the number of comorbid diagnoses, $t(\text{df} = 21.66) < 1$. Deteriorated patients: M = 1.8 diagnoses in addition to PTSD (SD = 0.8); improved patients: M = 1.9 (SD = 1.6). A series of χ^2 tests indicated that deteriorated and improved patients did not differ in terms of the prevalence of any particular comorbid diagnosis, *p*s > .05.

Table 3 shows that improved and deteriorated patients did not differ on most pretreatment variables. These groups differed on only two variables. Compared to patients who deteriorated, those who improved tended to be older and have fewer days of pain-related bedrest. These variables were entered into a discriminant analysis. Both had salient loadings on the discriminant function (absolute value of loadings > .60). They performed moderately well in predicting who would improve versus deteriorate. The hit rate for discriminating groups was 79%. The sensitivity in predicting deterioration was 62% and the specificity was 93%. These findings should be interpreted with caution, given the large number of statistical tests performed in order to identify predictors of improvement versus deterioration.

Although we had moderate success in identifying who would improve or deteriorate in treatment, the predictors do not necessarily indicate why some patients would get better or worse during treatment. The less time patients spend in pain-related bedrest, the greater their opportunity to attempt in vivo exposure exercises. This helps us understand why some patients improved, but it does not tell us why some deteriorated. Why should greater bedrest and younger age be associated with a worsening of PTSD symptoms? It may be that age and frequency of bedrest are simply correlates of the variables causing these patterns (clusters) of treatment outcome.

To further explore the reasons for these patterns we conducted a series of analysis of variables pertaining to events occurring during treatment (Table 4). Although they cannot be used as pretreatment predictors of treatment response, these variables may shed light on the reasons for the response

Table 3. Comparison of patients who improved versus deteriorated: Pretreatment assessment.

	Deteriorated ($n = 13$)		Improved ($n = 15$)		t-test for unequal variances or χ^2	df
	M	SD	M	SD		
Demographics						
Age (years)	33.6	6.5	40.5	8.2	2.45*	25.81
Female (%)	69		60		0.26	1.00
Caucasian (%)	69		87		1.26	1.00
Single, separated, or divorced (%)	46		53		0.14	1.00
Education level	5.4	1.8	5.1	1.8	0.47	25.38
Yearly family income	2.6	1.6	2.9	1.6	0.45	23.84
Unemployed or on disability support (%)	54		33		1.20	1.00
Background variables						
Number of serious MVAs (ie, someone injured)	2.2	1.2	2.3	1.3	0.08	25.92
Duration of PTSD (years)	2.9	3.6	3.2	3.9	0.20	25.85
Loss of consciousness in most severe MVA (%)	38		40		0.01	1.00
Current litigation for MVA (%)	77		47		2.67	1.00
Dissatisfaction with previous medical treatment	142.9	34.0	135.6	19.9	0.66	17.15
Satisfaction with social support	31.4	6.7	25.5	8.3	2.04	24.51
Current antidepressant or anxiolytic meds (%)	23		40		0.91	1.00
Analgesics (%)	85		60		2.07	1.00
Symptom variables						
PTSD symptoms (Penn PTSD Scale)	37.9	14.0	40.3	15.7	0.43	25.97
PTSD symptoms (PTSD Symptom Scale)	35.7	8.2	34.9	6.9	0.29	23.71
Anxiety	22.6	12.9	24.5	13.9	0.38	25.86
Depression	24.3	9.9	24.0	13.2	0.07	25.56
Anger proneness (trait anger)	22.0	7.6	16.6	5.1	2.08	18.70
Anger about accident & aftermath	3.6	2.8	4.1	3.1	0.47	25.95
Guilt about accident & aftermath	10.7	6.8	11.0	3.7	0.14	18.01
Pain severity	3.8	1.0	3.4	1.0	1.26	25.39
Frequency of pain-related bedrest	2.8	1.5	1.6	1.5	2.21*	25.07
Perceived loss of control over life	3.3	1.4	2.5	2.1	1.28	24.52
Stressfulness of insurance claim	6.5	3.3	6.6	4.3	0.05	25.57

* $p < .05$ (2-tailed).

patterns. Table 4 shows that patients who deteriorated, compared to those who improved, attended fewer therapy sessions. Regarding homework compliance, mean compliance was computed across sessions for each patients and then the mean of these means was computed for each cluster. The clusters did not differ in terms of homework compliance (see Table 4). The grand mean (across clusters) was 4.7 (a score of 4 indicates that the patient completed a portion of the assigned homework, and 5 indicates that the patient fully completed the homework).

Two patients had MVAs during the course of treatment; both were in the group of patients who deteriorated. Although this difference between groups was not statistically significant (Table 4), there were significant differences in the frequency of other stressful life events; such events were experienced by all patients who deteriorated, and in only half the patients who improved.

A discriminant function based on two variables – other stressors during the course of treatment and number of sessions attended – predicted deterioration (vs. improvement) with reasonably good success: hit rate = 83%, sensitivity in predicting deterioration = 63%, specificity = 100%. Loadings for both predictor variables were salient (> .64). Note that both variables significantly contributed to cluster discrimination, and both were largely unrelated to one another. This is shown in the following analyses. The point-biserial partial correlation between cluster (improvement vs. deterioration) and number of other stressors (controlling for number of sessions attended) was .53, $p < .05$. The point-biserial partial correlation between cluster and number of sessions attended (controlling for number of other stressors) was .55, $p < .05$. Number of sessions and number of other stressors were not significantly correlated, $r = .24$, $p > .1$.

Discussion

The present study has several limitations and so the results should be regarded as provisional. For most analyses, sample sizes tended to be small, resulting in low statistical power. Moreover, we conducted a large number of statistical tests, and so some of the results may be Type I errors. Nevertheless, the results are provocative and encourage further research into the treatment of MVA-PTSD. Compared to other CBT outcome studies (van Etten & Taylor, 1998), we had a comparable number of dropouts but a poorer treatment response. The reason for the latter is unclear. One possibility is that our patients were more severe than patients in previous treatment-outcome studies. Recall that most previous studies included few patients with MVA-PTSD. Most had PTSD arising from other sources (e.g., combat, rape, assault). There was a great deal of psychiatric morbidity in our sample.

Table 4. Comparison of patients who improved versus deteriorated: Treatment-related variables and stressors during the treatment period.

	Deteriorated ($n = 13$)		Improved ($n = 15$)		t-test for unequal variances or χ^2	df
	M	SD	M	SD		
Number of treatment sessions attended (out of 12)	8.8	2.3	10.7	1.2	2.52*	17.61
Homework compliance (mean rating/session)**	4.5	0.5	4.8	0.4	1.80	21.25
Change in medication during treatment (%)	17		33		0.44	1.00
Another MVA during treatment (%)	22		0		2.48	1.00
Other stressful life event during treatment (%)	100		50		5.54*	1.00

* $p < .05$ (2-tailed).
** Mean ratings across sessions were computed for each patient, and then the mean (and SD) of these means was computed for each cluster, as shown in the table.

Our patients had a mean of two disorders in addition to PTSD. They tended to have recurrent pain (albeit of generally insufficient severity to meet DSM-IV criteria for pain disorder) and were involved in litigation or other stressful dealings regarding their MVA-related insurance claims. It may be that these additional problems make PTSD especially difficult to treat.

We found that treatment dropouts tended to have more severe psychopathology than those who completed treatment. This finding is of clinical importance because it may be argued that the patients who are most severe are in the greatest need of treatment. Thus, it is important to find ways of improving these patients' abilities to tolerate CBT. We identified several predictors of who is likely to complete treatment. Further research is needed to determined which of these are most consistently predictive.

Two patterns of treatment outcome were identified. Surprising, one pattern was where patients tended to deteriorate from pre- to posttreatment. We identified predictors of deterioration versus improvement, although their clinical utility remains to be further explored. Our results suggest that patients are most likely to deteriorate if they have ongoing stressful life events during the course of therapy. One of these patients, for example, described his life as being "like living in a war zone." He experienced frequent stressful altercations in his job as a hospital security guard, only to return home to deal with a physically and verbally abusive alcoholic neighbour. Ongoing stressors made it difficult for therapists to work directly on reducing our patient's MVA-PTSD. Another patient lived in a chaotic family, which was the source of ongoing distress. To top it off, one of her family members was brutally murdered and dismembered part way through treatment. The patient had a very close relationship with this family member and knew the perpetrators. This traumatic experienced produced a major setback in the treatment of her MVA-PTSD. Yet another patient suffered a series of stressors throughout the course of treatment, including ongoing financial and legal problems, the overdose-related death of a close friend, and threatened eviction from his landlord because the patient had fallen behind in rental payments.

Therapists reported that for these types of patients it was often necessary to devote part of treatment to crisis management, and to help them cope with ongoing life stressors. This was needed because these stressors appeared to be exacerbating the patient's PTSD, in the same way that stressors can exacerbate other anxiety reactions such as fears and phobias (Jacobs & Nadel, 1985; Rachman, 1990).

The question arises as to why some patients are more likely to experience stressful life events. A variety of factors may be at work. We found no evidence that patients had a "compulsion to retraumatize" themselves. Patients who experienced stressors during treatment did not differ from patients did not experience stressors in terms of the number of previous MVAs or number of other previous traumatic stressors. If there was a compulsion to repeat then we would expect that the patients experiencing ongoing stressors would be more likely to have experienced more frequent traumatic events in the past.

MVAs and MVA-PTSD can cause stressors such as ongoing financial difficulties (including bankruptcy) and protracted litigation and related stressors (e.g., examinations for discovery). Irritability and chronic anger are common symptoms of MVA-PTSD. These hyperarousal symptoms can result in interpersonal stressors such as conflicts with friends spouses, and coworkers. The MVA and MVA-PTSD are not the only sources of ongoing stressors. Some patients, compared to others, live in more dangerous neighbourhoods or have more hazardous occupations, which increases their risk for stressful events. Some patients, such as those who are impulsive risk-takers, may be tend to create stressful life situations. Other patients do not seem to be risk-takers but live in chaotic families in which some members take impulsive risks. Still other patients may be simply the victims of bad luck (e.g., being diagnosed with cancer during a medical evaluation that happened to occur during the course of PTSD treatment). To improve treatment outcome for MVA-PTSD it would be important to examine these possibilities in future research, and to develop methods for reducing the risk for experiencing recurrent stressors. It may also be useful to extend the duration of treatment to permit more time for generic stress-management training.

References

American Psychiatric Association (1994). *Diagnostic and statistical manual of mental disorders* (4th ed.). Washington, DC: Author.

Beck, A. T. & Emery, G. (1985). *Anxiety disorders and phobias.* NY: Basic Books.

Beck, A. T. & Steer, R. A. (1987). *Manual for the revised Beck Depression Inventory.* San Antonio, TX: Psychological Corporation.

Beck, A. T. & Steer, R. A. (1990). *Manual for the Beck Anxiety Inventory.* San Antonio, TX: Psychological Corporation.

Blake, D., Weathers, F. W., Nagy, L. M., Kaloupek, D. G., Charney, D. S. & Keane, T. M. (1997). *Clinician administered PTSD scale (revised).* Boston, MA: Behavioral Science Division, Boston National Center for Post-Traumatic Stress Disorder.

Blanchard, E. B., Hickling, E. J., Taylor, A. E. & Loos, W. (1995). Psychological morbidity associated with motor vehicle accidents. *Journal of Nervous and Mental Disease, 183,* 495–504.

Blanchard, E. B., Hickling, E. J., Taylor, A. E., Loos, W., Forneris, C. A. & Jaccard, J. (1996). Who develops PTSD from motor vehicle accidents? *Behaviour Research and Therapy, 34,* 1–10.

Davidson, J., Foa, E. B., Blank, A. S., Brett, E. A., Fairbank, J., Green, B. L., Herman, J. L., Keane, T. M., Kilpatrick, D. L., March, J. S., McNally, R. J., Pitman, R. K., Resnick, H. S. & Rothbaum, B. O. (1996). Post-traumatic stress disorder. In T. A. Widiger, A. J. Frances, H. A., Pincus, R. Ross, M. B. First, & W. W. Davis (Eds.), *DSM-IV sourcebook, vol. 2* (pp. 577–605). Washington, DC: American Psychiatric Association.

First, M. B., Spitzer, R. L., Gibbon, M. & Williams, J. B. W. (1996). *Structured Clinical Interview for Axes I and II DSM-IV disorders – Patient edition.* New York: Biometrics Research Department, New York State Psychiatric Institute.

Foa, E. B., Steketee, G. S. & Rothbaum, B. O. (1989). Behavioral/cognitive conceptualizations of post-traumatic stress disorder. *Behavior Therapy, 20*, 155–176.

Foa, E. B., Rothbaum, B. O., Riggs, D. S. & Murdock, T. B. (1991). Treatment of posttraumatic stress disorder in rape victims: A comparison between cognitive-behavioral procedures and counseling. *Journal of Consulting and Clinical Psychology, 59*, 715–723.

Foa, E. B., Riggs, D. S., Dancu, C. V. & Rothbaum, B. O. (1993). Reliability and validity of a brief instrument for assessing post-traumatic stress disorder. *Journal of Traumatic Stress, 6*, 459–473.

Foa, E. B., Riggs, D. S., Massie, E. D. & Yarczower, M. (1995). The impact of fear activation and anger on the efficacy of exposure treatment for posttraumatic stress disorder. *Behavior Therapy, 26*, 487–499.

Frueh, B. C., Turner, S. M. & Beidel, D. C. (1995). Exposure therapy for combat-related PTSD: A critical review. *Clinical Psychology Review, 15*, 799–817.

Hammarberg, M. (1992). Penn Inventory for Posttraumatic Stress Disorder: Psychometric properties. *Psychological Assessment, 4*, 67–76.

Hickling, E. J. & Blanchard, E. B. (1997). The private practice psychologist and manual-based treatments: Post-traumatic stress disorder secondary to motor vehicle accidents. *Behaviour Research and Therapy, 35*, 191–203.

Jacobs, W. J. & Nadel, L. (1985). Stress induced recovery of fears and phobias. *Psychological Review, 92*, 512–531.

Kerns, R. D., Turk, D. C. & Rudy, T. E. (1985). The West Haven-Yale Multidimensional Pain Inventory. *Pain, 23*, 345–356.

Koch, W. J. & Taylor, S. (1995). Assessment and treatment of victims of motor vehicle accidents. *Cognitive and Behavioral Practice, 2*, 327–342.

Kuch, K., Cox, B. J., Evans, R. J. & Shulman, I. (1994). Phobias, panic, and pain in 55 survivors of road vehicle accidents. *Journal of Anxiety Disorders, 8*, 181–187.

Marshall, G. N., Hays, R. D., Sherbourne, C. D. & Wells, K. B. (1993). The structure of patient satisfaction with outpatient medical care. *Psychological Assessment, 5*, 477–483.

Mayou, R., Bryant, B. & Duthie, R. (1993). Psychiatric consequences of road traffic accidents. *British Medical Journal, 307*, 647–651.

Norris, F. H. (1992). Epidemiology of trauma: Frequency and impact of different potentially traumatic events on different demographic groups. *Journal of Consulting and Clinical Psychology, 60*, 409–419.

Öst, L-G. (1987). Applied relaxation: Description of a coping technique and a review of controlled studies. *Behaviour Research and Therapy, 25*, 397–409.

Peterson, K. C., Prout, M. F. & Schwarz, R. A. (1991). *Post-traumatic stress disorder.* NY: Plenum.

Pitman, R. K., Altman, B., Greenwald, E., Longpre, R. E., Macklin, M. L., Poire, R. E. & Steketee, G. S. (1991). Psychiatric complications during flooding therapy for posttraumatic stress disorder. *Journal of Clinical Psychiatry, 52*, 17–20.

Rachman, S. J. (1990). *Fear and courage* (2nd ed.). NY: Freeman.

Sarason, I. G., Sarason, B. R., Shearin, E. N. & Pierce, G. R. (1987). A brief measure of social support: Practical and theoretical implications. *Journal of Social and Personal Relationships, 4*, 497–510.

Spielberger, C. D. (1988). *State-trait anger expression inventory.* Odessa, FL: Psychological Assessment Resources.

Taylor, S. (1998, March). *Posttraumatic stress disorder due to motor vehicle accidents: Efficacy of cognitive behaviour therapy.* Paper presented at the 18th meeting of the Anxiety Disorders Association of America, Boston, MA.

Taylor, S. & Koch, W. J. (1995). Anxiety disorders due to motor vehicle accidents: Nature and treatment. *Clinical Psychology Review, 15*, 721–738.

van Etten, M. & Taylor, S. (1998). Comparative efficacy of treatments for posttraumatic stress disorder: A meta-analysis. *Clinical Psychology and Psychotherapy, 5*, 126–145.

Author Notes

The research reported in this chapter was supported by a grant from the British Columbia Health Research Foundation. Special thanks to Cindy Oxenbury for coordinating this study. Thanks also to the following people for their valuable assistance: Eva DeHaas, Lori Brotto, Derek Mitchell, Wendy Freeman, Quincy Young, and Nichole Fairbrother.

24

Treatment of PTSD in Children Following Road Traffic Accidents

WILLIAM YULE

Professor of Applied Child Psychology, University of London Institute of Psychiatry

Introduction

Motor vehicle accidents and road traffic accidents (RTAs) are a major cause of physical injury in children in all industrialized countries. Despite concerted efforts to improve the safety of vehicles, the safety of roads and to educate children in crossing roads, death and injury remain at unacceptably high levels. However, it is only in the past decade that there has been a focus on the psychological sequelae of RTAs on children.

Following our work with the survivors of major shipping disasters (Yule & Williams, 1990; Yule & Udwin, 1991) we were interested in pursuing further studies of the effects of disasters on children. But it seemed rather ghoulish to be waiting for the next disaster to happen. In any case, there is a considerable lead time between perceiving the need for research and having proper projects funded. Meanwhile, more and more children and adolescents were being referred to our specialist Child Traumatic Stress Clinic for evaluation and treatment following road traffic accidents. Many of these presented with Posttraumatic Stress Disorder (PTSD) and so the question was raised as to what proportion of children developed stress and anxiety disorders following an RTA and how best to treat them.

Table 1. Estimated Incidence of PTSD following RTAs

Study	Age Range	Number	Est. % PTSD	Time
Canterbury et al, 1993	8–16	28	<21	11 months
Heptinstall, 1996	7–16	20	50	4–6 months
DiGallo et al, 1997	5–18	57	14	12–15 weeks
Mirza et al, 1998	8–16	119	45	4–7 weeks
Ellis et al, 1998	6–16	45	44	4–7 months
Stallard. 1998	5–18	119	35	3–11 weeks

Incidence of PTSD following RTAs to Children

Our first pilot study was undertaken at a busy South London Accident and Emergency Department (Canterbury, Yule & Glucksman, 1993; Canterbury & Yule , 1997). We found that it was difficult to gain the cooperation of RTA survivors many months after the accidents, with many parents saying that while they were willing to participate, their child was still too upset and they did not want to upset them by reminding them of what happened. Thus, we knew that any estimate of the incidence of PTSD we made in this small sample was likely to be an underestimate. Even so, when we estimated a rate of just over 20%, we were more than surprised. Surely if there was this level of major stress reactions, it would have been spotted hitherto. But of course, once the child's immediate physical needs have been seen to, it is rare for them to be followed up and the brunt of emotional reactions are borne by families and schools, as well as by the children themselves.

Our assessment methodology was followed by Stallard & Law (1993) in their pioneering study of treating child survivors of a school bus crash. It was also built on by others such as the Child Accident Prevention Trust (Heptinstall, 1996) in their study of three large Accident and Emergency Departments catering for children. This latter study established that emotional consequences were widely reported following other types of accidents as well. Parents were mainly satisfied with the physical care their children received but were unprepared and largely unhelped to deal with the emotional aftermath.

Other British studies focusing on the incidence of PTSD following RTAs are summarized in Table 1. Rates vary slightly as do the intervals between the accident and the assessment, but it is evident that around 33% of children who survive a RTA – without the complication of a head injury – are likely to develop a post traumatic stress disorder. Other sequelae are also possible. Casswell (1997) also reports high scores on IES on a subsample of children who survived a school bus crash.

Table 2. Psychological Consequences of RTAs in Children

- Specific Fears of Travelling
- (Short Term) Adjustment Disorder
- Other Anxiety Disorders
- Bereavement Disorders
- P.T.S.D.

Psychological Consequences of RTAs in Children

It is important to remember that children react to threats and accidents in a variety of ways. In part, this depends on the nature and severity of the threat, and in part on individual characteristics of the child. Here, I will focus briefly on some of the major reactions to be considered in relation to RTAs.

Specific fears of travelling may develop. The child may refuse to go in cars or other forms of transport, thereby severely disrupting family life. They may show distress when in a car, or may be very wary of particular routes, being passed by other cars and so on. The link between the symptoms and the precipitating accident is usually evident. While parents may manage to alleviate the distress using common sense methods akin to systematic desensitization with its emphasis on gradual reintroduction to the feared situation, in many instances professional help will be required. To date, there are no studies of the incidence of specific fears following RTAs involving children.

(Short Term) Adjustment Disorders also appear to be quite common. The distress goes beyond a circumscribed fear of cars and spills over into more generalized sleep disturbance, fears of dying, poor concentration and so on. While strongly resembling PTSD, the symptoms are often either not sufficiently severe or not there in sufficient numbers to sustain a formal diagnosis of PTSD.

Other anxiety disorders may also develop. It may be that a subclinical problem gets exacerbated or that new ones emerge. Separation anxiety is common, especially in younger children. They need to be close to their parents for comfort, although this can be very irritating to the parents. Such separation problems may be part of a PTSD or exist in isolation. In one of my clinic cases, a 17 year old adolescent developed a manic disorder after a serious crash. There had been no prior history of mania and the disorder settled with treatment within six months.

Bereavement disorders are possible where someone died in the crash. Being faced with death is increasingly rare for children in most industrialized societies so that to witness the death of a loved one in a car crash can be doubly unsettling. Where the child may also have been injured and have to remain in hospital, then it is possible that they miss out on the grieving rituals surrounding a funeral and this can further complicate their recovery (see the case of Mary below).

Post Traumatic Stress Disorders in children are now far better understood than they were at the beginning of the 1980s. Until 15 years ago, it was widely accepted that children mainly responded to frightening events with transient distress and that not all children who experience a potentially traumatic event react with disabling stress reactions (Garmezy & Rutter, 1985). One reason for the underestimation of the effects of traumatic events on children was that the evidence was incomplete. Put simply, the bulk of the then existing evidence came from data provided by parents and teachers. Few investigators had done what is now so obvious – *they had not asked the children themselves!*

Post traumatic stress disorder (PTSD) was first officially recognised as a syndrome by the American Psychiatric Association in 1980. It was classified as an anxiety disorder and three major groups of symptoms were seen as holding together: distressing and recurring recollections of the traumatic event; avoidance of stimuli associated with the trauma; and a range of signs of increased physiological arousal (American Psychiatric Association, 1994).

Following a traumatic event, children often need to be close to their parents for comfort and reassurance. This clinginess is understandable, but often extremely irritating to parents who are not let out of their child's sight for weeks. Even teenagers may need to be reassured at night and often regress to sharing the parental bed. But the most troublesome symptom from the child's point of view can be the *intrusive images* of the event. These can occur at any time, day or night and are notable for their vividness. Usually, the child "sees" the event replaying over and over again, but this can be accompanied by repetitive memories in any of the sensory modalities – sound, smell, touch and motion. Occasionally, children will report that the experience is so vivid that they truly believe it is happening all over again. Such dissociative experiences are called *flashbacks*. Bad dreams and nightmares are also very common.

The intrusive images often come to the children as they are settling down for the night. So upsetting can they be that children will fight against sleep and try to stay awake. It is ironic that children who are extremely tired still try to remain awake with the obvious consequence that they become tired, irritable and unable to concentrate. The irritability can lead on to anger that can be difficult to deal with. Children develop fears, especially of stimuli that were present when the traumatic event happened. Thus, following the sinking of the Cruise Ship, "Jupiter", teenagers reported a marked increase in fears of drowning, water in general, death and travel (Yule, Udwin & Murdoch, 1990). Following road traffic accidents, children are likely to find it difficult to get back into cars for some time. Obviously, these fears have a survival value, but when present in extreme, they can disrupt the child's and family's life.

In the immediate aftermath of an accident, children sometimes experience a great pressure to talk about what happened. Then, they often find it difficult to talk, especially with parents and friends. Anecdotally, many children report that they do not want to upset their parents when they talk about what happened and so they keep their feelings to themselves. In such circumstances, being able to talk to someone outside the family has obvious potential benefit.

Survivors have learned that life is very fragile. This can lead to a loss of faith in the future or a *sense of foreshortened future*. Their priorities change. Some feel they should live each day to the full and not plan far ahead. Others realise they have been over-concerned with materialistic or petty matters and resolve to rethink their values. Their "assumptive world" has been challenged (Janoff-Bulman, 1985).

Adolescent survivors report significantly high rates of *depression,* some becoming clinically depressed, having suicidal thoughts and taking overdoses in the year after a disaster. A significant number become very *anxious* after accidents, although the appearance of *panic attacks* is sometimes considerably delayed. When children have been *bereaved*, they may need bereavement counselling.

Preschool children also develop distress that lasts beyond being an adjustment disorder and probably qualifies for the diagnosis of PTSD. In general, the DSM system is inadequate to reflect the stress reactions of very young children (Scheeringa et al, 1995; Almqvist & Brandell-Forsbrg, 1997) which include playing out the traumatic event repetitively, drawing it repetitively and more unfocused aggression (Misch, et al, 1993).

Treatment of PTSD

While there have been a number of single case reports of treatment of children suffering PTSD, as yet there are no accounts of randomized controlled studies. For the most part, treatment approaches are predominantly cognitive-behavioural and appear to consist of adaptations of approaches used with adults (Yule, 1991; Smith, Perrin & Yule, 1998).

Critical Incident Stress Debriefing techniques have been adapted for use with groups of children following a variety of traumas (Dyregrov, 1991). Such a structured crisis intervention approach was used with some children following the Jupiter sinking, with good effects on lowering the levels of

Table 3. Interventions for PTSD in Children

- Crisis Intervention
  - Critical Incident Stress Debriefing
  - Variations
- Group Treatments
- Individual Treatments
  - Cognitive Behaviour Therapy – Exposure
  - Eye Movement Desensitization and Reprocessing

Table 4. Three Recent Treatment Cases

Name	Age at RTA	Age at Treatment	No of Sessions	I.E.S	
				Pre	Post
Geoff	7	11	2*	32	2
David	9	12	4*	63	25 (0)
Mary	10	16	4**	43	15

* EMDR
** Bereavement work plus exposure in vivo

intrusion and of fears (Yule & Udwin, 1991). Stallard & Law (1993) used two debriefing sessions to reduce distress in girls who survived a school bus crash. Casswell (1997) also reports good results from debriefing following a school bus crash, although data were not systematically gathered.

Group treatments are obviously to be preferred as a first line of intervention when large numbers are involved. Gillis (1993) suggests that groups of 6 to 8 are optimum, and advises that separate groups should be run for boys and girls. However, different types of incident surely require different responses from professional (Galante & Foa, 1986; Yule & Williams, 1990) and it is too soon to pontificate on what should be a standard approach.

Individual treatment centres mainly on cognitive behavioural therapies that aim both to help the survivor make sense of what happened and to master their feelings of anxiety and helplessness. Drug treatments, as in the rest of child psychopathology, have little place. Asking children to draw their experiences can be useful in helping them recall both the event and the emotions associated with it (Blom, 1986; Newman, 1976; Galante & Foa; 1986; Pynoos & Eth, 1986) but merely drawing the trauma is not a sufficient therapy. A recent study from former Yugoslavia where great emphasis was placed on getting children to express their emotions through drawing found that six months after having had very structured sessions on drawing and other expressive techniques, there was no measurable change in children's adjustment on a whole range of self-report measures of stress reactions (Bunjevac & Kuterovac, 1994).

Saigh (1986) was one of the first to provide clinical evidence that, as Rachman (1980) had predicted, there were dangers in using standard systematic desensitization approaches as the length of exposure sessions may be too short to permit adequate habituation of anxiety. It should also be remembered that where children are frightened by the vividness of their memories then relaxation may only serve to intensify the vividness. The theoretical aspects of exposure therapy in treating PTSD in children are discussed elsewhere (Saigh, Yule & Inamdar, 1995) and other suggestions of techniques to promote emotional processing are described in Rachman (1980), Yule (1991), Richards & Lovell (1999) and Saigh (1992).

There is considerable interest and scepticism in Eye Movement and Desensitization and Reprocessing (EMDR) treatment (Shapiro, 1991). To date there are few published accounts of its use with children and adolescents, although claims for its value are being made on the conference circuit! As with all techniques that have no clear rationale, caution has to be exercised. However, if symptomatic relief can really be attained in a few brief sessions, then the approach needs to be carefully evaluated. Since there does seem to be a different quality to the memories of a trauma that appear at the same time to be locked in, vivid and unchangeable by merely talking about them, then any technique that will allow emotional processing to proceed must be examined. Some examples of using EMDR with child survivors of RTAs are given below.

Contingency planning: When trauma affects a large number of children at once, as in an accident at school, then a public health approach to dealing with the emergency is required (Pynoos, Goenjian & Steinberg, 1995). Schools need to plan ahead not only to deal with large scale disasters, but also to respond to the needs of children after threatening incidents that affect only a few of them. Thus, there are now a number of texts written especially for schools to help them develop contingency plans to deal with the effects of a disaster (Yule & Gold, 1993; Johnson, 1993; Klingman, 1993). The Child Accident Prevention Trust has recently published leaflets containing advice for professionals, parents and the children themselves describing the main emotional reactions to accidents and some of the first-aid that can be followed in the hope that emotional difficulties will not become serious (Child Accident Prevention Trust, 1998).

Case examples

Geoff was aged 7 when he was badly frightened in an unusual car accident. He was seated in the back seat of the car driven by his mother, waiting in a queue to enter a park when a car behind went out of control and hit their car, causing quite a bit of damage but no injury to the occupants. Three years later he was referred for treatment.

The car was hit on his side, and Geoff thought he was going to be badly hurt, if not killed. Shortly afterwards, Geoff started to have nightmares and kept waking in the night. There were times he was scared to sleep. He kept seeing pictures of the other car that hit them. He also developed a very strong fear of death.

When seen, he still had worries about travelling by car. He still saw recurring pictures of what happened and these were upsetting. His nightmares occurred at least once per week. In the nightmare, the car turns over and goes into a ditch full of water. They fall down and with that he usually woke up shouting, with the bedcovers all over the place. He has occasionally had flashbacks when it felt as if it was all happening all over again. He did not like watching programmes on television that involve car crashes. He felt shaky and scared.

He did not lose interest in hobbies nor revert to bed-wetting, but he often had to sleep in his parents' bed. He never felt emotionally cut off from other people. He felt that the accident had not really affected his future, although it may affect him when he is older and starts to drive.

Sleeping was a problem and he was waking up at least once a month. He denied being unduly irritable or having any concentration problems. He had become much more aware of dangers when he was in a car or walking on a pavement. He tried to stay in the middle of the seat when in the car.

He said that he did not feel miserable or depressed, but was anxious. He worried about death. He got upset by sudden loud noises. Geoff completed some questionnaires and scored as follows:

Scale	July	September
Impact of Event	32	2
Birleson Depression	14	6
Child Anxiety	21	1

There were no concerns about his development prior to the accident. It was followed immediately by the appearance of many symptoms of stress reactions and anxiety. As a direct consequence of the accident, Geoff developed a positive psychiatric disorder, namely a Post Traumatic Stress Disorder of moderate severity but which ran a chronic course and he still met criteria for the diagnosis three and a half years later.

Fortunately, following only two sessions of "Eye Movement Desensitization and Reprocessing", during which he recalled many details of the accident very vividly, there was a remarkable drop in the level of reported symptoms. His mother confirmed that he was greatly improved and he no longer met criteria for a diagnosis of PTSD.

David was aged 12 when first seen in our clinic, some three years after he had been involved in a road accident in which his grandmother was killed. In many ways, he was still grieving for her, as was his mother. He was haunted and upset by intrusive images of what happened when a car hit her right in front of him. He avoided talking about it and avoided going near the road where it happened. He fulfilled the formal criteria for a diagnosis of PTSD.

He was given four sessions of EMDR. He quickly focused on the accident and whilst he was upset at recalling some of the details, in fact he described many things graphically that he had seen, even seeing his grandmother lying on the road, blood coming out of her nose and mouth, and her false teeth lying nearby. As he recalled these images, so the subjective distress diminished rapidly. At follow-up three months later, he reported that he was sleeping well, had no intrusive images and was much less avoidant. His scores on the IES had gone from 63 to 25 to 0.

Mary was aged 15 when referred to our clinic, some 5 years after being in a car when her grandfather, who was driving, died at the wheel. The car crashed; she suffered a head injury and had to be hospitalised for ten days; she missed her grandfather's funeral. At evaluation, she had both a PTSD and a complex grief reaction. However, she declined the offer of treatment. She was re-referred a year later and accepted the offer of help.

I was in two minds whether to offer CBT or EMDR, when she announced that, following the diagnostic session, she knew what she had to do – she had to return to the scene of the crash and say goodbye properly to her grandfather. I supported her in this approach and although it took four sessions of reinforcing her resolve to go there, she managed it and, as her self-report questionnaires show, her symptoms largely resolved.

These are only illustrative cases and one cannot draw firm conclusions about the effectiveness of treatment from such small numbers. However, one can say that in some cases, even after 3 to 5 years after the accident, treatment can be effective and also fairly quick. I do not know whether I have unwittingly selected the appropriate treatment in each case but as the last case shows, I followed my maxim of listening to the child and following her lead.

A few other points can be made about these three cases before looking at general conclusions:

1. In my experience, solicitors are fairly good at sending me cases where the children do have an anxiety disorder, usually PTSD.
2. In many cases, the PTSD has lasted many years.
3. Whilst for legal reasons in cases of personal injury, solicitors are often concerned when bereavement reactions are mentioned (as such, they are not directly compensable under English law), these do occur and have to be dealt with.
4. I know of no evidence that non-directive counselling helps in cases of PTSD. Indeed, I have seen many cases where that has only prolonged the distress.
5. In these three cases, I did not have to involve the parents. However, particularly where the parents have also been involved in the accident, careful thought must be given as to how best to work with them. To date the evidence on how parental involvement affects the onset of PTSD is contradictory, with Ellis et al (1998) claiming that children whose parents were involved in the same accident were at highest risk, and Perrin et al (1996) finding the opposite.
6. There is general agreement that whatever the objective threat present in the accident, one of the most important factors in producing PTSD is whether the child thought he or she was going to die. It is important for clinicians to ask about this explicitly as often children are diffident about volunteering this worst fear.

General Conclusions

It is now well established that PTSD is a common reaction among children following RTAs. Other, predominantly anxiety reactions may also develop. PTSD can last for many years. Currently, few children and their families get help and advice on the emotional reactions they may develop. The scene is changing as the extent of the psychopathology is increasingly recognised and the psycho-educational leaflets produced by organizations such as the Child Accident Prevention Trust are greatly welcomed.

There is some evidence that early intervention helps. Despite the current controversy surrounding the effects of early intervention with adults following disasters, the few studies with children are more promising. However, there is no evidence that non-directive counselling and art therapy work at all.

To date, there are no random control trials of any form of treatment for children with PTSD, let alone PTSD following RTAs. Such evidence is urgently needed. Rather, evidence from single case studies, of the sort reported above and from uncontrolled interventions (Stallard & Law, 1993) indicate that interventions based on cognitive behavioural treatments, including EMDR, can help in some cases. As yet, it is far from clear which cases are helped by which treatment.

The role of the family remains unclear, but cannot be ignored. Further studies are required to establish whether the involvement of a parent in the same accident impedes or helps the child's recovery. Ways of helping parents to help their own children are also needed.

References

Almqvist, K. & Brandell-Forsberg, M. (1997). Refugee children in Sweden: Post-traumatic stress disorder in Iranian preschool children exposed to organized violence. *Child Abuse and Neglect, 21,* 351–366.

American Psychiatric Association (1993) *Diagnostic and Statistical Manual of Mental Disorders* (Fourth Edition). Washington, DC: APA

Blom, G.E. (1986) A school disaster – intervention and research aspects. *Journal of the American Academy of Child Psychiatry, 25*, 336–345.

Bunjevac, T. & Kuterovac, G. (1994) Report on the results of psychological evaluation of the art therapy program in schools in Hercegovina. Zagreb: UNICEF

Canterbury, R., Yule, W., & Glucksman, E. (1993) *PTSD in child survivors of road traffic accidents.* Paper presented to Third European Conference on Traumatic Stress, Bergen, 6–10 June 1993.

Canterbury, R. & Yule, W. (1997) The effects on children of road traffic accidents. Chapter 5 in M. Mitchell (Ed.) *The Aftermath of Road Traffic Accidents: Psychological, social and legal consequences of an everyday trauma.* London: Routledge (pages 59–69).

Casswell, G. (1997) Learning from the aftermath: The response of mental health workers to a school-bus crash. *Clinical Child Psychology and Psychiatry, 2,* 517–523.

Child Accident Prevention Trust (1998) *Providing emotional support to children and families after an accident.* Child Accident Prevention Trust, 18–20 Farringdon Lane, London E1R 3HA, UK.

DiGallo, A., Barton, J. & Parry-Jones, W. (1997) Road Traffic Accidents: Early psychological consequences in children and adolescents. *British Journal of Psychiatry, 170,* 358–362.

Dyregrov, A (1991) *Grief in Children: A Handbook for Adults.* London: Jessica Kingsley Publishers.

Ellis, A. J., Stores, G. & Mayou, R. A.(1998) Psychological consequences of road traffic accidents in children. *European Child and Adolescent Psychiatry, 7,* 61–68.

Galante, R. & Foa, D. (1986) An epidemiological study of psychic trauma and treatment effectiveness after a natural disaster. *Journal of the American Academy of Child Psychiatry, 25*, 357–363

Garmezy, N. & Rutter, M. (1985) Acute reactions to stress. In Rutter, M. & Hersov, L. (Eds.), *Child and Adolescent Psychiatry: Modern Approaches* (2nd Edition, pp. 152–176), Oxford, Blackwell.

Gillis, H. M. (1993) Individual and small-group psychotherapy for children involved in trauma and disaster. Chapter 9. In C.F. Saylor (Ed.), *Children and disasters.* (pp 165–186). New York: Plenum. .

Heptinstall, E. (1996) *Healing the Hidden Hurt: The emotional effects of children's accidents.* London: Child Accident Prevention Trust.

Janoff-Bulman, R. (1985) The aftermath of victimization: Rebuilding shattered assumptions. In C. R. Figley (Ed.), *Trauma and its Wake.* (Vol. 1). New York: Brunner/Mazel.

Johnson, K. (1993) *School crisis management: A Team Training Guide.* Alameda, CA: Hunter House.

Klingman, A. (1993) School-based intervention following a disaster. Chapter 10. In C. F. Saylor (Ed.), *Children and disasters.* (pp 187–210). New York: Plenum.

Mirza, K. A. H., Bhadrinath, B. R., Goodyer, I. & Gilmour, C.(1998) Post-traumatic stress disorder in children and adolescents following road traffic accidents – a preliminary study. *British Journal of Psychiatry, 172,* 443–447.

Misch, P., Phillips, M., Evans, P. & Berelowitz, M. (1993) Trauma in pre-school children: A clinical account. In G. Forrest (Ed) *Trauma and Crisis Management.* ACPP Occasional Paper.

Newman, C. J. (1976) Children of disaster: Clinical observation at Buffalo Creek. *American Journal of Psychiatry, 133*, 306–312.

Perrin, S., Yule, W. & Smith, P. (1996) Post Traumatic Stress in children as a foundation of sibling and parental exposure of the trauma. Paper presented at sympossium "Family influences on PTSD in children and adolescents." at Twelfth Annual Meeting of the International Society for Traumatic Stress Studies, San Francisco, November 1996.

Pynoos, R. S. & Eth, S. (1986) Witness to violence: The child interview. *Journal of the American Academy of Child Psychiatry, 25*, 306–319.

Pynoos, R. S., Goenjian, A. & Steinberg, A. M. (1995) Strategies of disaster interventions for children and adolescents. In S. E. Hobfoll and M. de Vries (Eds.), *Extreme Stress and Communities: Impact and Intervention.* Dordrecht, Netherlands: Kluwer

Rachman, S. (1980) Emotional processing. *Behaviour Research and Therapy, 18,* 51–60

Richards, D. & Lovell, K. (1999) Imaginal and in-vivo exposure in the treatment of PTSD. Chapter in Yule, W (Ed) *Post Traumatic Stress Disorder* Chichester: Wiley

Saigh, P. A. (1986). In vitro flooding in the treatment of a 6-yr-old boy's posttraumatic stress disorder. *Behaviour Research and Therapy, 24*, 685–688

Saigh, P. A. (1992) The behavioural treatment of child and adolescent posttraumatic stress disorder. *Advances in Behaviour Research and Therapy,* **14,** 247–275.

Saigh, P. A., Yule, W. & Inamdar, S. C. (1996) Imaginal flooding of traumatized children and adolescents. *Journal of School Psychology, 34*, 163–183.

Scheeringa, M. S., Zeanah, C. H., Drell, M. J. & Larrieu, J. A. (1995) Two approaches to the diagnosis of Posttraumatic Stress Disorder in infancy and early childhood. *Journal of the American Academy of Child and Adolescent Psychiatry, 34,* 191–200.

Shapiro, F. (1995) *Eye movement desensitization and reprocessing: Basic principles, protocols and procedures.* New York: The Guilford Press.

Smith, P. A. & Yule, W. (1999). Eye movement desensitization and reprocessing therapy (EMDR) and other rapid treatments. Chapter in Yule, W (Ed) *Post Traumatic Stress Disorder*. Chichester: Wiley

Smith, P., Perrin, S. & Yule, W. (1998) Post Traumatic Stress Disorders. Chapter in P. Graham (Ed.), *Cognitive Behaviour Therapy for Children and Families*. Cambridge Monograph Series in Child and Adolescent Psychiatry. Cambridge: Cambridge University Press.

Stallard, P. & Law, F. (1993) Screening and psychological debriefing of adolescent survivors of life-threatening events. *British Journal of Psychiatry, 163*, 660–665.

Stallard, P. (1998) The psychological consequences of everyday road traffic accidents. Paper presented to Conference: "*Road Accidents and the Mind*", 1–3 September, 1998; Bristol

Yule, W. (1991) Work with children following disasters. Chapter 20 in M. Herbert (Ed.), *Clinical Child Psychology: Social Learning, Development and Behaviour*. (pp.349–363). Chichester: John Wiley. .

Yule, W. & Gold, A. (1993) *Wise before the event: Coping with Crises in Schools*. London: Calouste Gulbenkian Foundation.

Yule, W. & Udwin, O. (1991) Screening child survivors for post-traumatic stress disorders: Experiences from the Jupiter sinking. *British Journal of Clinical Psychology, 30,* 131–138.

Yule, W., Udwin, O. & Murdoch, K. (1990) The Jupiter sinking: Effects on children's fears, depression and anxiety. *Journal of Child Psychology and Psychiatry, 31*, 1051–1061.

Yule, W. & Williams, R. (1990) Post traumatic stress reactions in children. *Journal of Traumatic Stress, 3,* 279–295.

25

Psychological Debriefing – Does it Work?

DR. JONATHAN I. BISSON BM MRCPsych Dip Clin Psychotherapy, Consultant Liaison Psychiatrist

Gabalfa Clinic, 213 North Road, Cardiff, CF4 3AG

Introduction

Attempts to prevent the development of psychological sequelae following traumatic events have focused on early intervention. These strategies are based on the hypothesis that the earlier intervention occurs, the less opportunity there is for maladaptive and disruptive cognitive (thinking) and behavioural patterns to become established (Rachman, 1980). Trauma psychology suggests that the majority of victims of severe trauma will experience some distressing experiences as they assimilate their experience. In 1983 Mitchell described Critical Incident Stress Debriefing as a semi-structured group intervention with emergency personnel. Others (e.g. Dyregrov, 1989) have described the process as Psychological Debriefing (PD) and the terms have come to be used interchangeably although there are some differences in the interventions (Rose, 1997). (The term PD will be used in this paper). In more recent years other workers have adapted the Mitchell/Dyregrov model to debrief individuals (e.g. Lee, Slade & Lygo, 1996; Hobbs, Mayou, Harrison & Warlock, 1996). It has been argued that PD should be used as one part of a comprehensive traumatic stress management programme but it has been widely used as a single session intervention.

A Psychological Debriefing (PD) is a semi-structured crisis intervention designed to prevent psychological sequelae following traumatic events by promoting emotional processing through the ventilation and normalisation of reactions and preparation for possible future experiences. Its purpose is to review the impressions and reactions of those involved shortly after a traumatic incident. It has been used with survivors, victims, emergency care workers and providers of psychological care. Its aim is to reduce immediate distress, prevent unwanted psychological sequelae, identify individuals' needs, facilitate engagement if future help is required and to provide support. The focus of a PD is on the present reactions to the traumatic event, psychiatric labelling is avoided and the emphasis is placed on normalisation. The participants are assured that they are normal people who have experienced an abnormal event.

Factors That May Affect Outcome

It has been suggested that PD may help to prevent avoidance behaviour, adoption of a sick role, isolation, enable individuals to recognise that they are not on their own with their experiences, offer the opportunity to release emotions in a "safe" setting, mobilise support systems and help an individuals' mind to emotionally process the trauma. A key hypothesis is that by "reliving" what actually happened the mind can habituate to the levels of distress this invokes (cf getting back on a horse having fallen off one). The risk is that in some individuals such reliving may increase distress and merely serve to retraumatise the individual. Other factors that may affect outcome include whether the PD occurs in an individual or group setting, how it is conducted and by whom. There may also be issues concerning the nature of the traumatic event under consideration (it was originally advocated for emergency workers in the USA who probably represent a very different population to road traffic accident victims in Bristol). Personality factors and the ways that individuals naturally deal with stressful situations may affect outcome (some individuals seem to cope better by talking about what happened, others enter a phase of denial which may be helpful to them). Proximity to the event may influence outcome as may medicalisation of what is essentially a normal reaction. For some individuals focusing on the trauma alone may not address some of their key emotional difficulties (e.g. when major traumatic events from the past have been reignited by a recent trauma).

Criticisms of PD

The routine use of early interventions following traumatic events has become widespread, fuelled by anecdotal reports of its effectiveness despite reviews of the literature cautioning against this (e.g. Raphael et al, 1995, Bisson & Deahl, 1994). It has also been argued that overzealous attempts to normalise emotional reactions following traumatic events may delay individuals presentation for more proactive treatment (McFarlane, 1989). Concerns have also been raised over individuals feeling forced to partake in PDs leading to resentment and the fact that debriefers may become traumatised themselves by the traumatic nature of the material discussed (Talbot, 1990). Finally, given the limited resources available to provide psychological input following traumatic events it would appear prudent to prioritise their use for interventions that have been shown to work.

Systematic Review of PD

Wessely, Rose & Bisson (1998) have recently completed a systematic review of all randomised controlled trials (RCTs) of psychological debriefing and other one off early interventions. A systematic review involves searching (through electronic databases, journals, articles and personal contacts for RCTs of an intervention (RCTs are widely accepted as being the most methodologically sound way of testing the effectiveness of a specific intervention). In the case of PD and other early interventions of one session only this involved searching for studies in which individuals who had been involved in a similar traumatic event were randomly allocated to receive PD/one session early intervention or no intervention at all. There are seven such studies currently published.

1. *Bunn & Clarke (1979)*. Bunn & Clarke studied 30 relatives of seriously ill/injured patients who had presented for treatment to a hospital in Australia less than twelve hours earlier. Half the relatives received twenty minutes of supportive counselling during which individuals were encouraged to express their feelings and concerns about the crisis, the others received nothing. Interview immediately after the counselling revealed the intervention group to be less anxious than the control group. A major problem with this study was the absence of proper follow-up and therefore no conclusions can be made about any lasting effect of the intervention.

2. Bordow & Porritt (1979). Bordow and Porritt studied 70 male victims of road traffic accidents who were treated at another hospital in Australia. Individuals were randomly allocated to no intervention, a one off immediate intervention described as "a structured interview to review the experience of injury and hospitalisation and the subject's emotional reactions to these" less than one week post trauma or to a more prolonged social work input over three months. Follow up interviews three months after the RTAs considering variables such as mood and anxiety revealed the social work group to fare better than the immediate intervention group which fared better than the no intervention group.

3. Hobbs, Mayou, Harrison & Warlock (1996). Hobbs and his colleagues studied 106 victims of road traffic accidents. They were randomised to no intervention or to individual PD which occurred 24 to 48 hours after the RTA. The PD combined a review of the traumatic experience, encouragement of emotional expression and promotion of cognitive processing of the event. Follow-up four months later using the Impact of Event Scale (IES) (Horowittz et al, 1979) and the Brief Symptom Inventory (Derogatis & Melisaratos, 1983) revealed the PD group to be faring slightly worse overall although the injury severity was higher in the PD group.

4. Lee, Slade & Lygo (1996). Lee and her colleagues considered women shortly after a miscarriage. Randomisation was to no intervention or individual PD based on the Mitchell and Dyregrov methods two weeks after the miscarriage. Follow-up at four months using the IES and the Hospital Anxiety and Depression Scale (HADS) (Zigmond & Snaith, 1983) revealed no difference in outcome between the groups. However, those who received the PD perceived it as being helpful as judged by a mean score of 74 on a 100mm scale from 0 (extremely unhelpful) to 100 (extremely helpful).

5. Stevens & Adshead (1996). Stevens and Adshead (in Hobbs & Adshead, 1996) studied individuals who presented to an Accident and Emergency Department following traumatic injury sustained through a road traffic accident, assault or a dog bite. Randomisation was to no intervention or to single session individual counselling which occurred less than 24 hours after the trauma. Follow-up at one week, one month and three months revealed no overall differences between the groups using the IES, Beck Depression Inventory (Beck et al, 1961) and the Spielberger Self Evaluation Questionnaire (Spielberger, 1983). A major drawback to this study was that individuals who became "unduly distressed" during the counselling session were excluded. This introduced bias in favour of the intervention group because individuals distressed during the session would be expected to do worse at follow-up.

6. *Bisson, Jenkins, Alexander & Bannister (1997)*. Bisson and his colleagues studied 130 acute burn trauma victims admitted to a regional burns unit. Individuals were randomly allocated to no intervention or to PD following Dyregrov's description adapted for individuals which occurred 2–19 days post burn trauma. Follow-up using the Clinician Administered PTSD Scale (Blake, Weathers & Nagy, 1990), a semi-structured interview and questionnaire measures of traumatic stress (the IES), anxiety and depression (the HADS) at three and thirteen months revealed the PD group to fare worse than the no intervention group. A limitation to this study was that the PD group were slightly more traumatised than the no intervention group. It was also found that level of initial distress was more predictive of outcome than the presence or absence of PD.

7. *Chemtob, Tomas, Law & Cremniter (1997)*. Chemtob and his colleagues combined single session group PD with education. The total intervention lasted five hours and was administered to secondary victims six and nine months after a hurricane. The intervention resulted in a significant reduction in IES scores which could not be accounted for by the passage of time. Unfortunately it is difficult to determine which component of the intervention was useful (PD, education or both). It is also difficult to compare the results of this study with other studies due to the time that had elapsed from the trauma to the intervention.

Other Studies

There are many anecdotal reports and open trials of PD and other one-off early interventions. Such reports are often very difficult to interpret and more susceptible to bias than RCTs. For this reason only three such studies will be considered. Robinson & Mitchell (1993) studied 172 emergency workers who were contacted two weeks after group PD. Sixty percent completed questionnaires and in common with other studies there was marked subjective evidence for the helpfulness of PD. Deahl, Gillham, Thomas, Searle & Srinivasan (1994) studied British regular soldiers who volunteered for war grave duty in the Gulf War. For operational reasons, only part of the sample received PD and so the rest formed the control group. Twenty (50%) of the PD sample reported that they had found the intervention helpful but psychological measures showed no significant difference between the PD and control group at 9 month follow-up. Kenardy et al (1996) performed a naturalistic study of 195 helpers following an earthquake in Australia. Sixty-two individuals were debriefed, the remaining 133 were not. There was no evidence of improved rate of recovery in either group according to psychological questionnaires on four occasions over the next two years.

Everly, Flannery & Mitchell (1998) have performed a non-systematic review of studies. They concluded positively about the effectiveness of debriefing although it is apparent that the studies quoted have significant shortcomings. Amongst the positive studies cited include Western Management Consultants in Canada who reported positively about a comprehensive Critical Incident Stress Management (CISM) programme for nurses. Twenty four percent of those involved in a PD reported a decline in personnel turnover and 99% reported a decline in sick leave days. Dyregrov (1998) anecdotally reported similar experiences with PD as part of a CISM programme in Norway and commented that the effectiveness seemed related to the experience of the facilitator.

Conclusions

The studies discussed vary greatly in their quality but overall the quality of the studies is poor. Common methodological shortcomings include small sample size, lack of randomisation, lack of control group, varying degrees of trauma, other confounding variables ignored, low response rates, sampling bias, lack of uniformity of intervention and timing variance. Overall the studies provide little evidence that PD or other one-off early psychological intervention for individuals prevents psychopathology following trauma despite it being well received overall by participants. Some negative outcomes following individual PD were found but overall the impact of the single early psychological interventions when considered collectively was neutral. At present the routine use of PD can not be advocated nor can it be argued that PD should be discontinued as a possible intervention following trauma. Indeed it can be strongly argued that there should be some form of early intervention to provide support, education and screening to detect those individuals who may benefit from more complex intervention. There is an urgent need for randomised controlled trials especially of group PD as part of a Critical Incident Stress Management Programme and of more complex early interventions.

References

Beck, A., Ward, C., Mendelson, M., Mock, J. & Erbaugh, J. (1961). An Inventory for Measuring Depression. *Archives of General Psychiatry*, *4*, 561–571.

Bisson, J. & Deahl, M. (1994). Psychological Debriefing and Prevention of Post-traumatic Stress – More Research is Needed. *British Journal of Psychiatry, 165*, 717–720.

Bisson, J., Jenkins, P., Alexander, J. & Bannister, C. (1997). A Randomised Controlled Trial of Psychological Debriefing for Victims of Acute Burn Trauma. *British Journal of Psychiatry*, *171*, 78–81.

Blake, D. D., Weathers, F. W. & Nagy, A. G. Y. (1990). A Clinician Rating Scale for Assessing Current and Life-time PTSD: the CAPS-1. *Behaviour Therapist*, *18*, 187–188.

Bordow, S. & Porritt, D. (1979). An Experimental Evaluation of Crisis Intervention. *Social Science and Medicine*, *13*, 251–256.

Bunn. T. & Clarke. A. (1979). Crisis Intervention: An Experimental Study of the Effects of a Brief Period of Counselling on the Anxiety of Relatives of Seriously Injured or Ill Hospital Patients. *British Journal of Medical Psychology*, *52*, 191–195.

Chemtob, C. Tomas, S., Law, W. & Cremniter, D. (1997). Postdisaster psychosocial interventions: a field study of the impact of debriefing on psychological distress. *American Journal of Psychiatry*, *154*, 415–417.

Deahl, M., Gillham, A., Thomas, J., Searle, M. & Scrinivasan, M. (1994). Psychological Sequelae Following the Gulf War-Factors Associated with Subsequent Morbidity and the Effectiveness of Psychological Debriefing. *British Journal of Psychiatry*, *165*, 60–65.

Derogatis, I. & Melisaratos, N. (1983). The Brief Symptom Inventory: An Introductory Report. *Psychological Medicine*, *3*, 595–605.

Dyregrov, A. (1989). Caring for Helpers in Disaster Situations: Psychological Debriefing. *Disaster Management*, *2*, 25–30.

Dyregrov, A. (1998). Psychological debriefing – an effective method? *Traumatologyc*, 4, Article 1.

Everly, G. S., Flannery, R. B. & Mitchell, J. T. (1998). Critical Incident Stress Management (CISM): A Review of the Literature. In Press.

Hobbs, M. & Adshead, G. (1996). Preventive Psychological Intervention for Road Crash Survivors. In Mitchell, M., (ed) *The aftermath of road accidents: psychological, social and legal perspectives*. (pp. 159–171). Routledge, London, UK.

Hobbs, M., Mayou, R., Harrison, B. & Warlock, P. (1996). A Randomised Trial of Psychological Debriefing for Victims of Road Traffic Accidents. *British Medical Journal*, *313*, 1438–1439.

Horowitz, M., Wilner, N. & Alvarez, W. (1979). Impact of Events Scale: A Measure of Subjective Stress. *Psychosomatic Medicine*, *41*, 209–218.

Kenardy, J., Webster, R., Lewin, T., Carr, V., Hazell, P. & Carter, G. (1996). Stress debriefing and patterns of recovery following a natural disaster. *Journal of Traumatic Stress*, *9*, 37–49.

Lee, C., Slade, P. & Lygo, V. (1996). The Influence of Psychological Debriefing on Emotional Adaption in Women following Early Miscarriage: A Preliminary Study. *British Journal of Medical Psychology*, *69*, 47–58.

McFarlane, A. (1989). The prevention and management of the psychiatric morbidity of natural disasters: an Australian experience. *Stress Medicine*, *5*, 29–30.

Mitchell, J. T. (1983). When Disaster Strikes.... *Journal of Emergency Medical Services*, *8*, 36–39.

Rachman, S. (1980). Emotional Processing *Behaviour Research and Therapy*, *18*, 51–60.

Raphael, B., Meldrum, L. & McFarlane, A. C. (1995). Does Debriefing after Psychological Trauma Work? *British Medical Journal*, *310*, 1479–1480.

Robinson, R. & Mitchell, J.T. (1993). Evaluation of Psychological Debriefings. *Journal of Traumatic Stress*, *6*, 367–382.

Rose, S. (1997). Psychological Debriefing: History and Methods. *Counselling–The Journal of the British Association of Counselling*, *8*, 48–51.

Spielberger, C. (1983). *The State Trait Anxiety Questionnaire: A Comprehensive Bibliography*. Palo Alto, California Consultant Psychologist Press, USA.

Talbot, A. (1990). The importance of parallel process in debriefing crisis counsellors. *Journal of Traumatic Stress*, *3*, 265–277.

Wessely S., Rose S. & Bisson J. (1998) *A Systematic Review of Brief Psychological Interventions ('debriefing') for the Treatment of Immediate Trauma Related Symptoms and the Prevention of Posttraumatic Stress Disorder*. The Cochrane Library, published on CD-ROM Update Software Inc, CA, USA and Oxford, UK.

Zigmond, A. S. & Snaith, R. P. (1983). The Hospital Anxiety and Depression Score. *Acta Psychiatrica Scandinavia*, *67*, 361–370.

26

A Cognitive Approach to the Understanding and Treatment of Posttraumatic Stress Disorder

PROF. DR. ANKE EHLERS, Wellcome Trust Principal Research Fellow

Department of Psychiatry, University of Oxford, UK

In the immediate aftermath of traumatic events such as road traffic accidents (RTA), many people experience some of the symptoms of posttraumatic stress disorder (PTSD), including involuntary reexperiencing of aspects of the event, hyperarousal, or loss of interest in previously significant activities. About half of the people who initially develop PTSD recover within the first year after a road traffic accident (RTA, e.g., Blanchard et al., 1997; Ehlers et al., 1998b). It is estimated that a third of the people who develop PTSD after a traumatic event will not recover for many years (Kessler et al., 1995). This raises the question of what factors determine the persistence of PTSD symptoms in these individuals. The present chapter reviews our group's cognitive approach to this question, and studies that have tested predictions and treatment procedures derived from this approach.

A Cognitive Model of Persistent PTSD

Ehlers & Clark (in press) suggested that persistent PTSD occurs only if individuals process the traumatic experience in a way which produces a sense of a serious current threat. Once activated, the perception of current threat is accompanied by intrusions and other reexperiencing symptoms, symptoms of arousal, and strong emotions such as anxiety, anger, shame or sadness. The model proposes that two key processes lead to a sense of current threat.

First, it is suggested that individual differences in the personal meaning (appraisal) of the trauma and its sequelae determine whether persistent PTSD develops. Some people are able to see the trauma as a time-limited terrible experience that does not necessarily have negative implications for the future, and may also be able to find some element of personal growth in it. These people are likely to recover quickly. Individuals with persistent PTSD are characterized by excessively negative appraisals of the event and/or its sequelae.

Second, it is suggested that the trauma memory differs from other autobiographical memories. Autobiographical memories are normally organised in a way that prevents triggering of very vivid and emotional reexperiencing of an event. Recall is driven by themes and personal time periods, and it is relatively abstract (Conway, 1997). Ehlers & Clark (in press) propose that trauma memories do not have this level of organisation. The traumatic event is insufficiently elaborated at the time of the trauma, so that the resulting memory is inadequately integrated into its context in time, place, subsequent and previous information, and other autobiographical memories. At the same time, stimuli that occurred during the traumatic event are perceptually primed (i.e. the threshold for their perception is reduced) and, by classical conditioning, associated with strong affective responses. Because of the nature of the trauma memory, retrieval is mainly cue-driven. Stimuli that bear resemblance to those occurring shortly before and during the traumatic event trigger reexperiencing symptoms, and the threat that the person experienced during the event is reexperienced as if it was happening right now rather than being a memory from the past.

Why do the negative appraisals and nature of trauma memory persist? It is proposed that the negative appraisals prompt a series of dysfunctional cognitive and behavioural responses that have the short-term aim of reducing distress, but have the long-term consequence of preventing cognitive change and therefore maintain the disorder. Ehlers & Clark (in press) propose that these behaviours and cognitive strategies maintain PTSD in three ways. First, some behaviours directly lead to increases in symptoms, e.g., thought suppression leads to paradoxical increases in intrusion frequency. Second, other behaviours prevent changes in the problematic appraisals, e.g., constantly checking one's rear mirror (a safety behaviour) after a car accident prevents change in the appraisal that another accident will happen if one does not check the mirror. Third, other behaviours prevent elaboration of the trauma memory and its link to other experiences. For example, avoiding thinking about the event prevents people from incorporating the fact that they did not die into the trauma memory, and they thus continue to reexperience the fear of dying they originally experienced during the event.

Negative Appraisals of the Traumatic Event and/or its Sequelae

Effect of trauma on beliefs about the self and the world

A traumatic event threatens the person's view of the self and the world. Several theorist propose that this threat to basic inner models is at the core of PTSD, or of responses to trauma in general (e.g., Ehlers & Clark, in press; Foa & Riggs, 1993; Janoff-Bulman, 1992; Horowitz, 1976; Resick & Schnicke, 1993). For example, Janoff-Bulman (1992) proposed that traumatic events "*shatter*" previously held beliefs (e.g., "The world is a safe place"), and that post-trauma adjustment requires rebuilding of basic beliefs about the self and the world. Foa & Riggs (1993) and Resick & Schnicke (1993) have pointed out that PTSD is quite often associated with a *confirmation* of previously held negative beliefs rather than shattering of positive beliefs (e.g., "Bad things always happen to me") and that recovery requires the modification of these beliefs. Several studies have found empirical evidence for a relationship between PTSD and negative beliefs concerning the self and the world (Dunmore et al., 1997, 1999; Resick et al., 1991; Wenninger & Ehlers, 1998). In a prospective study of assault victims, such negative beliefs predicted persistence of PTSD (Dunmore et al., 1998).

Appraisals of trauma sequelae

Appraisals of trauma sequelae have been a particular research interest of our group. We assumed that the power of appraisal processes in predicting persistent PTSD can be enhanced if trauma sequelae are included.

Appraisal of PTSD symptoms. Ehlers & Steil (1995) observed that people differ widely in the meaning they assign to the occurrence and content of intrusive recollections of traumatic events. Whereas many individuals see them as a normal part of recovery from an upsetting event, others interpret them in a more negative way, for example as an indication that they are going mad. Ehlers & Steil (1995) proposed that such negative interpretations are important in explaining the maintenance of intrusive recollections and PTSD in general because they determine: (1) how distressing the intrusions are; (2) the extent to which the patient engages in strategies to control the intrusions which then prevent change in meaning of the trauma and posttraumatic intrusions. They provided evidence for these hypotheses in correlational studies of RTA victims (Steil & Ehlers, in press) and of ambulance workers (Clohessy & Ehlers, 1999), and in a large-scale prospective longitudinal study of 967 RTA survivors (Ehlers et al., 1998b). The latter study found that negative interpretations of intrusive memories were among the most important predictors of PTSD severity at 1 year after the accident. They predicted PTSD severity over and above what could be predicted from symptom severity at 3 months.

People with persistent PTSD do not only interpret intrusive memories in a negative way, but also other PTSD symptoms such as irritability (e.g., "I will lose control and harm somebody"), poor concentration (e.g., "I must have a brain injury"), or emotional numbing (e.g., "Feeling numb means that I will never have normal emotions again"). In a series of studies of assault victims, Dunmore et al. (1997, 1998, 1999) found that such negative interpretations of PTSD symptoms, including interpretations of intrusive memories, were related to PTSD severity, and were among the most important predictors of persistence of PTSD. Similarly, in a recent study that we conducted in collaboration with Foa's group in Philadelphia, negative interpretation of PTSD symptoms distinguished between trauma survivors (many of whom had experienced accidents) with and without PTSD (Foa et al., in press).

Appraisal of other people's responses. Many people with persistent PTSD describe that others responded in a negative way after the traumatic event, or that their responses were less supportive than expected. For example, a RTA survivor was very distressed because she had felt that the hospital staff was uncaring and she had felt left alone when in hospital. She interpreted this experience as meaning "Nobody is there for me". Sometimes, well-meant or positive behaviours can also be interpreted by the traumatized individual in a negative way. For example, another RTA survivor interpreted her friend's offer to help her after the accident as meaning that the friend thought she was unable to cope on her own. Studies have shown that such negative appraisals of others' responses are related to PTSD, and that they predict the persistence of PTSD (Dunmore et al., 1997, 1998, 1999).

Perceived negative responses of other people or a perceived inability to relate to others after trauma can give rise to an overall feeling of alienation. We have found that an overall feeling of alienation impedes recovery in rape victims and in survivors of torture (Ehlers et al., 1998a; Ehlers et al., in press). Furthermore, alienation is related to PTSD in trauma survivors, including those who have experienced RTAs (Foa et al., in press).

Perceived permanent change. Traumatic events can have long-term negative consequences. For example, many RTA survivors suffer long-term physical problems such as pain and financial hardship. Persistent health problems were among the most important predictors of persistent PTSD after RTA (Blanchard et al., 1997; Ehlers et al., 1998b; Mayou et al., 1993, 1997), and were more important in predicting persistent PTSD than injury severity. Some traumatized individuals interpret such longstanding problems that result from the trauma as meaning that their lives were destroyed completely. Others interpret their initial reactions to the trauma, including the initial PTSD symptoms, as indicating a permanent change for the worse in their personality. Such perceived permanent change predicted PTSD studies of assault and torture victims (Dunmore et al., 1997, 1998; 1999; Ehlers et al., in press). It was related to PTSD in people who had experienced a wide range of trauma including RTA (Foa et al., in press) and to poor outcome in exposure treatment of rape victims (Ehlers et al., 1998a).

Assessment of problematic appraisals of the traumatic event and its sequelae

On the basis of the studies described above, we have developed a comprehensive questionnaire, in collaboration with Foa's group, that assesses problematic appraisals of the traumatic event and its sequelae. The 33-item Post-traumatic Cognitions Inventory (PTCI) had very good internal consistency and test-retest reliability, and showed good sensitivity (.78) and excellent specificity (.93) in discriminating trauma survivors with and without PTSD. In comparison, the World Assumptions Scale that Janoff-Bulman developed to test the shattering of beliefs hypothesis (Janoff-Bulman, 1992), only had specificity of .26 (Foa et al., in press).

Nature of the Trauma Memory

Memory in PTSD is rather puzzling. On the one hand, patients with persistent PTSD often have difficulty in intentionally retrieving a complete memory of the traumatic event. Their *intentional* recollection is fragmented, details may be missing, and they have difficulty recollecting the temporal order of events (e.g., Foa & Riggs, 1993; Amir et al., 1998; Koss et al., 1996;

van der Kolk & Fisler, 1995). On the other hand, there is evidence that in some respects they appear to have a strong memory for the trauma. In particular, they *involuntarily* reexperience aspects of the trauma in a very vivid and emotional way. In addition, many patients with persistent PTSD show a phenomenon which we have called "affect without recollection" (Ehlers & Clark, in press). This refers to the triggering of intense affect by the presence of stimuli that were associated with the trauma, without simultaneous recollection of the traumatic event. For example, a PTSD patient who had experienced a severe car accident reported that he became extremely anxious and felt something terrible was going to happen when riding on a train (he was not at all afraid of traveling by train). At the time, he was not able to put his finger on what triggered the anxiety. Only afterwards he realised that he had heard a baby cry shortly before he became anxious. The pitch of the baby's voice was the same as that of the sound of the impact during his accident. At the time he became anxious on the train, he was not aware of this link and did not recall the accident.

In order to explain these rather puzzling phenomena, Ehlers & Clark (in press) have suggested that part of the problem in persistent PTSD may be a dissociation in memory with poor initial elaboration leading to weak intentional recall (explicit memory) and retrieval being dominated by the basic memory mechanisms that operate through cue-driven retrieval (implicit memory), as outlined above. This could explain, (1) the nature of intrusions (strong sensory impressions with the original emotions and a 'here and now' quality), (2) easy cuing of intrusions by stimuli that may have been temporarily associated with the trauma, even if they do not have a strong meaning link, and (3) the fragmented nature of recall.

In a preliminary test of Ehlers & Clark's (in press) model, Ehlers et al. (in prep.) presented students with a sequence of three pictures which made up a story. The initial pictures were neutral and the last picture showed either a traumatic or a neutral outcome of the story. In a trauma sequence, the first picture shows a woman standing by a table with a drinking glass and a table lamp. The next picture shows a man's hands holding a bathrobe cord and the final picture shows the woman strangled. In a parallel neutral sequence, the first picture is rather similar but the final picture shows a woman looking thoughtful after making a telephone call. Following presentation of the 'picture stories', memory for objects shown in the initial pictures was assessed in two different ways. First, in order to assess perceptual priming (implicit memory), participants were presented with blurred objects and asked to identify them. Some of the objects had been presented in the "stories" and others had not. Perceptual priming would be evidenced by better identification of the objects that had been presented. Second, explicit memory was assessed by asking participants to recognise non-blurred objects from the story pictures within a set of similar distractor objects. There were no differences in explicit memory between objects from the traumatic and non-traumatic stories. However, as predicted, perceptual priming was better for the objects shown in the trauma stories. To assess whether enhanced perceptual priming (implicit memory) might be plausibly linked to PTSD-like symptomatology, participants in the experiment were followed up after four months and asked whether they had any unwanted intrusive recollections of the material that had been presented within the experiment. As predicted, there was a significant positive association between perceptual priming for objects from traumatic stories and the presence of subsequent intrusions.

The promising preliminary results obtained in this analogue experiment study have recently been extended in a larger scale, naturalistic, prospective study of road traffic accident victims. This study focussed on fragmentation of intentional recall and found that degree of memory fragmentation predicted PTSD at both one month and six months post accident (Murray et al., in prep.). Other experiments are underway to more rigorously test the suggestion that PTSD symptomatology is partly a result of a dissociation between explicit and implicit memory processes.

Behaviours and Cognitive Responses that Maintain PTSD

It is well known from research on phobias that *avoidance behaviour* maintains anxiety disorders. Several studies have demonstrated that avoidance also plays a crucial role in maintaining PTSD (e.g., Bryant & Harvey, 1995; Dunmore et al., 1998). Avoidance includes situational avoidance, e.g., of places, people, conversations, and other stimuli that remind the individual of the trauma, and cognitive avoidance, i.e. efforts not to think about the trauma. Situational avoidance is not restricted to avoidance of reminders of the traumatic event. People who perceived negative responses from others in the aftermath of the event, or those who feel that other people will not understand their response to the trauma, often withdraw from a wide range of social situations. This has the negative effect that they are less likely to receive social support, to correct negative beliefs about themselves and others, and to benefit from the therapeutic effects of talking about their emotions with others (e.g., Pennebaker, 1989), and thus contributes to the maintenance of PTSD.

Even if there is no obvious situational avoidance, people with PTSD commonly show subtle avoidance behaviours ("*safety behaviours*") that prevent change of problematic appraisals, and maintain anxiety. For example, a RTA survivor who had been trapped in her car after the accident because her seat belt could not be opened, kept checking whether her seat belts were still functioning. This prevented her from testing the appraisal "If I do not check my seat belt, I will be trapped again". Other common safety behaviours in RTA survivors include driving very slowly, stepping on the brakes repeatedly, checking the mirrors repeatedly, or holding onto one's seat. In line with their hypothesized role in maintaining PTSD, safety behaviours predicted persistent PTSD in a prospective longitudinal study of assault victims (Dunmore et al., 1998).

Several authors have pointed out that maintenance of PTSD cannot be solely explained by avoidance, and have suggested that cognitive responses play a crucial role (e.g., Ehlers & Steil, 1995; Foa & Riggs, 1993; Horowitz, 1976).

Research on the effects of *thought suppression* (e.g., Wegner, 1989) suggests that efforts to suppress memories of the traumatic event may increase their frequency (Ehlers & Steil, 1995). Two studies of RTA survivors and a study of ambulance workers (Clohessy & Ehlers, 1999; Steil & Ehlers, in press), found that suppression of memories of the traumatic event was related to PTSD. These retrospective findings were confirmed in a prospective longitudinal study of RTA survivors. Suppression of memories assessed at 3 months after the accident predicted PTSD severity at 1 year (Ehlers et al., 1998b). Furthermore, recent experimental studies demonstrated that thought suppression increased the frequency of trauma-related intrusions in RTA and rape survivors (Harvey & Bryant, 1998; Shepherd & Beck, 1999), and in volunteers who had seen a traumatic film (Davies & Clark, 1998).

People with PTSD commonly *ruminate* about aspects of the traumatic event and its sequelae (e.g., "*if only* the accident had not happened or I had done something differently", or why did it happen to me?). Rumination appears to play a role in maintaining PTSD. Steil and Ehlers (in press), and Clohessy & Ehlers (1999) showed that rumination about intrusive memories correlated with PTSD severity in RTA survivors and ambulance workers. Warda & Bryant (1998) showed that rumination distinguished between RTA survivors with and without acute stress disorder, a precursor of PTSD. In several prospective studies of RTA survivors, rumination was one of the most important predictors of PTSD, and of delayed onset of PTSD (Ehlers et al., 1998b; Murray et al., in prep.). At this stage, it is unclear what exactly the mechanisms are by which rumination maintains PTSD. It probably strengthens problematic appraisals of the trauma (e.g., The trauma has ruined my life), and is probably similar to cognitive avoidance in interfering with the formation of a more complete trauma memory because it focuses on "what if . . ." questions rather than on the experience of the trauma itself. Finally, it may also directly increase feelings of nervous tension, dysphoria, or hopelessness, and, because it provides internal retrieval cues, intrusive memories of the traumatic event.

Some of the cognitive processes that maintain PTSD symptoms are not intentional. Patients with PTSD have an *unintentional attentional bias* to stimuli that are reminiscent of the traumatic event (see McNally, in press, for a review). Involuntary selective attention to reminders may be one of the reasons why these patients have frequent reexperiencing symptoms.

Dissociation is another yet poorly understood cognitive style that interferes with recovery in PTSD. Both, dissociation during the traumatic event and when reminded of the trauma seem to play a role in PTSD. Dissociation is defined as a "disruption of the usually integrated feelings of consciousness, memory, identity, or perception of the environment" (American Psychiatric Association, 1994, p. 477). As the definition suggests, dissociation is a complex process that has several components, e.g., feelings of derealisation and depersonalisation, emotional numbing, and distorted time perception. Dissociation can occur as an unintentional response to extreme distress, but can also represent a habitual response to stress that can be intentionally activated. Several prospective longitudinal studies that included large numbers of RTA survivors have found that dissociation during and shortly after a traumatic event predicts PTSD (Ehlers et al., 1998b; Murray et al., in prep.; Shalev et al., 1996). Continuing dissociation in response to intrusive memories was a predictor of persistence of PTSD in prospective studies of RTA survivors (Murray et al., in prep.). It remains to be studied what mechanisms underlie the relationship between dissociation and PTSD. Aspects of dissociation may be related to the way the trauma is laid down in memory (Ehlers & Clark, in press; Foa & Hearst-Ikeda, 1996; van der Kolk & Fisler, 1995).

A Cognitive-Behavioural Treatment of PTSD

Imaginal reliving, combined with in vivo exposure to reminders of the traumatic event, is an effective treatment of PTSD (Foa & Meadows, 1997; Foa & Rothbaum, 1998). However, the treatment is stressful and not acceptable to all patients. On the basis of the Ehlers & Clark (in press) model, our group has developed a version of cognitive-behavioural treatment that integrates imaginal reliving with cognitive therapy techniques such as modification of dysfunctional appraisals of the trauma and initial symptoms, restructuring of images, and thought suppression experiments. By using cognitive therapy methods to change problematic appraisals of the trauma and its sequelae directly, we were able to reduce the number of imaginal reliving sessions substantially. In a pilot study of the treatment, 20 consecutive cases (many of whom had experienced traffic accidents) received a mean of eight weekly treatment sessions plus two booster sessions over the next three months (Ehlers, 1998). Only three of the sessions included some imaginal reliving. The treatment was effective. At the end of treatment eighteen (90% of the original sample) no longer met diagnostic criteria for PTSD. One patient dropped out, and one improved substantially, but continued to meet diagnostic criteria. The treatment is currently being evaluated in two randomized controlled trials to test whether the promising results can be replicated.

References

American Psychiatric Association (1994). *Diagnostic and statistical manual of mental disorders* (4th ed.). Washington, DC: Author.

Amir, N., Stafford, J., Freshman, M.S. & Foa, E.B. (1998). Relationship between trauma narratives and trauma pathology. *Journal of Traumatic Stress, 11*, 385–392.

Blanchard, E. B., Hickling, E. J., Barton, K. A., Taylor, A. E., Loos, W. R. & Jones-Alexander, J. (1996). One-year prospective follow-up of motor vehicle accident victims. *Behaviour Research and Therapy, 34*, 775–786.

Bryant, R. B. & Harvey, A. G. (1995) Avoidant coping style and post-traumatic stress disorder following motor vehicle accidents. *Behaviour Research and Therapy, 33*, 631–635.

Clohessy, S. & Ehlers, A. (1999). PTSD symptoms, response to intrusive memories, and coping in ambulance service workers. *British Journal of Clinical Psychology, 38*, 251–265.

Conway, M. A. (1997). Introduction: What are memories? In M.A. Conway (Ed.), *Recovered memories and false memories* (pp. 1–22). Oxford, UK: Oxford University Press.

Davies, M. I. & Clark, D.M. (1998). Thought suppression produces a rebound effect with analogue post-traumatic intrusions. *Behaviour Research and Therapy, 36*, 571–582.

Dunmore, E., Clark, D. M. & Ehlers, A. (1997). Cognitive factors in persistent versus recovered post-traumatic stress disorder after physical or sexual assault: a pilot study. *Behavioural and Cognitive Psychotherapy, 25*, 147–159.

Dunmore, E., Clark, D. M. & Ehlers, A. (1998, July). *The role of cognitive factors in posttraumatic stress disorder following physical or sexual assault: findings from retrospective and prospective investigations.* Paper presented at Annual Conference of British Association of Behavioural and Cognitive Therapies. Durham, UK.

Dunmore, E., Clark, D.M. & Ehlers, A. (1999). Cognitive factors involved in the onset and maintenance of posttraumatic stress disorder after physical or sexual assault. *Behaviour Research and Therapy.*

Ehlers, A. (1998, July). *Posttraumatic stress disorder: A cognitive approach to understanding an treatment.* Keynote address presented at Annual Conference of British Association of Behavioural and Cognitive Therapies. Durham, UK.

Ehlers, A. & Clark, D. M. (in press). A cognitive model of persistent posttraumatic stress disorder. *Behaviour Research and Therapy.*

Ehlers, A., Clark, D. M., Dunmore, E. B., Jaycox, L., Meadows, E. & Foa, E.B. (1998a). Predicting response to exposure in PTSD: The role of mental defeat and alienation. *Journal of Traumatic Stress, 11*, 457–471.

Ehlers, A., Maercker, A. & Boos, A. (in press). PTSD following political imprisonment: The role of mental defeat, alienation, and perceived permanent change. *Journal of Abnormal Psychology.*

Ehlers, A., Mayou, R. A. & Bryant, B. (1998b). Psychological predictors of chronic posttraumatic stress disorder after motor vehicle accidents. *Journal of Abnormal Psychology, 107*, 508–519.

Ehlers, A., Michael, T. & Chen, Y.P. (in preparation). *Perceptual priming for stimuli that occur in a traumatic context.*

Ehlers, A. & Steil, R. (1995). Maintenance of intrusive memories in posttraumatic stress disorder: a cognitive approach. *Behavioural and Cognitive Psychotherapy, 23,* 217–249.

Foa, E., Ehlers, A., Clark, D. M., Tolin, D. F. & Orsillo, S. M. (in press). The post-traumatic cognitions inventory (PTCI): development and validation. *Psychological Assessment.*

Foa, E. B. & Hearst-Ikeda, D. (1996). Emotional dissociation in response to trauma: An information-processing approach. In L. K. Michelson & W. J. Ray (Eds.), *Handbook of dissociation: Theoretical, empirical, and clinical perspectives.* New York: Plenum Press.

Foa, E. B. & Riggs, D.S. (1993). Post-traumatic stress disorder in rape victims. In J. Oldham, M. B. Riba & A. Tasman (Eds.), *Annual review of psychiatry.* Vol. 12 (pp. 273–303). Washington, DC: American Psychiatric Association.

Foa, E. B. & Meadows, E. A. (1997). Psychosocial treatments for posttraumatic stress disorder: A critical review. *Annual Review of Psychology, 48,* 449–480.

Foa, E. B. & Rothbaum, B. O. (1998). *Treating the trauma of rape: a cognitive-behavioural treatment manual for PTSD.* New York: Guilford.

Harvey, A. G. & Bryant, R. A. (1998). The effect of attempted thought suppression in acute stress disorder. *Behaviour Research and Therapy, 36,* 583–590.

Horowitz, M. J. (1976). *Stress response syndromes.* New York: Aronson.

Janoff-Bulman, R. (1992). *Shattered assumptions: Towards a new psychology of trauma.* New York: The Free Press.

Kessler, R. C., Sonnega, A., Bromet, E., Hughes, M. & Nelson, C. B. (1995). Posttraumatic stress disorder in the National Comorbidity Survey. *Archives of General Psychiatry, 52,* 1048–1060.

Koss, M. P., Figueredo, A. J., Bell, I., Tharan, M. & Tromp, S. (1996). Traumatic memory characteristics: a cross-validated mediational mode of response to rape among employed women. *Journal of Abnormal Psychology, 105,* 421–432.

Mayou, R. A., Bryant, B. & Duthie, R. (1993). Psychiatric consequences of road traffic accidents. *British Medical Journal, 307,* 647–651.

Mayou, R. A., Tyndel, S. & Bryant, B. (1997). Long term outcome of motor vehicle accident injury. *Psychosomatic Medicine, 59,* 578–584.

McNally, R. J. (in press). Posttraumatic stress disorder. In T. Millon, P.H. Blaney, and R.D. Davis (Eds.), *Oxford textbook of psychopathology.* Oxford, UK: Oxford University Press.

Murray, J., Ehlers, A. & Mayou, R. M. (in preparation). *Information processing and posttraumatic stress disorder after motor vehicle accidents: Results of two prospective studies.*

Pennebaker, J. (1989), Confession, inhibition, and disease. *Advances in Experimental Social Psychology, 22,* 211–244.

Resick, P. A., Schnicke, M. K. & Markway, B. G. (1991, November). *The relationship between cognitive content and posttraumatic stress disorder.* Paper presented at the Annual Meeting of the Association for Advancement of Behavior Therapy, New York.

Resick, P. A. & Schnicke, M. K. (1993). *Cognitive processing therapy for rape victims: A treatment manual.* Newbury Park: Sage Publications.

Shalev, A., Peri, T., Canetti, L. & Schreiber, S. (1996). Predictors of PTSD and injured trauma survivors: a prospective study. *American Journal of Psychiatry, 153,* 219–225.

Shepherd, J. C. & Beck, J. G. (1999). The effects of suppressing trauma-related thoughts on women with rape-related post-traumatic stress disorder. *Behaviour Research and Therapy, 37,* 99–112.

Steil, R. & Ehlers, A. (in press). Dysfunctional meaning of posttraumatic intrusions in chronic PTSD. *Behaviour Research and Therapy.*

Van der Kolk, B. A. & Fisler, R. (1995). Dissociation and the fragmentary nature of traumatic memories: overview and exploratory study. *Journal of Traumatic Stress*, *8*, 505–525.

Warda, G. & Bryant, R. A. (1998). Thought control strategies in acute stress disorder. *Behaviour Research and Therapy*, *36*, 1171–1175.

Wegner, D. M. (1989). *White bears and other unwanted thoughts: suppression, obsession, and the psychology of mental control.* New York: Viking.

Wenninger, K. & Ehlers, A. (1998). Dysfunctional cognitions and adult psychological functioning in child sexual abuse survivors. *Journal of Traumatic Stress*, *11*, 281–300.

Subject Index

Author Index